Occupational Cancer

Occupational Cancer

Michael Alderson

Chief Medical Statistician, Office of Population Censuses and Surveys, London

Butterworths   London   Boston   Durban   Singapore   Sydney   Toronto   Wellington

First published 1986

© Butterworth & Co. (Publishers) Ltd, 1986

British Library Cataloguing in Publication Data

Alderson, Michael
    Occupational cancer.
    1. Cancer   2. Occupational diseases
    I. Title
    616.99′4071   RC262
    ISBN 0–407–00297–9

Library of Congress Cataloging in Publication Data

Alderson, M. R. (Michael Rowland)
    Occupational cancer.

    Bibliography: p.
    Includes index.
    1. Cancer. 2. Occupational diseases. 3. Carcinogens
—Environmental aspects. 4. Industrial toxicology.
I. Title. [DNLM: 1. Carcinogens, Environmental.
2. Neoplasms—chemically induced. 3. Occupational
Diseases. QZ 202 A362o]
RC262.A376 1985   616.99′4071   85–19030
ISBN 0–407–00297–9

Typeset by Scribe Design, Gillingham, Kent
Printed in Great Britain by The Garden City Press Ltd, Letchworth, Herts

Preface

This book provides an up-to-date review of the occurrence and causes of occupational cancer. The intention has been that the text should assist all those involved with the health of workers (including medical and safety staff, management, and health and safety representatives). The material should be of particular interest to those mounting studies on the health hazards of specific work processes and the carcinogenicity of the work environment.

Chapter 1 provides a description of the main classes of epidemiological study that can be used to investigate any potential cancer hazard to which a group of workers is exposed. This is (a) to enable the reader to have sufficient understanding about the advantages and disadvantages of the various methods so that he can judge the weight to be placed upon any specific findings, and (b) to guide those planning specific studies.

Chapter 2 provides a detailed review of present knowledge on the causes of occupationally induced cancers; the sections are restricted to specific chemical or physical agents, for which there is evidence of an association with increased risk of cancer. A major contribution of this chapter is from the tables which provide a synoptic view of reported studies on workers exposed to these specific agents. The text mentions evidence from animal and other laboratory tests of carcogenicity, where these have provided guidance in the absence of relevant epidemiological data. The main thrust of the reviews is on epidemiological studies (and case reports) that have clarified knowledge of the actual situation. The general issues of toxicology and product safety are beyond the scope of the present work. However, it must be remembered that plant engineering to reduce worker exposure may be crucial in removing a potential hazard from cancer, although actually being carried out for the more immediate aim of avoiding discomfort or toxic effects.

Chapter 3 complements the preceding one on carcinogenic agents, with a review of those industries in which an increased incidence or mortality from cancer has been reported. Industries are included when there is no obvious non-occupational confounding factor operating and also no indication that the increased cancer is associated with exposure to any specific agent in the work environment. Again synoptic tables are provided when a number of studies have been reported. The text also concentrates on epidemiological studies and case reports. Should the reader, in searching for discussion of a particular topic, not immediately find an entry where expected, the index should be consulted, where generous cross-reference is provided. Many topics are indexed under several synonyms, as well as under both the agent and the industry in which this occurs.

Chapter 4 provides a brief note of the major known causative agents of malignant disease at each main site. In the space available only limited discussion is provided, but key references are provided. The intention is that anyone concerned about the occurrence of a particular cancer in a group of subjects can readily check on the present knowledge of aetiology. This should help consideration of whether there may be some non-occupational factor leading to excess risk of the cancer.

The final chapter discusses the general approaches to prevention of occupational cancer. Sections deal with the contribution from research, the general approaches suitable for prevention, the impact of legislation, and the contribution from national and international bodies. The final section discusses action taken to control a number of specific carcinogens.

The initial work on the reviews of occupational cancer was carried out when the author held the

Cancer Research Campaign chair of epidemiology at the Institute of Cancer Research. Grateful thanks are due to the Campaign for the generous funding of this post. The work has been extended and revised; it is now presented as a personal view of the published literature on the subject.

Michael Alderson
Southampton

Abbreviations

BCME	bis(chloromethyl)ether	OPCS	Office of Population Censuses and Surveys
BLV	bovine leukaemia virus		
CEC	Council of European Communities	OSHA	Occupational Safety and Health Administration
Ci	curie (old unit of radiation activity)	P	probability
		PAH	polyaromatic hydrocarbons
CL	confidence limits	PCBs	polychlorinated biphenyls
CME	chloromethyl ether	PMR	proportional mortality ratio
CMME	chloromethyl methyl ether	ppm	parts per million
CNS	central nervous system	PRR	proportional registration ratio
2,3-D	dichlorophenoxyacetic acid	PVC	polyvinyl chloride
DBCP	dibromochloropropane	rem	rem (old unit of radiation dose equivalent)
DDT	dichlorodiphenyltrichloroethane		
DNOC	dinitro-*o*-cresol	RES	reticulo-endothelial system
E	expected (deaths)	RR	relative risk
FLV	feline leukaemia virus	SE	standard error
GRO	General Register Office	SMR	standardized mortality ratio
Gy	gray (absorbed dose of radiation)	SRR	standardized registration ratio
HCH	hexachlorocyclohexane	STT	short-term tests
HLA	histocompatibility antigens	Sv	sievert (new unit of radiation dose)
HSC	Health and Safety Commission		
HSE	Health and Safety Executive	2,4,5-T	trichlorophenoxyacetic acid
IARC	International Agency for Research on Cancer	TCDD	tetrachlorodibenzo-*p*-dioxin
		TCP	trichlorophenols
ICD	International Classification of Diseases	TLV	treshold limit value
		TWA	time-weighted average
ILO	International Labour Organisation	UNSCEAR	United Nations Scientific Committee on the Effects of Atomic Radiation
LET	linear energy transfer		
MCPA	chloromethylphenoxyacetic acid	UK	United Kingdom
NHSCR	National Health Service Central Register	US	United States
		UV	ultraviolet light
NIOSH	National Institute of Occupational Safety and Health	VC	vinyl chloride
		VCM	vinyl chloride monomer
nm	nanometre (10^{-9} m)	WHO	World Health Organisation
O	observed (deaths)		

Contents

1

Epidemiological method

Epidemiology is one of the disciplines that can help in the investigation of occupationally induced cancer. It can contribute to (a) identifying possible hazards, (b) testing hypotheses on cause, (c) quantifying dose–response relationships, and (d) evaluating preventive measures. Studies on these aspects utilize the conventional methods of epidemiology, but certain adaptations are required for this particular field of cancer epidemiology. The present chapter, in the space available, can only provide an introduction to the methods used; standard texts on the subject should be consulted for further detail. (A list of recommended reading is given at the end of the chapter.) However, the following should provide a basic guide to the principles involved. This should be sufficient to assess the results from studies reported in the literature, and provide enough information to mount preliminary studies.

Though this chapter deals with method, the consideration of occupational mortality and incidence statistics is supplemented by an appendix on national publications of such statistics.

1.1 Different types of study

This section describes briefly 8 different types of study. These studies are in an order that goes from simple use of routine data through analytical studies of increasing complexity to prospective studies (the latter being the studies of longest duration and usually the definitive studies prior to preventive action).

1.1.1 Routine occupational mortality and incidence statistics

This section describes the development of regular analyses of occupational mortality. The section covers the generation of statistics from the national system of death notification, with or without the use of census statistics, to provide estimates of the population at risk within different occupations. Some countries extend the method to the data available from population cancer registries. A brief comment on the background for presenting statistics is given, followed by a discussion of some of the method issues of use, analysis and interpretation of the data, validity of the material, and possible extensions of the basic method.

In introducing a brief glimpse of the historical aspects of occupational mortality statistics, it is worth remembering that Paracelsus—the first to describe an industrial disease—said: 'Science cannot look back to the past'. Hunter (1957) recorded that Rammazzini wrote in the eighteenth century about disease occurring in over 60 occupations. Increasing attention was paid to the effect of occupation on health in the early part of the nineteenth century. Thackrah (1832) published his work *The Effects of Arts, Trades and Professions on Health and Longevity*. Chadwick (1842) stressed in his report on the sanitary condition of the labouring population of Great Britain the need for the collection and examination of facts. A few years later, Engels (1845) wrote of the condition of the working class in England. Farr (1875) pointed out that these previous writers employed methods which could render no precise results except in cases where the influences they dealt with were very powerful.

It was a major advance when the Registrar General (1855) first collated such information from the 1851 census with the mortality returns for that year. He wrote:

'The previous investigations of the various rates of mortality in the districts of the Kingdom have shown how much the health and life of the population are affected by fixed local influence.

The professions and occupations of men open up a new field of enquiry on which we are now prepared to enter, not unconscious, however, of peculiar difficulties that beset all enquiries into the mortality of limited, fluctuating, and sometimes ill-defined sections of the population.'

Subsequent analyses of occupational mortality have been produced following each decennial census. In recent decennial reports, the mortality data have been based on deaths in 5 or 3 years around the time of the census, in order to provide a larger number of deaths in any individual occupation. The occupation used for the numerator in calculating the rates is the final occupation recorded at death registration. Enhancement of the method has been by:

(a) Selection of well-defined jobs for examination.
(b) Combination of allied or easily confused occupations.
(c) Cross-classification of job by geographical region.
(d) Use of occupation and industry to provide increased specificity.

The first detailed discussion of the problems involved in the interpretation of occupational mortality data was by Ogle (1885); he gave a clear description of the selection process into and out of occupations. Further attention was paid to this problem of selection into and out of occupation by Tatham (1902; 1908). Stocks (1938) presented evidence suggesting that variation in male mortality in England and Wales was influenced by housing, and to a lesser extent by social class and latitude. Attempts were made to distinguish the influence of a man's work, the industry in which he worked, and his general environment. Separate analyses of mortality by occupation and industry were carried out. The 1930–32 Decennial Supplement attempted to permit examination of the influence of job, independently of industry and locality, by presenting cause-specific mortality for wives. It was suggested that the study of the direct influence of occupation was possible from comparison of the standardized mortality ratio (SMR) of men and their wives. For example it was suggested that the influence of selection might be responsible for farmers having a lower SMR than their wives, rather than from benefit of their actual work.

Alderson (1972) indicated the following problems by using the following data:

(a) The validity of the cause of death—does knowledge of the job bias the wording of the certificate?

(b) Validity of occupation recorded at death registration—does the informant inflate the importance of the job of the deceased?
(c) Use of denominator from a different source—how is someone temporarily out-of-work from sickness or redundancy or prematurely retired classified?
(d) Selection biases—into and out of certain occupations in relation to physique, mental stamina, health.
(e) Use of last-held occupation, instead of job held longest.
(f) Relation of occupation to work environment—is there dilution due to aggregation of very different types of work?
(g) Confounding with non-occupational factors—do individuals in certain jobs smoke more, eat foods with high fat content etc.?

One of the problems that has had most attention devoted to it is the concern of the validity of the denominator; this is discussed further in 1.1.1.3.

1.1.1.1 Uses of occupational mortality statistics

Initially the statistics may be used for descriptive purposes: to indicate the numbers of deaths and the patterns of mortality for different categories of workers. The material may also be used to look at the variation in mortality from one occupation to another, or variation in one occupation from earlier periods in time. An extension of the simple descriptive use of statistics is as a source of fresh hypotheses ('fishing' for variation that stimulates some line of thought about possible aetiology). A very different application is the calculation of incidence or mortality by specific occupation in hypothesis testing. In general, descriptive and hypothesis generation studies will involve relatively broad categories of work, whilst hypothesis testing will be related to specific groups of workers— wherever possible identifying those exposed to a specific agent and preferably distinguishing categories of workers with variation in degree of exposure (both intensity or level and duration of exposure).

Hunches may be derived from clinical experiences, from other direct experiences, from laboratory investigation and from epidemiology. A milestone in the identification of carcinogenic factors was the work of Pott (1775), who identified the relationship between scrotal cancer and chimney sweeping. There are many other examples in the field of malignant disease where clinicians have been the first to suspect a hazard. It is important to acknowledge that laboratory investigation has contributed as much to the identification of fresh hazards as has epidemiology. In the past, epidemiology has usually relied on analysis of routine national statistics in the generation of fresh leads, although as the following sections indicate, fresh approaches are now being explored.

Stevenson (1923) pointed out that the influence of occupation on health could be indirect, as well as via the direct influence of a hazard upon mortality risk. He began the use of comparison of husbands' and wives' mortality, in order to distinguish the extent of the indirect component, i.e. where the SMR of both husbands and wives was greater than 100, the indirect component could be gauged by the excess of the female SMR over 100. However, Fox and Adelstein (1978) pointed out that (*a*) the percentage of wives aged 15–64 economically active and retired had risen from about 10% in 1931 to nearly 50% in 1971, and (*b*) many working wives will be in a job related to that of their husband and thus exposed to similar work and home environment. Fox and Adelstein (1978) go on to suggest that social class standardization of the occupational SMRs can assist by (*a*) allowing for general social class differences in mortality that are independent of work environment, (*b*) adjusting for specific patterns of behaviour such as smoking that show a clear social class gradient, and (*c*) distinguishing area from social class contributions to certain diseases.

Fox and Leon (1982) reviewed the use made of the 1970–72 report for England and Wales (Registrar General, 1978). Enquiry to potential users suggested the material was of value (*a*) as reference on occupation hazards, (*b*) for collation studies, (*c*) in consideration of health risks, (*d*) to distinguish occupational and non-occupational effects, (*e*) to generate hypotheses. However, the authors do not provide a single example where the latest or an earlier report has been the first lead to the identification of a fresh occupation hazard.

The *Lancet* (1983a) appeared to suggest that insufficient effort is devoted to following up clues about occupational cancer generated by routine statistics. It fails to discuss the relative advantages and disadvantages of this use of routine statistics. Moriyama (1984) suggested that there was ample evidence to show that occupational mortality data do not shed much light on occupational risk. He said that their chief use had been to present mortality differentials by social class, but it was not possible to make inferences about occupational risks from these data. He argued that if every death certificate had been occupation and industry coded, analytical studies could not produce risk factors from the data. Frazier *et al.* (1984) agreed with Moriyama's point that the occupational mortality did not permit a direct inference about disease or workplace hazard.

1.1.1.2 SMR and proportional mortality ratio (PMR)

There is a close relationship between age of an individual and the probability of dying. Thus when comparing observed mortality in two occupational groups with different age structures, some method is required to take account of this age effect. One approach to this problem is to examine the mortality by specific age groups. Although this enables direct comparisons to be made irrespective of any variation in age distribution, it can result in the presentation of a large amount of material (if, for instance, the age-specific mortality rates for 15 5-year age groups are examined). This creates a problem in the preparation and presentation of the material, and the sheer number of separate sets of data creates difficulties in interpretation.

Standardization is a technique that may be used for producing an index of mortality, which is adjusted for the age distribution in the particular occupational group being examined. One approach is to apply the age-specific rates for a 'standard' population to the age-specific numbers of individuals in the study population and then to derive an expected figure for the numbers of deaths.

When the denominator comes from a different statistical system (such as the census), there are major differences in the circumstances of recording the occupation. This has long been recognized as a problem in the method used by the Registrars General in England, Wales and Scotland. For a study in the United States (US), Stocks suggested the use of a PMR as a screening device, to identify SMRs that were not raised because of numerator/denominator biases (*see* Guralnick, 1962). The same type of approach was discussed by Logan (1982), who used two indices that were comparable to a PMR for comparison against the SMR.

Wang and Decoufle (1982) derived the algebraic relationship between the SMR and and PMR. This showed that the validity of the PMR depended upon the homogeneity of the age-specific overall SMRs and the value of the average SMR. They related this to a number of epidemiological studies and pointed out that incomplete death ascertainment can lead to biased estimates.

As indicated in the worked example (*see* 1.5.5), the SMR can be based upon any chosen age range. Doll and Cook (1967), when discussing presentation of data on cancer incidence, advocated (*a*) the use of a truncated age-standardized index, with different age ranges and weights depending upon the age-specific incidence of the particular cancer, and (*b*) the use of the ratio of the rates at ages 55–64 : 35–44 as an index of the rate at which the incidence increases with age.

1.1.1.3 Validity of occupational mortality and incidence statistics

Three rather different aspects need to be considered: (*a*) the validity of the cause of death on the certificate, (*b*) the validity of the occupations recorded for the denominator and numerator, and (*c*) the effect of small numbers especially when using the material for hypothesis generation.

Cause of death

Some general points of the validity of this item are discussed and then the possible specific biases in relation to occupational mortality. The cause of death is a crucial item of occupational mortality statistics, and the main statistic examined in historical prospective studies (*see* 1.1.7); the following general note on validity is equally applicable to this other use of the material on cause of death.

Any routine data collection system is liable to inaccuracies. This problem is best discussed by considering the separate steps in the chain leading to the production of mortality statistics, which are:

Conversion of basic information about the patients into the diagnosis by the clinician → Completion of the death certificate → Transcription onto the death notification → Classification of underlying cause of death → Coding → Processing → Analysis → Interpretation of the statistics.

A number of studies have examined the accuracy of the diagnostic information available at the time of death; usually this has been compared with data derived from autopsy. A major study was sponsored by the General Register Office (GRO) (Heasman and Lipworth, 1966). Alderson (1981a) has reviewed the literature on this topic, and pointed out that some studies indicate a worrying degree of variation between autopsy and clinical diagnoses. Other recent studies using this approach were by Busuttil, Kemp and Heasman (1981), and Cameron and McGoogan (1981).

Another approach has been to use 'dummy' case histories and obtain 'mock' death certificates from clinicians, e.g. Reid and Rose (1964), McGoogan and Cameron (1978), and Gau and Diehl (1981).

Others have compared death certificates with a review of detailed case histories (*see*, for example, Moriyama *et al.*, 1958; Alderson, 1965; Puffer and Griffith, 1967; Alderson and Meade, 1967; Pole *et al.*, 1977; Clarke and Whitfield, 1978).

Wingrave *et al.* (1981) compared the coding of the death certificates for 205 deaths by staff in (*a*) a Royal College of General Practitioners research unit, and (*b*) the Office of Population Censuses and Surveys (OPCS) and GRO Scotland.

It is generally accepted that mortality statistics, because of these problems, must be interpreted with caution. Obviously there are some conditions where the medical knowledge and facilities for diagnosis

have altered markedly over time, or may vary from place to place. This will have a major impact on interpretation of the data—similar to situations where there have been major alterations in the International Classification of Diseases (ICD) with splitting or amalgamation of various cause groups. It has been suggested that approximately 20% of coded causes of death involve relatively minor errors and 5% major errors (where a major error is a change from one chapter of the ICD to another, which generally implies alteration from one body system to another).

The possibility that knowledge of an occupational risk might influence certification in workers was discussed by Mole (1982) and Kneale and Stewart (1982)—the former suggesting that doctors near a plant might 'overcertify' and the latter that doctors further away might 'undercertify' a particular cancer. No hard evidence to support either contention was presented.

Occupation recorded for numerator and denominator

Heasman, Liddell and Reid (1958) carried out a study which provided some facts relevant to a discussion of the accuracy of occupational mortality data, though this work was restricted to a survey on the accuracy of job descriptions on records used for the calculation of indices of occupational mortality and morbidity in the mining industry. These authors comment on errors in the descriptions of occupations used in the numerator and denominator of the occupational mortality rates, including errors introduced by the coding system. Following the 1961 census a postenumeration survey was carried out for the first time to check the accuracy of the information collected at the census; results of this are provided in the General Report of the 1961 Census (General Register Office, 1968). Some of the occupation questions had been differently phrased, and thus comparisons between the census and the postenumeration survey are difficult to interpret; however, the survey did support the earlier suggestions that there was overstatement of the number economically inactive. The second study discussed in the General Report of the 1961 Census concerned the matching of the information recorded at the death registration with the census schedule for a sample of deaths occurring shortly after the census. Out of 2196 males, 63% were assigned to the same occupation unit at death registration and, at census, 10% were assigned to different units within the same occupational order, whilst 27% were assigned to different orders.

Alderson (1972) has reported a study amongst a representative sample of males dying in Bristol during 1962–63. A chronological history was obtained of all occupations held since leaving school for each deceased person in the study; this information was obtained by interview with the next of kin. These occupation histories have been coded, and compared with the coding of the occupations recorded at death registration. Comparison showed that there was complete agreement between the two sets of data regarding the final occupation for 79% of the subjects; there were negligible discrepancies for 6%, minor discrepancies at unit level for 5% of the subjects, and major discrepancies for 10% of the subjects.

Where an individual has developed a fatal chronic disease (whether or not occupationally induced) and has had to change his occupation because of impaired ability, mortality will be shown against the final occupation. Should the change of job have been due to onset of occupationally induced disease, this will not be reflected in the mortality rate for the principal occupation; there will also be an erroneously high mortality rate for the final occupation.

Swanson, Schwartz and Burrows (1984) compared occupation and industry obtained from (*a*) 2000 death certificates, (*b*) 2000 cancer registrations, (*c*) 352 interview results in Detroit in 1980–81. The death certificates had data completed on occupation for a higher proportion than the registration material. The death certificate occupation and industry were an exact match with the interview data for 76%.

Number of events

Though there were 273 129 deaths in males aged 15–64 in England and Wales in 1970–72, when the topic of interest is a relatively rare cancer, in a small occupational unit the number of observed and expected deaths may be very low. For example, the SMR for laryngeal cancer was 146, but this was based on the observed deaths (O) = 16, and the expected deaths (E) = 10.96, which were not significantly different.

When scanning tables of SMRs, some approach is required to indicate the likelihood of the value differing from 100 by chance. A simple test which calculates chi-squared (χ^2) is described in 1.5.6. It is suggested that a conservative test, when scanning many hundreds of results, should only identify those where the probability (*P*) < 0.01 and O $\geqslant$ 20. *Table 1.3* sets out the associated values of O, E, and the SMR to identify such significant results.

1.1.1.4 Extensions of the basic method: extended occupational history

It is sometimes suggested that the value of occupational mortality statistics would be enhanced by the collection of an extended occupational history at death registration. For example, this point is included in the Royal College of Pathologists and

Physicians (1982) report on death certification; it was one of the recommendations made by the House of Lords select committee on occupational health (Gregson, 1984). However, there are a number of points that need to be borne in mind in considering this suggestion: (*a*) the informant at death registration may be distressed by the recent bereavement, may not know the details of the occupations held by the deceased, and may inflate the importance of the job held by the deceased; (*b*) this collection of detail will not necessarily overcome the issue of the numerator/denominator bias in the statistics; (*c*) the effort involved in the data collection and more detailed analysis may not be justified in relation to other ways of monitoring the health of employees.

One alternative to the collection of the information at death registration was selected in the US, as part of the Third National Cancer Survey. In this study, information was collected from all patients with cancers of sites, except superficial skin, for 9 geographical locations in the US in 1969–71. The population covered was just over 21 million (10% of the US population). Details were obtained from medical records for 181 027 incident cancers; this was supplemented by interviews with 10% of the patients, at which details such as occupation and smoking were obtained (Williams, Stegens and Goldsmith, 1977).

Combined use of PMR and SMR

Reference has already been made to the use of the PMR as a tool for searching for those SMRs that are raised and do not reflect numerator/denominator bias in the data. This can be extended by the use of the SMR to determine the overall force of mortality of an occupation, and weight the PMRs for specific diseases, so that the all-cause PMR is not 100, but the value of the SMR. This might have the advantage that the SMRs could be generated every decade, or be based on a sample of deaths, whilst the cause-specific PMRs (from which large numbers of deaths are required) could be based on continued coding of all deaths.

This suggestion would utilize the power of the linked studies to obtain a valid all-cause SMR without bias, and the value of the PMRs for exploring specific causes. This should overcome the defect of the PMR that in general use one cannot distinguish, from an internal examination of the material, whether a value is genuinely raised, or reflects a decrease in the force of mortality from some other major cause of death.

1.1.2 Record linkage

A more powerful probe of an occupational influence may be provided by record linkage. One example is the longitudinal study carried out in England and Wales, which permits linkage of job details provided at census to subsequent patterns of mortality through national linkage (Office of Population Censuses and Surveys, 1973). A recent report (Fox and Goldblatt, 1982) presented a wide range of results from mortality of the 1971 cohort over the period 1971–75. Chapter 12 of this report provided results by occupational order; there are marked overall differences from the decennial supplement, with the linked study showing relatively low rates for all occupational orders and a high SMR for men unoccupied at the time of the census. The relatively low SMR for the occupational orders is due to the 'selection' of those fit for work and is another aspect of the 'healthy-worker effect' (*see* 1.3.9). Comparison between occupational orders showed some with relatively high SMRs, which were in agreement with the direction of the differences found in the decennial supplement. Though the longitudinal study overcomes the numerator/denominator biases, insufficient deaths have accumulated to permit examination of cause of death for occupational units (Fox and Leon, 1982). The national systems described for Canada, Denmark, Norway, and Sweden all depend on record linkage. The former links occupational data from social security records to deaths, whilst the Scandinavians are all linking census to cancer incidence and mortality (*see* Appendix).

Instead of organizing record linkage as a routine, and then periodically using the linked file for special studies, an alternative approach is to carry out a specific record-linkage study in order to probe a particular problem. Mancuso and Coulter (1959) described how the US Bureau of Old-age and Survivors Insurance records could be used to identify individuals with specific long-term work histories. Linkage with deaths from vital records permitted examination of the mortality patterns of those in particular occupations. Alderson (1980a) arranged for OPCS staff to link records from the 1961 census with subsequent mortality. The census files were searched for codes compatible with an occupation as hairdresser. This enabled the census staff to identify the original census schedules, check the occupation and abstract full identification particulars for each individual. About 2000 men were identified (a 10% sample of the occupation in 1961); the identification particulars were used to trace each individual on the National Health Service Central Register (NHSCR), and thus find the death entries for those who had died. These data were used to calculate expected mortality and contrast this with observed numbers of deaths for 5 malignancies which other studies had suggested might be associated with exposure to hair dyes.

The main conceptual difference of an *ad hoc* study of this nature is that the effort of linkage is devoted solely to the individuals of particular interest, rather than using routine record linkage for the total population. Also it was possible to go back to the 1961 census, because the computer records that still existed for this could provide the cross-index to the hard-copy original schedules for all hairdressers.

A special example of record linkage is the establishment of registers of patients with specific rare cancers that may be of occupational origin— such as registers of hepatic angiosarcoma or mesothelioma patients. The use of the latter is discussed in 2.31.9.4 and 2.31.13. Falk and Baxter (1981) reviewed the use of hepatic angiosarcoma registries and pointed out: (*a*) the lengthy time to establish the register, (*b*) the effort required to confirm diagnoses, (*c*) the difficulty of getting information from next-of-kin spread across the country, (*d*) the absence of retrievable job records, (*e*) the constraint from lack of a control group. They emphasized the need to obtain information from several sources; death certificate review was inadequate without review of pathology.

1.1.3 Collation studies

A less precise probe, but one readily carried out, is to compare the distribution of cancer mortality (or incidence) with that of indices of variation in occupation geographically or over time. For example, cancer mortality by specific site was prepared and mapped for the counties in the US for 1950–69. At the same time these counties had been classified by industrial activity. Blot *et al.* (1977) compared 39 petroleum industry counties with 117 counties matched for geographical region, population size and various demographic indicators. The definition of a petroleum county was one where (*a*) at least 100 persons were employed in the industry, and (*b*) at least 1% of the county's population was estimated to be petroleum employees. Age-adjusted mortality rates during 1950–69 for 23 cancer sites were calculated for white residents. Males in the petroleum industry counties experienced significantly more cancer for 7 sites of malignancy: stomach, rectum, nasal cavity and sinuses, lung, testis, skin including melanoma, brain. The excesses for cancer of the stomach, rectum and testis occurred in the more highly populated petroleum industry counties. The paper commented that other industries are generally to be found in the same location as the petroleum industry, but no attempt was made to define which other industry, if any, might have contributed to the high mortality from various disease groups.

1.1.4 Proportional mortality analysis

A relatively simple check of an issue can be carried out where records are available that identify the cause of death in a group of workers. The analysis merely requires the following information for each individual who had died: sex, date of birth, date and cause of death. The technique tests whether the proportion of deaths from the cause of interest is greater or less than one would expect in relation to deaths from all causes. The expected figure is usually calculated by applying the proportion of deaths by cause for the county as a whole to the distribution of actual deaths, taking age, sex and calendar period into account.

Boyd and his colleagues (1970) cross-checked the initial observations of a pathologist in Cumberland that iron-ore miners appeared to have a higher prevalence of lung cancer at autopsy than one would expect (bearing in mind the relative frequency of this as a cause of death in males in England and Wales). They had access to the death certificates issued for all males dying in Cumberland in 1948–67. These were sorted to identify all decedents recorded as being iron-ore miners; the deaths of all other individuals were used as the comparison group. Taking age and calendar period into account, the relative proportion of deaths from lung cancer, other cancers, respiratory disease and all other causes were examined. They observed 42 deaths from lung cancer in the miners, with an expected of 27.7 based on national data and 28.8 based on local mortality.

Their results thus supported the initial observations of the pathologist, though no definitive cause of the malignancy was identified. (A suggestion was made that the atmosphere in the mine was contaminated with radon, which might have accounted for the enhanced risk, rather than this being due to the dust from the iron-ore.)

Although an identical technique may be used to examine cancer registrations, it may not be so easy to identify all diagnoses of cancer. In a workforce, there may not be any employer or union mechanism for recording such material, and there may be great difficulty in obtaining particulars for those who leave the industry or retire. In addition, not every country has available national cancer registration statistics that can be used for calculation of the expected events.

For a condition that is relatively common, it may be possible to use local rather than national statistics in order to estimate the expected distribution of events; this may have an advantage of correcting for any regional, social class, or other local factor that influences the pattern of mortality other than that possibly due to the specific occupation.

A brief description of the statistical technique for handling such data is provided in 1.5.2.

Ad hoc studies using this technique have usually obtained the event data for the occupation being investigated from (*a*) company records, (*b*) union records, (*c*) insurance schemes (including those operated by companies or unions), (*d*) professional societies or registers of accredited professionals and (*e*) details recorded at death or cancer registration in a defined locality. Routine national systems may also use this approach, where there is doubt about the validity of estimates of the exposed population, e.g. in England and Wales for annual analyses of cancer registrations by occupation.

1.1.5 Cross-sectional studies

It is a relatively simple matter to identify subgroups of workers in industries where irradiation or benzene exposure may have occurred, and to classify the groups by extent of exposure. Samples of the men may then be approached and, in addition to collecting data on non-occupational factors causing chromosome abnormality, the men may be requested to give an appropriate sample so that detailed chromosome analyses may be carried out. Such a study was carried out on workers exposed to benzene; the initial findings of a highly significant excess of abnormalities in the benzene workers was not confirmed in a follow-up study, which showed an even higher abnormality rate in the control population selected (Tough and Court Brown, 1965; Tough *et al.*, 1970). The prevalence of chromosome aberrations was determined in the peripheral blood lymphocytes of dockyard workers exposed to mixed neutron γ-radiation. Exposures were mostly below the accepted permissible level of 0.05 gray (Gy) per year, but a significant increase in chromosome damage was noted with increased exposure (Evans *et al.*, 1979).

Such cross-sectional studies are only suitable for investigating carcinogenesis when there is some valid measure of a precursor of malignant neoplasms. Surveys of chromosome aberration, *in situ* cancer, or prevalence of benign lesions may be suitable. The prevalence of cancer will usually be so low that it would be impossible to mount an adequately sized survey of an exposed and non-exposed workforce to obtain interpretable results.

1.1.6 Case-control studies

Conventional case-control studies may be used to probe for occupational exposures with cancer. There are two conceptually different approaches: type 1 chooses one or more sites of malignancy and explores a range of aetiological factors including occupation, searching for differences between the cases and the controls. Type 2 is much more focused on one site of malignancy, estimating the risk for those exposed to a particular occupation.

Type 1 study

In the United States Third National Cancer Survey interviews were obtained from 7518 persons with cancer in 8 areas (a response of only 57%). Information was collected on alcohol and tobacco use as well as on employment history. The analyses consisted of two-times-two tables of counts of persons with/without a particular cancer against having/not having a specific employment; with 29 sites and 202 employment categories, this generated 5858 comparisons. This use of 'intercancer comparisons' has the problem that a cancer in the control group may be exposure-biased (under or over-represented); unless this cancer was more than a small proportion of the total, this effect would be minimal. Williams, Stegens and Goldsmith (1977) suggested that a major advantage of the study was that it permitted use of smoking, alcohol and socio-economic status as control variables.

Type 2 study

Damber and Larsson (1982) identified 604 males dying from lung cancer in northern Sweden, an equal number dead from other conditions, and 467 living controls. History of occupation and smoking were obtained from next-of-kin. The particular focus of interest was the influence of work underground in the local iron-ore mines, and the relative effect of such work and smoking on risk of lung cancer.

The important point in distinguishing between these two approaches is that the former (study 1) is an exploratory or 'fishing' study, which can only be used to generate hypotheses for further study, whilst the latter (study 2) may quantify the risk or evaluate aspects such as dose–response.

A more restricted study may only collect data from a sample of index patients, and then compare the distribution of occupation reported with those published from the census. Though this involves a lower cost per case than in conventional case-control studies, there may be bias in the two sources of information. Lee, Alderson and Downes (1972) used this approach in a study of scrotal cancer and Acheson, Cowdell and Rang (1972; 1981) in studies on nasal cancer.

1.1.7 Historical prospective studies

Rushton and Alderson (1981a) used industry records to identify men employed for at least a year in 8 oil refineries in the UK in the period 1950–75. Those who had left their company's employment and retirees whose vital status was not known were traced through central Social Security and the NHSCR records. All deaths were thus identified, the causes obtained, and compared with the calculated expected value based on national mortality rate with adjustment for regional variation. A statistical test was then applied to the comparisons between O and E. The results are presented in *Table 3.5*.

Where there are available records of individuals' work histories, with a complete file of data on mortality that has occurred among these individuals, it should be possible to relate the data on the 'population at risk' to the identifiable outcome, i.e. mortality. The occupational records are used to identify each individual in the study. It is essential to know the following: each individual's date of birth (or age at starting work), the date of entry to the occupation, some indication of potential environmental exposure, the follow-up status. The latest date known to be alive should be obtained for all individuals, including those still in the workforce and those who have retired. Individuals who have left the industry should be traced in order that their status can be obtained. Such leavers are likely to be different in a number of ways from those staying in the industry; without follow-up information on such individuals, the statistics may produce an incomplete or biased result. Rushton (1982) compared the results from a study which included tracing all those leaving the industry prior to retirement with results excluding this group. There were no appreciable differences and it was pointed out that avoidance of the lengthy and costly tracing should be considered, bearing in mind the age of these premature leavers, their length of service, and the proportion of deaths they are likely to contribute to the study results. For all deaths that have occurred in the study population, the date of death and cause of death is required. This material can be manipulated in a standard fashion to generate 'person-years at risk', which are tabulated by age and calendar period (*see* 1.5.3). By applying national age, sex and calendar period cause-specific mortality rates, the expected numbers of deaths by cause may be calculated. A comparison is then made between the respective numbers of observed and expected deaths for particular causes; the statistical aspects of this comparison are discussed in 1.5.4.

This approach can be used to explore the risk of a specific cancer, or to examine patterns of mortality of the workers in more general terms.

Occasionally, full details of each member of the workforce are not available, but company records may be able to provide estimates of the numbers of employees and pensioners by age group over the period for which death details are available. Using such material, Dean *et al.* (1979) were able to calculate expected deaths by cause and to compare these with observed deaths for the blue-collar workers at a Dublin brewery in 1954–73. This technique is less precise than using the calculated person-years at risk based on data for each individual, but it provided a sounder statistic than proportional-mortality analysis.

There are three 'types' of cohort that may be followed in such studies: (a) a group in post at a particular point in time (which will usually include individuals of varying age, and mixed duration of exposure), (b) a study confined to new entrants to a workforce over a defined period, (c) a combination, with staff in post supplemented by new entrants over succeeding years. These different approaches introduce appreciable differences in the age structure of the study population, the duration of exposure, and the time periods at which exposure occurred. If there have been major changes in the environment of the plant over time, there will be confounding between duration and intensity of exposure.

Many studies fail to distinguish these aspects both in description of the study and in the interpretation of the data.

1.1.8 Prospective studies

In 1953 the National Coal Board began a survey of working coal miners; in 1953–58 men at 24 collieries in the UK were interviewed and had a chest X-ray. Subsequent surveys involved medical examination and assessment of respiratory function, and respondents completed a questionnaire on respiratory symptoms and smoking habits. Work histories and measurements of respirable dust concentrations permitted calculation of cumulative exposure for individuals. Analyses of mortality in relation to these factors were reported by Miller, Jacobsen and Steele (1981). As an example, there were 19 550 men in England and Wales for whom reliable information on cumulative exposure to mine dust was available; the exposures were divided into 4 groups. Because older men predominated in the higher exposure categories, analyses were by age group at first survey. Two tables provided mortality from stomach and other digestive organs; there was a significant trend in mortality with increasing dust exposure. However, there was also a close association between dust exposure and pneumoconiosis, and between pneumoconiosis and mortality from digestive cancers. It was not possible to distinguish between a direct effect of dust or an indirect effect via pneumoconiosis on risk of these cancers.

The distinction from historical prospective studies is that, after the study design has been confirmed, *ad hoc* arrangements are made to collect detailed data on (a) exposure to agents in the work environment, (b) confounding factors, (c) long-term outcome. Rather than retrieve details of occupation held by individuals and relate this to subjective assessment of exposure, the work environment is surveyed at intervals to quantify 'dose'.

During the study design phase, the important confounding factors should be listed and consideration given to collecting relevant data from the subjects in the study. This is especially important for an aetiological factor known to play an appreciable part in the cause of the cancer, or where there is suspicion of interaction between the occupational environment and this second factor.

1.2 Principles of occupational studies

The following subsections discuss some of the general aspects of occupational studies. In addition to the points made here reference should be made to a textbook on epidemiological method to obtain more information, e.g. Alderson, 1983.

1.2.1 Who is at risk of an occupational hazard?

It is not only workers involved in primary production who may be at risk of cancer from exposure to carcinogens. An obvious example of the chain is that associated with asbestos; this involves those working in the mines, handling the 'raw' asbestos in factories, applying asbestos as in lagging and insulating, even stripping insulation out of various articles at breakers' yards etc. In addition to this chain of exposures, it has been shown that the families of workers and those living in the vicinity of an asbestos factory had an increased mortality from mesothelioma (Newhouse and Thompson, 1965). This was thought to be due to (a) contamination of the workers' clothes which then exposed the wives who washed these, and (b) contamination of the locality surrounding the factory with fibres transmitted in the air. This indicates the expanding ring of contacts who need to be considered when assessing any hazard from a particular industrial process.

Rather more difficult to investigate is the possibility that the next generation may be at risk—from fetal loss, excess stillbirths, congenital malformations, or cancers. This has been tackled in 1.4.6.

1.2.2 Which individuals are eligible for inclusion in a study?

A number of points of eligibility need to be considered in planning a study. It is often desirable to exclude workers with a minimum duration of employment (to restrict those transients with limited relevant exposure). This may be excluding those who have worked for only 1 month, 3 months, 1 year or perhaps 5 years. It is recommended that individuals with employment over the minimum (such as a year) should be included, even though their exposure is relatively limited, as they help provide estimates of a dose–response relationship.

If a hazardous agent is extremely potent and the

latent interval for generating the hazard is less than 20 years, then an adequate indication of this may come by studying just those in employment. However, if the condition is rare, and the latent interval is long, then it is unlikely that the hazard will be clearly identified in those under the age of 65. If the turnover in the occupation is high, then it is even more important that not only pensioners, but also those leaving prior to retirement, are followed up. It is usually possible to organize retrieval of vital status for pensioners, but it is much more expensive to trace the leavers. However, if the number who have worked on a particular plant or process is small, it may be crucial to trace these individuals in order to obtain enough numbers of events for statistical analysis. Rather different is the point that, if the workers who leave the industry are a biased group of those who have been exposed to risk, it is extremely important to trace them—for example were they the dirty workers who had a higher than average exposure? Were they individuals who were in some way sensitive to the environment? In the past, many studies of occupational hazards have excluded women, because of the small numbers involved. However, with the advent of legislation against sexual discrimination, the inclusion of women becomes more appropriate. It is also possible that the exposure and reaction to exposure differs between the sexes and again this argues for inclusion of women. One particular aspect of this is if the hazard influences the risk, not to the exposed person, but to the next generation; ionizing radiation may, for example, have an effect on the pregnant woman which it cannot have on the exposed male.

In many industries, contractors may come onto the site and have an environmental exposure entirely different from that of the normal plant operators. However, because the organization of their employment records is different, it is often difficult to include contractors' personnel in an occupational study. Rather different are 'visitors'— for instance in some fields of work it may be customary to have individuals coming from abroad to work for a limited period of months or years. It is an important issue to consider whether such individuals also need to be included in the study.

Other reasons for difficulty in studying specific groups of men are: (*a*) maintenance staff, who have not only the exposures specific to their craft, but work in many parts of a plant, often with higher potential exposure than process workers; (*b*) management systems with flexible manning and workers moving between plants of different environments; (*c*) movement of staff in complex installations from plant to plant, for increasing experience or on promotion; (*d*) progression of long-stay workers from the 'dusty or dirty' end of a process, to more popular jobs with lower exposure levels.

1.2.3 Factors influencing initiation of a study

With finite resources and the likelihood of a stream of fresh leads to consider, it is not possible to launch a definitive study on each 'hunch'. Less tangible issues may be critical to the decision, such as the enthusiasm of the research workers, the degree of collaboration available for the project, or even the very implausibility of a new and previously unsuspected health hazard. Having selected the appropriate research topic, there is then need to ensure that appropriate research facilities are available; these may be the techniques, the ideas, the equipment, and other facilities required. Providing the facilities are available, there must be access for the study to be carried out. The specific points requiring clearance will depend upon the design of the study, but many require access to retrievable records, or the investigation of individuals. As far as retrievable records are concerned, this may need access to (*a*) personnel records, (*b*) environmental data and (*c*) follow-up data on individuals who have left the industry. Such access requires the approval of management and union, with permission to disclose the identity and release information required to trace individuals who have left the industry. The tracing of leavers raises the issue of confidentiality of personal records; the Medical Research Council (1973) has provided guidelines for research in this field. The Faculty of Occupational Medicine (1982) has also produced notes of guidance on the ethics for occupational physicians.

1.2.4 Tracing individuals

Particularly with historical prospective studies, there is a need to trace subjects to determine their vital status. The actual approach used will depend on the employer's records, and the avenues open in different countries.

As far as employer's records are concerned, the study may initially identify all men ever employed. The tracing will usually be required for (*a*) those leaving prior to retirement, and (*b*) at least some of the retirees, i.e. those not known to the pension fund to be alive or dead. In the United Kingdom (UK), it is possible to trace individuals through the central Social Security records to identify the fact of death, or through the NHSCR to obtain fact and cause of death. The former is simpler if the National Insurance Number is known; the latter is facilitated by the NHS number and has the great advantage that once a group of workers have been identified on the register, their entries can be 'flagged' and the research worker informed as future deaths occur. For either system, identification must include surname, forenames, and date of birth in order to distinguish individuals in these national files.

Transfer of the names from the industry, via the researcher, to the central registers must comply with accepted ethical agreements on confidentiality of such information. Since 1971 in England and Wales and also in Scotland, cancer registrations have been annotated on the NHSCR. With appropriate safeguards on confidentiality, this information may be released to the research worker for workers who develop cancer.

Equivalent systems exist in Scandinavia, whilst the newly established death index in the US will provide an alternative source. In other countries *ad hoc* local follow-up is required.

1.2.5 Validity

This section covers a number of points that are particularly relevant to studies of occupational cancer. However, there is an extensive literature on general aspects of validity of the different types of occupational study (*see* Alderson, 1983, for review).

1.2.5.1 Bias in subjects studied

A preliminary consideration is whether all employees 'at risk' were covered in the study. Marsh and Enterline (1979) stressed the importance of independent check of the completeness of occupational cohorts. In a validation of records for 6 plants in the United States, additional records for 21% further subjects were found by cross-checking against Inland Revenue records. The reason for the emphasis on requiring a complete cohort is the worry that those missing are atypical in respect of exposure, other risk factors, or development of disease.

Rather different is the consideration of the selection process involved; Ogle (1885) gave a clear description of some of the biases associated with selection into and out of occupations. For example, some jobs can only be done by the physically strong and active; these characteristics of the workforce may determine their patterns of morbidity and mortality, rather than any aspect of the work environment. An associated aspect is the influence of non-occupational factors on risk of disease that may also be linked to work. For example, many occupational studies have involved examination of the (potential) hazard of lung cancer—a lung cancer for which there is a known major behavioural risk factor (smoking). If smoking habits have not been recorded for the employees in a specific occupation, it is always questionable whether variation in smoking could account for any difference in lung cancer mortality in the workers. Of course, if information is available on intensity and duration of chemical exposure and a dose–response relationship is found with lung cancer, this is less likely to be due

to confounding with smoking; however, such results do not rule out a multiplicative or interactive effect between the smoking habits of the workers and their occupational environment.

1.2.5.2 Dilution of environmental effects

When a work hazard only directly affects a restricted group of individuals, the impact of this may be diluted or lost by studying a broader group of the workforce. In general terms this was well recognized over 100 years ago (Registrar General, 1855); it is a point that warrants consideration whenever it is not known precisely what is the specific hazard responsible for the health problem being studied. Without clear definition of the discrete group of workers 'exposed to risk', there may be loss of precision in the study; this may also be an inevitable consequence of those studies using routine or retrievable data, when job titles cover broad categories of workers.

1.2.5.3 Validity of exposure data

There is bound to be considerable difference in the quality of exposure for the different types of study. Occupational mortality and incidence statistics rely on job descriptions obtained at one point in time and processed in a routine statistical system (with potential bias between the numerator and denominator for rates, and SMRs). Very different is the quality of data that are collected in prospective studies. It also appears that in the past the degree of recording has been higher when physical measures are involved (asbestos, dusts in general, irradiation) rather than levels of chemicals in the work environment.

With a process involving a single suspect agent, it may be satisfactory merely to document whether or not exposure was likely to have occurred. More suitable data for analysis are provided by the quantification of the intensity of exposure and the duration of exposure. It may be difficult to gauge in which broad category of exposure level individual workers should be placed; in many industries, no records exist of environmental or personal monitoring for specific chemicals. This difficulty is exacerbated where a complex chemical works has many plants and workers move from one plant to another. Sometimes the range of chemicals involved in some of the plants and processes might be unknown, let alone their levels in the environment monitored. Indirect assessment of potential exposure of process workers may be possible. This becomes much more difficult, if not impossible, for maintenance staff who move throughout a site; often, because of the nature of their work, exposure may be very difficult to gauge and very different from that of the normal working of the plants. Smith, Waxweiler and

Tyroler (1980) developed a method which calculated the expected yearly exposure for each case from the work histories of controls matched on year of birth and year of hire. They suggested that this permitted exploration of exposure level, latency and interaction in such studies.

Obviously the scope for the research worker to handle valid data will depend on the type of study being carried out. Where routine or retrievable data are used, the issue has to be dealt with by cautious interpretation of available material. In a planned survey or prospective study, steps should be taken to ensure that the data collected are of adequate validity.

1.2.5.4 Validity of 'outcome' data

In surveys and case-control studies, the researcher should be able to control the quality of the diagnostic information. In prospective studies, an important primary task is to check that all the study groups are correctly followed up and the 'endpoints' identified, i.e. development of disease, death or emigration. Providing complete ascertainment can be achieved, the next step is to consider the validity of the diagnostic information. Obviously when using some form of record linkage, and calculating expected events, thought must be given to possible biases and confounding factors that can account for the differences between observed and expected deaths, e.g. differences in social class, region, behaviour, non-work environment etc., that could be responsible.

The validity of cause of death from death certificates has already been discussed (*see* 1.1.1.3). In a historical prospective study, it is possible to check the cause of death in the cohort, but not for the expected figures when these are based on 'external' rates. Enterline (1976a) has emphasized the bias from adjusting the causes for the observed deaths alone.

1.2.6 Inference

Alderson (1983) discussed the strategies for drawing the correct inference from one or more sets of results. This is based on logic, such as Mill's canons or methods of scientific inquiry. Hill (1965) discussed the distinction between association and causation, when examining the influence of environment on disease. He stressed the need to consider: the strength of the relationship, consistency of result, specificity, temporality, dose–response, plausibility, coherence of evidence, the impact of change in exposure, and presence of analogous relationships. Statistical tests help to rule out the play of chance and can indicate the magnitude of the effects; appropriate methods may help to consider the

influence of multiple factors, but they do not result in proof of a cause-and-effect relationship from observational data.

Rothman (1982) pointed out that Kant distinguished: (*a*) analytical judgements which were logical truisms unrelated to empirical judgements, from (*b*) synthetic judgements that extended knowledge, sometimes without reference to experience. Identification of causation was a synthetic *a priori* judgement.

A crucial aspect in the interpretation of a study is to distinguish those findings stemming from planned testing of an hypothesis from 'associations' derived from sifting through a complex set of results. This issue has already been touched upon in discussing the use of mortality statistics and case-control studies. Unfortunately, many published papers do not clearly distinguish these two approaches. However, when risk for different sites of cancer is probed for, in a wide range of occupations (whether in routine data, a case-control, or a historical prospective study), the results should be treated as pointers to further work and not indicators of a confirmed hazard. A particular difficulty exists in even determining the significance of results where multiple comparisons have been made (*see* Alderson, 1983).

1.3 Advantages and disadvantages of different types of study

General texts on epidemiological method discuss the relative power of different types of epidemiological study. The following brief notes concentrate on aspects particularly relevant to studies of occupational cancer. In considering this, it is important to bear in mind that studies may be: (*a*) descriptive—indicating the patterns of mortality or cancer incidence in categories of worker; (*b*) hypothesis generating—by demonstrating variation in risk and leading to consideration of possible factors involved; (*c*) hypothesis testing—examining the risk in relation to specific exposures, preferably seeking dose–response effects; (*d*) method studies, required as a preliminary to further studies of types (*a*)–(*c*).

In general, descriptive studies and hypothesis-generating ones will involve relatively broad categories of occupation. Occasionally, routine statistics may be used to examine the disease-specific incidence or mortality for a particular occupation in hypothesis testing. However, hypothesis testing will be predominantly by *ad hoc* studies of specific groups of workers—wherever possible identifying those exposed to a specific environmental agent, and distinguishing categories of worker with variation in degree of exposure (both intensity or level and duration of exposure).

It is unusual for enquiry on a particular topic to follow through the types of study described in 1.1, exactly in the order described there. Alderson (1983), in discussing the general principles of study design, suggested that selection of the appropriate design will depend on:

(*a*) The opportunities available for the study.
(*b*) The available facilities.
(*c*) The time by which an answer is required.
(*d*) The assessment of the importance of the topic.
(*e*) The required level of validity in the results.

The factors affecting detection of risk should be borne in mind. It has been suggested (Alderson, 1979) that these are: the size of the relative and absolute risks, the specificity of the risk, the number of individuals exposed, the degree of job stability, the latent period for generation of disease, and the contribution of confounding factors. These points affect the relative efficiency of different methods of studying the same problem. As a rule of thumb, for relative risk (RR) of different magnitude if:

RR > 1000 Clinical observation should recognize the hazard.
RR > 100 Clinical observation may recognize the hazard, especially for rare tumours; routine data should indicate the association.
RR > 10 Careful *ad hoc* study (case-control or historical prospective) should demonstrate the risk.
RR ≃ 2 There may be great difficulty in quantifying the hazard with carefully conducted studies especially in the presence of variable exposure to non-occupational factors.

The planning of the study to provide valid results includes consideration of the power of the study. Power is defined as the probability that a study: (*a*) will detect in a population an increase in disease or death over that expected, if such an increase has in fact occurred, or (*b*) will not provide a false negative result.

Thus calculation of the power to detect a doubling (or other increase) in RR provides a more direct statement of the adequacy of that study for evaluating the carcinogenicity of an exposure.

1.3.1 Routine data

The ready availability of routine data and low cost to the user are the principal advantages, which have to be balanced against lack of precision of environmental exposure and inflexibility. Routine data are primarily a tool of descriptive studies, to be followed by analytical work using other approaches.

Although 1.1.1 dealt with occupational analyses, simpler approaches may also be of value. For example, Gardner, Acheson and Winter (1982) examined the geographical distribution of pleural mesothelioma in England and Wales in 1966–78. They identified high areas for men where shipbuilding and repairing were concentrated, and for women where gas mask manufacture was predominant—together with high rates for both sexes in East London (a focus for asbestos factories). Nearly all the high mortality areas had known major industrial use of asbestos.

1.3.2 Record linkage

The power of record-linkage studies, including historical prospective studies, may be relatively greater than in other fields of work, as there may be data on potential aetiological exposure that is of higher quality than for other behavioural and environmental agents.

1.3.3 Collation studies

Collation studies have the same advantages of other studies that use routinely available data—the material should be immediately available for the proposed use (providing that any relevant data are collected in the national or other systems). However, the available information may not readily permit the exclusion of confounding effects, e.g. the production of organic chemicals may be a marker of many aspects of 'behaviour' rather than a specific environmental hazard. Also, when the studies are carried out without any prior hypothesis in mind, the results have to be interpreted with caution; the vast number of comparisons that can be made permit the research worker to fully probe so many permutations of the material that the chance of a number of intriguing (but false) hypotheses being generated is high.

Siematycki *et al.* (1981) suggested that such studies were suitable for identifying those isolated localities where there was a single-process industry with a particular health hazard.

1.3.4 Proportional-mortality analyses

The basic drawback, on finding an excess proportion of deaths, is that one does not know if the overall mortality from another cause is low, or if the actual death rate from the disease being studied is high. The approach can only be used as a pointer to further work, rather than as a definitive examination of a particular issue.

A proportional-mortality analysis is very simple to carry out, provided the basic records on the deaths exist; such records may be available through the pension fund or union records, or obtainable from the system for registering mortality in the population. The ease of carrying out such a study is obviously an advantage, but must be balanced against the difficulty in interpreting the data (*see* 1.5.2). Such a study may be used to provide a check of suggestions of a hazard from clinicians or workers; the findings from a proportional-mortality analysis provide a quick appraisal, but will often require confirmation from a definitive study.

1.3.5 Cross-sectional studies

These are suitable for studying disease where there is a high prevalence of the condition in the workforce, and a clearcut method of identifying early abnormality or disease. The advantage will be enhanced if this information can readily be associated with information about 'present' exposure, and this is thought to reflect variation in the potential hazard of the environment. Obviously the converse will apply, so that the method will not be of any use to study disease that is rare, or only occurs after a long latent interval—conditions that usually apply to occupational cancer. Investigation of benign conditions, chromosome abnormalities, or *in-situ* cancer may be more suitable, if the prevalence of these changes is higher and the latent interval shorter.

1.3.6 Case-control studies

The distinction from the cross-sectional surveys is that the case-control studies are usually concerned with aetiological factors that operated in the past. The validity will therefore depend to a great extent on the degree to which it is found possible to quantify the past exposure of the individuals in the study and also to assess the influence of confounding factors. When the starting point of the study is deaths from a given cancer, information will have to be obtained from either relatives or retrievable occupational records. This restricts the depth of information that can be obtained.

The relative advantage is that the studies can be quite quickly mounted and they do not require even as large numbers as the cross-sectional surveys, let alone prospective studies. The data collection is usually dependent upon questioning the subjects, rather than examination or investigation; the costs of data collection are thus usually low.

1.3.7 Historical prospective studies

Such studies depend upon the quality of the retrievable data on past exposure, and then the efficiency of the linkage process that determines the outcome in the cohort. The other crucial issue is the appropriateness of the comparison statistics used. Case and Lea (1955) acknowledged that an external standard may not be applicable to men in a particular study, and demonstrated how 'industrial comparisons' could be made. In a series of papers, Mancuso and his colleagues (Mancuso and Coulter, 1959; Mancuso, 1963; Mancuso and El-Attar, 1966; Mancuso, Ciocco and El-Attar, 1968) raised a number of topics: dilution due to imprecise job descriptions; bias in follow-up with loss of deaths in some categories of individuals; multiple-cause coding; the use of morbidity as an alternative end-point; the 'healthy-worker effect' and use of workers' rates to calculate expected figures; the influence of age at entry, length of follow-up, age at death, and latent interval on the results. A number of other authors have discussed the advantages of internally based expected deaths (Redmond and Breslin, 1975; Enterline, 1976b; Ott, Holder and Langer, 1976). This issue is further discussed in 1.5.7.

Many historical prospective studies commence with a list of all employees engaged at a point in time, to which are linked recruits over the ensuing years. Person-years are only accumulated from the starting date, but there may be some information about the initial cross-section of employees prior to the date of the study start—such as the date of joining the company or the jobs performed. Care must be taken in analysing such material, as those subjects may not be typical of all those who had previously been employed; some of those who had left may have suffered from ailments (whether or not caused by their occupation) making them unfit to continue in the industry, or else may have left on promotion to other more mentally challenging or physically demanding work. In the absence of information about all employed prior to the start date of the study, it is difficult to interpret any analyses for those who remained.

1.3.8 Prospective studies

These are usually reserved for the definitive study of a known hazard, when it is important to quantify the dose–response effect of the agent, and examine other specific points about the aetiology. The method is suitable for a stable industry, where facilities exist for assessing the changes that occur in the work environment over time. Usually the method will be reserved for those conditions that have a relatively high incidence.

Such studies are not lightly undertaken, and the expenditure of time and effort may be justified when there is some hope that early recognition of the disease in the workforce will result in medical intervention that is of benefit to the individuals concerned.

A historical prospective study will give a relatively quick probe of a topic, but with limited specificity, while a genuine prospective study will explore the problem slowly, but with much greater power to quantify the exact aetiological relationships.

1.3.9 'Healthy-worker' effect

An issue that is of particular relevance to historical prospective studies, but that should be borne in mind when trying to interpret other types of study, is now commonly referred to as the 'healthy-worker' effect. Seltzer and Jablon (1974) analysed the 5345 deaths of 85 491 Second World War white male veterans followed from 1946 to 1969; expected mortality was calculated from United States national death rates. In particular, they looked at the trend in deficiency of deaths over time; malignant-disease deaths were about 55% of the expected in the first 5 years and then gradually rose to about 90% (no difference for 6, 10, 16 or 21–23 years of follow-up was significant). There were even more prolonged effects for other main causes of death. They emphasized the protracted effect of selection on any subsequent mortality and stressed that many sub-groups of the population might differ in both known and unknown ways. Follow-up of a cohort for a few years does not, therefore, lead to abolition of the differential in mortality between the worker and the total population.

There has been increasing disquiet about the suitability of national rates to generate a valid expected number of deaths. In many studies this has resulted in a ratio of O/E considerably less than one; often, the all-cause figure is about 0.75 and some recent studies have reported even lower figures. This creates confusion in the interpretation of the data, because the lower figure should not automatically be interpreted as indicating absence of a health hazard. Also, when specific causes of death are examined, it has been suggested that the all-cause ratio may be used as a yardstick against which to measure results from specific causes. Thus, with an all-cause figure of 0.75, it has been claimed that a ratio of 1.0 for cancers is raised, i.e. represents an increment of one-third over the expected figure of 0.75. This can produce considerable argument over the interpretation of the data, especially where the results are based upon large numbers of deaths and such differences are statistically significant. A number of authors have discussed this topic (Enterline, 1975; Gaffey, 1975; Goldsmith, 1975; McMichael, Hagues and Tyroler, 1975; McMichael, 1976).

Ogle (1885) had indicated that occupational cohorts demonstrate properties of selection, survival and length of follow-up. Fox and Collier (1976a) presented data for workers engaged in vinyl chloride manufacture and demonstrated that the reduced risk of death compared with the general population diminished with the lapse of time after entry to the industry. There was also an indication that those who left the industry had a relatively higher risk of death compared with those who remained.

Vinni and Hakama (1980) linked 1960 and 1970 census records for 20 000 Finnish workers and then followed the individuals to 1976. This enabled them to quantify the selection and survival effects. They suggested that the mortality of those who stayed within the same industry was 60% of those who retired prior to age 65, while the mortality of those who changed their job was 90% of those who stayed in the same job. There were also differences in this 'survivor' effect in various occupational categories.

1.4 Extension of method of occupational studies

The following notes describe various extensions to the classic methods described in 1.1, that are specifically associated with exploration of occupational hazards. The first two indicate ways in which data on occupational environment and health effects may be made available; the second pair cover different approaches to case-control studies, whilst the final section indicates a technique for converting job history to potential exposure.

1.4.1 An historical data-base

Many industries are paying increasing attention to the practicality of carrying out various forms of prospective study. The identification of exposed individuals from 'old' occupational records is a time-consuming task and the validity of this material is questionable. Where (*a*) such records exist for a large workforce, (*b*) they contain details of chronological job histories and (*c*) the industry is relatively complex, then it is appropriate to consider the suitability of making such historical records more easily retrievable. Conceptually this is in order to carry out a series of historical prospective studies; having once established the file of relevant data, it can be used to explore subsequent queries as they arise. This will avoid having to go back to the manual records every time a specific query is raised about the mortality of past employees in relation to particular chemicals. Providing follow-up status is available, including the cause of death for those who have died, the observed and expected mortality should be readily examined (*see* Hoar *et al.*, 1980). A system for recording, storing and retrieving occupational exposure data and linkage with medical information for individuals working in the chemical plants in Europe and the United States was described by Baxter and Henshaw (1982). It should be emphasized that the data-base is used to cross-check leads from other sources, not to carry out regular analyses searching for aberrant results (as discussed in the next subsection).

A rather different use of such material is where there is need to cross-check on past exposures of workers dying from a specific and relatively rare disease. If the historical file incorporates a mechanism for accumulating the cause of death for each decedent, it is a relatively simple matter to identify those dying from the particular cause of interest (for example, brain tumours). A sample of control subjects can be obtained from the occupational data-base. Using this material as a starting point, much more detailed enquiry could be made about the occupational histories of the small sample of subjects dying from brain tumours and of the controls. Such a case-control approach has been discussed in the previous section; the historical data-base merely facilitates such a study.

1.4.2 Occupational monitoring systems

An important issue to consider is whether industrial health records can be so organized that they can assist in the establishment of monitoring schemes to detect environmental hazards. The expression 'monitoring' is used to indicate the collection and regular analysis of information in an attempt to identify fresh hazards, not previously recognized. This should be distinguished from 'surveillance', which involves the regular review of material on a known hazard to check on the functioning of control measures. Support for the introduction of monitoring systems comes from the World Health Organisation (WHO, 1974) and the Council of European Communities (CEC, 1979). Their reports indicated the need to collect data on environment, on the population classified by exposure to agents, and on follow-up of the health of employees. In order to set up a monitoring system one requires an enlightened management, a labour force which appreciates the value of such an approach, and the availability of a sound industrial-hygiene service. These elements are essential prerequisites; then comes the need to collect, analyse and interpret relevant data.

It does not follow automatically that because more sophisticated data are being fed into a monitoring system that it will automatically provide valuable fresh leads. There are major statistical problems in the analysis and interpretation of such data; when more complex material is fed in (even assuming it is accurate data and up to date), there may be greater difficulty in interpretation. This is because the number of separate analyses and the range of factors that have to be taken into account increase geometrically; with this increase in complexity of the data-base, there is increase in the difficulty of distinguishing between false and genuine positive leads of equal statistical significance. The greater the number of separate comparisons that are carried out, the greater the number of results that will be 'statistically significant' at any chosen level. It may be possible to identify fresh leads and distinguish them from false leads by replication and comparison of subsets of data, taking into account the relationship between risk and dose, and time trends. It is important to remember that relative risk, absolute risk, specificity of risk, number of men exposed, job stability, latent period, and the influence of confounding factors are important in determining whether hazards can be readily identified. In planning such systems, consideration needs to be given to the availability of data, the feasibility of data collection, the interpretation of data, the process of 'decision making' on results from the system, costs and benefits, and confidentiality.

The items that might be recorded in such a system cover: (*a*) employee history (personal data, work history, reason for leaving); (*b*) medical events (medical history, morbidity on follow-up, mortality); (*c*) environmental exposure (potential exposure, area monitoring, individual exposure); (*d*) biomedical data (clinical history, examination, clinical chemistry, investigation of respiratory and cardiovascular function, chromosome analysis). The range of items that has been suggested (e.g. *see* Epidemiological Project Study Group, 1979) is very comprehensive, when one considers the material presently available for the majority of workers in any form of retrievable record system.

It is sometimes suggested that a surveillance scheme should concentrate on lung cancers occurring in younger men—to exclude the influence of smoking, which has a long median latent interval (Albert *et al.*, 1979). However, Depue and Menck (1980) showed that even using data for all deaths from lung cancer in the US, it would require 10 years to identify 100 deaths in male non-smokers.

Beebe (1981) emphasized the need for an efficient national surveillance system to detect hazards from occupational carcinogens. He discussed the various routine data sets in the US that might be linked to provide a surveillance instrument: (*a*) census records and subsequent deaths; (*b*) the industry from the Continuous Work History Sample, the occupation from the tax return, and subsequent deaths; (*c*) information from the Current Population Survey and subsequent deaths. He acknowledged problems from: legal barriers, especially of confidentiality, administrative organization of records, lack of full identification, lack of full information on occupation, and relationship of recorded occupation to environmental exposure.

The *Lancet* (1983a) suggested an early warning system analogous to the 'yellow-card' warnings of possible adverse reactions that practitioners send to the Committee on the Safety of Medicines. However, the tightening of analysis of routine data, plus improved facility to carry out *ad hoc* enquiry for a lead from any sources, and consideration of follow-up of workers exposed to new industrial agents may be a surer way forward.

Rutstein *et al.* (1983) drew up a table relating diagnosis to occupation (industry and agent involved). Only conditions which were either preventable or treatable were included. They suggest that such a table might increase the physicians' awareness of occupational disease; also, regular analysis of occurrence of such 'Sentinel Health Events (Occupational)' might form a base for public health surveillance.

Whorton (1983), from the US viewpoint, briefly indicated the possibility of using: (*a*) workers' compensation schemes; (*b*) mortality statistics, perhaps with associated occupations of the decedent; (*c*) cancer registration material; (*d*) company 'health surveillance systems'; (*e*) hospital discharge statistics. He suggested that any of these sources of data might be used to examine conditions with known occupational causes.

A recent supplement of the *Journal of Occupational Medicine* (1982; **24**, 781–866) provides a description of the use of various medical information systems in 14 American companies. Some of the method issues have been discussed by Paddle (1981). Because of the complexity of work in this field, it is suggested that further research is still required in order to clarify the optimum approach. This needs to look at the two rather different aspects of (*a*) the desirable level of detail on environment, potential exposure, and morbidity; (*b*) improved techniques for analysis of such complex files.

1.4.3 Case-control studies—'fishing'

The distinction between hypothesis testing and general exploration of variation in occupational exposure has already been made (*see* 1.1.6). As a wider range of factors is probed, and with increase in the number of sites of malignancy investigated, the study requires a very different approach from that of a classic case-control study. Siematycki *et al.* (1981) described their case-control system used to 'fish' for occupational hazards. They advocated the use of several hospitals as a source of cases, and controls with other cancers. It appears that they recommended several sites, so that even if an agent causes multiple-site cancer, this may still be identified from the site having the greatest relative risk. They stressed the advantage of using chemists and/or engineers to review the job histories and identify agents to which each subject is likely to have been exposed.

The International Agency for Research on Cancer (IARC, 1983) have recently initiated a programme entitled 'Surveillance of Environmental Aspects Related to Cancer in Humans' (SEARCH), with a network of collaborating centres. Case-control studies on pancreas, bile duct, and gallbladder cancers are underway, with the aim of improving the method for eliciting occupational histories from the subjects. Though the programme has the word surveillance in its title, the main thrust appears to be via these internationally coordinated case-control studies.

A rather different approach was the accumulation of occupational histories for patients attending a major cancer centre. During 1956–65, 25 416 patients were admitted to Roswell Park (a major cancer treatment centre in New York). All were asked to complete a detailed questionnaire which included demographic, social, medical, occupational, and smoking items. This information was recorded prior to a definitive diagnosis being made. A special analysis was made of the material for 6434 white male and 7515 white female patients with cancer of one of 22 different sites. The patients with non-neoplastic disease formed the control group. Relative risks were calculated by comparison of the numbers with (*a*) the site of interest in a given occupation and clerical occupations, (*b*) non-neoplastic disease in the same occupation or clerical occupations. The report had a brief discussion, but consisted chiefly of the statistical results; these were published by the National Institute for Occupational Safety and Health (NIOSH, 1977).

1.4.4 Case-control within a cohort study

A very different approach is to use a historical prospective study to identify cancers of a specific site developing in individuals; the individuals can then be matched from within the data file to other workers. Enquiries are then instituted about the detailed work histories of each of these subjects, with attempts being made to quantify the exposure to specific agents. For example, a study of over 30 000 workers in 8 oil refineries in the UK showed no overall excess of leukaemia. However, in order to explore the possible association with benzene exposure, the 30 deaths from leukaemia, together with 6 where leukaemia was a contributory cause, were used for a case-control study (Rushton and Alderson, 1981b). Each of these 36 deaths was matched with two sets of controls: the first set of three controls being matched for refinery and year of birth, and the second set of three controls being matched for refinery, year of birth and length of service. The detailed job histories of each individual were abstracted; in the absence of measurement of benzene in the work environment the job histories were used to allocate each man to one of three categories of benzene exposure ('low', 'medium' or 'high'). Logistic models were fitted to the cases and controls matched on year of birth. The risk for those men identified as having had 'medium' or 'high' exposure relative to the risk of those with 'low' exposure reached the formal level of significance when length of service was taken into account, either in the matching of cases and controls, or in the analysis. It was suggested that if there was an increased risk of leukaemia due to benzene exposure, it could have only been one that affected a very small proportion of the men within the total refinery workforce. It must be emphasized that the estimation of benzene exposure was not based on environmental or personal measurements.

Further discussion of this approach can be found in Liddell, McDonald and Thomas (1977), McDonald *et al.* (1980) and Darby and Reissland (1981).

1.4.5 Job titles indexed to chemical exposure

An American list which catalogued different occupations exposed to specific chemicals was used to identify 14 occupations thought to involve benzene exposure (Vianna and Polan, 1979). Deaths in the period 1950–69 in males in New York State were classified and the relative risk of lymphomas in these workers examined. A significant excess of deaths was found, though the possible importance of aromatic hydrocarbons could not be excluded, benzene being the only chemical used by all the occupational groups studied.

Though there were some questions about the method of the above study, it does indicate the way in which a cross-index of job titles to potential chemical exposure may be used to probe an issue. It would provide a preliminary cross-check of any hypothesis where (*a*) the chemical in question was identified in the chemical-job listing, and (*b*) the outcome data such as cancer incidence or mortality recorded jobs in sufficient detail.

Alderson (1980a) pointed out that if there was a list of all job terms in common use on the UK cross-indexed against chemicals to which workers were potentially exposed, one could consider periodic examination of the file of cancer deaths to look for possible chemical exposure indexed under job terms. It was accepted that there were many problems with such a suggestion: the validity of the recorded job, the cross-reference from job to chemical, and the calculation of the expected figure. However, this approach has been discussed more generally recently, using the expression 'job-exposure matrix'. A symposium at the MRC Environmental Epidemiology Unit (Acheson, 1983) discussed some of the conceptual and practical issues involved. Though the general approach may

be more relevant to the analysis of case-control studies, an example of the *ad hoc* application to mortality data was provided by Coggon, Pannett and Acheson (1984). Death certificates for all men under 40 dying of lung cancer and all men under 50 dying of bladder cancer in England and Wales in 1975–79 were matched with 2 control deaths. The occupations recorded at death registration were coded into 223 occupational units, and then the units grouped into likelihood of exposure to 9 potential carcinogens. This matrix was then used to examine the relative risk of the 2 types of tumour for each of the carcinogens. It was concluded that use of the job-exposure matrix added considerably to the conventional analysis of cancer risk in individual occupational categories.

1.4.6 Hazard to next generation

Hemminki, Sorsa and Vaino (1979) discussed ways of studying genetic risks caused by occupational chemicals; the long-term effects were spontaneous abortions, malformation and cancer. They noted that abortion rates varied with the method of study, it being difficult to determine loss in the early weeks of pregnancy. Morphological inspection may be a useful approach to teratological monitoring (there may be malformations in 5–10% of abortions). There was some evidence that exposure to copper smelters, laboratory environment, operating rooms, or vinyl chloride increased the risk of abortion. It was considered that malformation registers should help clarify the role of environmental factors.

Transplacental carcinogenesis had been observed in exposure to anaesthetic gases, diethylstilbestrol given in early pregnancy, possibly barbiturate, chlorinated pesticides, and smoking exposure.

Hemminki, Sorsa and Vaino (1979) suggested that occupational carcinogenesis may be more readily detected in childhood cancers, where the latent interval must be shorter than in some cancers occurring in workers.

The actual technique used to study this issue will depend on the specific outcome being considered and the information collected in the national or local registration system for that outcome. The following are the main options:

1.4.6.1 Spontaneous miscarriage

If the majority of subjects with clinically recognized miscarriage are admitted to hospital, it may be possible to (*a*) analyse the frequency of miscarriage by recorded occupation of the women from hospital discharge record systems, (*b*) link exposure data on a group of women, or mens' wives to hospital discharge for miscarriage.

1.4.6.2 Stillbirth

If the registration system records the occupation of both parents, proportional registration ratios (PRRs) or standardized registration ratios (SRRs) can be calculated by occupation (the latter using denominators from the census). Again case-control or prospective studies may be required.

1.4.6.3 Fertility

If the birth registration system records the occupation of both parents, SRRs or PRRs can be calculated. A particular aspect of fertility analyses are tabulations of the distribution of birth weight by parental occupation—which are possible if birth weight is one of the registration items.

1.4.6.4 Congenital malformations

Where these are registered for a defined population and parents' occupation is recorded, PRRs or SRRs can be calculated.

1.4.6.5 Childhood cancers

The same considerations apply as for congenital malformations.

For each of the above outcomes, the routine data system may permit linkage of a nominal roll of exposed women to the event data. This can provide automatic calculation of event rates in exposed women (and unexposed controls). In the absence of named outcome data, or by reasons of confidentiality, such linkage studies will be impossible. Absence of registration systems, e.g. for congenital malformation, will require *ad hoc* case-control, 'exposed'–'not exposed', or prospective studies. These pose problems of validity of data and, in case-control and exposed–not exposed studies, of biased recall for the case of exposed subjects.

Shilling and Lalich (1984) used the US National Nationality and Fetal Mortality Surveys of 1980 to study the association of maternal occupation with pregnancy outcome. This permitted tabulation of the percentage births with low birth weight, congenital malformation, and fetal death by occupational order. This was thought to be suitable for indicating particular occupation or industries in which further research was required.

Starr and Levine (1983) discuss the calculation of expected fertility from national data specific to race, birth cohort, age and parity. They suggest that comparison with a non-exposed occupational group may be more preferable than attempts to calculate an expected value.

1.5 Statistical methods

This section provides an introduction to some of the statistical methods that are particularly relevant to occupational studies. This is only to serve as a brief guide to this topic; it (*a*) indicates how some of the simpler calculations can be performed, and (*b*) provides some background when considering published studies. (Have the appropriate statistics been presented? Are the results likely to be a chance effect?)

1.5.1 Do differences in numbers of deaths or death rates mean anything?

If it is known that, over a period of years, there have been about 25 cancers recognized annually in a workforce, it is useful to have some simple method of gauging the extent to which this number might fluctuate. Statistical method can indicate how widely this number could vary: once in 40 years, the figure might be higher than the average plus twice the 'standard error' (s.e.) and once in 40 years below the average $-2 \times$ s.e. This is an estimate of the 95% confidence limits (95% CL). An approximate s.e. for a small average number of events is the square root of the figure,

$$
\begin{aligned}
\text{i.e. 95\% CL} &= \text{average number deaths} \\
&\quad \pm 2 \times \text{s.e.} \\
&= 25 \pm 2\sqrt{25} \\
&= 15\text{–}35
\end{aligned}
$$

Thus increase in the number from 25 one year to 34 or 35 the following year does not indicate more than a chance fluctuation in the figures. However, 'steady' increase, e.g. 25, 29, 31, 34, 37 would be good reason to mount an investigation—though initially aspects such as changing age structure of the workforce or improved diagnosis must be considered, as well as increased incidence from non-occupational or occupational cause.

When comparing the toll from cancer in different groups of workers, rates will usually be examined, or observed and expected events, which are discussed below. For rates, a comparable calculation to the above provides the s.e.,

$$
\text{i.e. s.e. of a rate} = \frac{\text{Rate}}{\sqrt{n}}
$$

where n = number of deaths on which rate is based

To compare the difference in two rates:

95% CL of difference =

$$
\text{Difference} \pm 2 \sqrt{\frac{(\text{Death rate})_1}{n_1} + \frac{(\text{Death rate})_2}{n_2}}
$$

Though this calculation is readily performed, the results can be read straight off the nomograms published by Rosenbaum (1963).

1.5.2 Proportional-mortality analysis

The application of this technique has already been discussed (*see* 1.1.4). The method of calculation requires, for the 'standard population', the number of deaths from all causes and from the cause of interest within appropriate age groups. The proportion of specific-cause to all-cause deaths is then applied to the number of deaths from all causes in the study population, to give the expected deaths. This is repeated for all the age groups involved. The proportional-mortality ratio is then given by:

$$\frac{\text{Sum of observed deaths}}{\text{Sum of expected deaths}} \times 100$$

The calculation is set out in *Table 1.1*, for the relatively simple data handled in this way in the decennial supplement on occupational mortality for 1959–63 (Registrar General, 1971).

This method can be used for national data, where the denominator is not readily available (in the example used in *Table 1.1*, there is appreciable variation in recording of occupation between census and death registration for persons aged 65–74 and indirect standardization using rates is not appropriate). The example in 1.1.4 used national and local data to calculate the proportional mortality of miners in Cumberland from various causes. The National Cancer Registration Scheme records occupation, where known, for each patient registered with cancer. As the information is not recorded for an appreciable number of patients and there are not readily available figures of the population at risk, proportional registration rates (PRRs) by occupation unit are calculated. The method is essentially the same as indicated in *Table 1.1*, but involves calculation for 12 5-year age groups from 15 to 74.

The principal drawback to this technique is that, as rates are not available, one does not know if the overall mortality is low or high in the study population. Thus when a specific cause has a low proportional-mortality ratio, this may be genuinely low, or 'apparently low' due to an actual excess from another cause. This dilemma in interpretation of the material means that the approach can only be used as a pointer to further work. Sartor (1982) discussed some of the problems of interpreting PMRs, and stressed that the PMR will only be equal to the SMR if the overall death rates are equal in the study and 'comparison' group.

1.5.3 Person-years at risk

In historical prospective and prospective studies, data are collected about subjects who have been exposed to aetiological risk at different times and are then followed over a period of time. Deaths or cancers may occur at any time in this period. A count can readily be made of the number of cancers (or deaths from cancer) that occur; to draw any conclusion some comparison is required. A very simple technique is to calculate the expected number of events. For this one requires to know: the date and age of entry into the study for each subject; the last date without cancer, or of development/ death from cancer for each subject; standard incidence or mortality rates for cancers, by age, sex, and calendar period. The dates enable the number of years of life lived in different age and calendar periods to be determined for all subjects. Applying the standard incidence or mortality rates to the person-years by age, sex, and calendar period, and then summing the products provides the number of expected events.

As Hill (1972) pointed out, when a large number of subjects are included in the study, even the simple calculation of the number of years at risk tabulated

Table 1.1 Calculation of proportional-mortality ratio (PMR) for stomach cancer in two occupational orders in England and Wales, 1959–63

		Age			
Occupation	*Cause*	*65–69*	*70–74*	*65–74*	*PMR*
All men	All causes	181 288	205 604		
	Stomach cancer observed	6477	6589		
	Proportion of stomach cancer	0.0357	0.0320		
Professional and	All causes	7613	9346		
technical	Stomach cancer observed	181	224	405	
	Stomach cancer expected*	271.8	299.1	570.9	71
Miners and	All causes	9318	11 190		
quarrymen	Stomach cancer observed	405	419	824	
	Stomach cancer expected*	332.7	358.1	690.8	119

Based on Registrar General, 1971.
*Expected deaths = All causes × Proportion of stomach cancer in all men in age-group,
e.g. = 7613 × 0.0357
   = 271.8.

by 5-year age groups is a laborious clerical task in which errors may occur. Many studies require consideration of the variation in incidence or mortality over time, and also the effect of latent interval since first exposure to the aetiological factor. Hill (1972) described a computer program he had devised to facilitate handling such material; a number of other comparable analysis packages are available.

The rates used in the calculation are usually national or regional rates for the total population. Also, those who have been employed for under 10 years may be used after a complete follow-up as a data-base from which to calculate occupation- or industry-specific expected figures. (The assumption being that such individuals have a more comparable basic mortality pattern than that obtained from the national data.)

1.5.4 Are the observed deaths raised?

A very common requirement in occupational studies is to check whether the observed number of deaths is significantly increased. This involves the concept of 'person-years at risk' which is used to calculate an expected number of deaths. The following note indicates how the results may be tested. There is need for some relatively simple system for checking the probability of obtaining the observed (or a greater) number of deaths in comparison with the expected deaths.

The actual technique will depend upon the numbers of events involved; if at least 5 deaths were expected, then the difference can be simply probed as follows:

$$\chi^2 = \frac{(O-E)^2}{E}$$

If O = 76, E = 105.56 then

$$\chi^2 = \frac{(76 - 105.56)^2}{105.56}$$

$$= \frac{(-29.56)^2}{105.56}$$

$$= 8.28$$

Check of the appropriate tables for the χ^2 distribution for one degree of freedom shows this value is very unlikely to be obtained by chance, i.e. $P<0.01$.

Another way to probe the same data is to examine the confidence limits of the ratio O/E; this is done by using the approach advocated by Bailar and Ederer (1964). For any given value of observed events, the factors for the comparison O/E can be read from a table they provide; these are then used as divisors to generate the 95% or 99% confidence limits for the particular ratio. For 70 observed events (76 is not tabulated), the factors are 0.791 and 1.28 for 95%

significance; these are used to divide the original ratio of O/E thus:

$$95\% \text{ confidence limits} = \frac{0.72}{0.791} \text{ to } \frac{0.72}{1.28}$$

$$= 0.91 \text{ to } 0.56$$

It can be seen that these results are asymmetrical about the original value of 0.72, but they do not encompass the value of 1.0; this agrees with the test of significance that the results are unlikely to be due to chance.

Instead of using the tables of Bailar and Ederer, an approximate formula for the 95% confidence limits may be used:

95% confidence limits

$$= \frac{(O - 2\sqrt{E})}{E} \text{ to } \frac{(O + 2\sqrt{E})}{E}$$

$$= \frac{(76 - 2\sqrt{105.56})}{105.56} \text{ to } \frac{(76 + 2\sqrt{105.56})}{105.56}$$

$$= 0.525 \text{ to } 0.915$$

Again, these values do not encompass 1.00 and support the contention that the results are statistically significant.

Where the expected number of events is less than 5, the data are treated as a Poisson variate. The test then examines the probability of obtaining the observed or a more extreme number of events, given that the expected value represents the mean value for the events in the parent population. The simplest way to examine this is to consult published tables, such as those of Pearson and Hartley (1970). Volume 1 of this work includes a table giving the probability of each increment in observed events for a given mean figure. For example, if there were 7 observed deaths in a subgroup of men with an expected figure of 2.3, entering the Pearson and Hartley table for this mean figure would show that the cumulative probability of observing 7 or more deaths was 0.00936. (Note: this may be obtained directly for some values of E by inspection of *Table 7*, or by summing the individual values of *Table 39* (both from Pearson and Hartley, 1970), which provides a finer gradation of values of E.) It must be remembered that the *P* value is obtained from a one-tailed test, quantifying the probability of obtaining the observed or a more extreme value. The confidence limits are obtained in the way set out above, as this method is valid for expected values of any size.

1.5.5 Calculation of an SMR

The general method of calculating an SMR is indicated in *Table 1.2*. The data are taken from a report on occupational mortality for the period 1959–63 (Registrar General, 1971).

If the observed mortality, after taking into account the age distribution of the specific population, is the same as that expected, an SMR of 100 will be obtained. If the mortality is high a figure of greater than 100 will be obtained, while if the mortality is low a corresponding reduction in the SMR will occur. The crude mortality rate for farmers was 5.9/1000 men per annum, and for the armed forces 2.8/1000 men per annum. This suggests a lower mortality in the armed forces. However, *Table 1.2(b)* shows that there are very few men in the older age groups in the armed forces and an age correction produces an SMR of 151 compared with that for farmers of 82 (*see Table 1.2(c)*). Standardization for age thus indicates a considerably lower mortality for the farmers. The mathematics involved are relatively simple; however, the important point at this stage is to grasp the broad outline of the approach and appreciate the indications for standardization and the situations in which it should be applied. A matter of judgement is whether to use age-specific rates or age-standardized rates for comparative purposes. The main consideration is the number of age groups for which a comparison is required; thus when comparing the mortality in different towns, to present the results of 15 5-year age groups would create difficulties, and it would be more appropriate to use age-standardized rates. The other extreme is consideration of the medical problems of a subgroup of the population defined by

age, such as infancy or middle age. In this kind of situation, it is more appropriate to use age-specific rates. Even when making use of an SMR it is advisable to check the age-specific rates for consistency. Kilpatrick (1962) discussed the problem of standardizing in a situation where an occupation has raised mortality at one end of the age range, and a low mortality at the other. Any index such as an SMR will be misleading in such a situation. Alderson (1981a) has reviewed a variety of indices and concluded that the indirectly calculated SMR is most suitable as the general technique.

The approach described in *Table 1.2* is known as indirect standardization. It is more generally suitable since it uses rates based on the standard population; this method has the advantages that these rates are usually easier to obtain than age-specific rates for the study population and, being based on larger numbers, they are less subject to chance variation and produce a better estimate of the SMR.

Liddell (1960) reviewed the application of four methods of age standardization and commented that no mortality index should be used without a knowledge of the inherent inadequacy due to variation in the relative death rates. Mantel and Stark (1968) showed how standard rates could be derived internally from the available data and used to carry out indirect standardization. They emphasized the need to treat with caution any results based

Table 1.2 Calculation of standardized mortality ratio for two occupational groups

(*a*) Original data 1959–63

Occupation	Number in occupational group	Observed deaths	Crude deathrate/ 1000 per annum
Farmers, foresters and fishermen	705 910	20 973	5.9
Armed forces	301 120	4282	2.8

(*b*) Calculation of expected number of deaths

Age	Annual deathrates/ 1000 men, England and Wales	Farmers, foresters, fishermen		Armed forces	
		Number in occupation	Expected deaths* 1959–63	Number in occupation	Expected deaths* 1959–63
15–24	1028	134 560	691.6	165 030	848.3
25–34	1118	124 100	693.7	73 240	409.4
35–44	2411	132 220	1593.9	42 250	509.3
45–54	7072	160 110	5661.5	15 930	563.3
55–64	21 710 .	154 920	16 816.6	4670	506.9
Total expected deaths			25 457.3		2837.2

*Expected deaths = number in occupation × national age-specific rate × 5. An annual death rate is being used and the expected deaths are required for the period 1959–63 (i.e. 5 years)

(*c*) Calculation of standardized mortality ratio

$$\text{SMR farmers, foresters, fishermen} = \frac{20\,973}{25\,457.3} \times 100 = 82$$

$$\text{SMR armed forces} = \frac{4282}{2837.2} \times 100 = 151$$

on indirect standardization. Cook (1979) drew attention to the age dependence of the SMR and the inability to compare rates for samples where the age distribution is different. There followed a dispute between Harnes (1980) and Cook (1980), in which various manipulations were suggested for trying to overcome this problem. Neither appeared to provide a generally acceptable solution to the problem. Alderson (1981b) has suggested that an alternative to comparison of the ratio of observed and expected deaths might be more detailed analyses based on the difference between the observed and expected deaths. This calculation provides something akin to an attributable risk; this may then be examined in relation to various estimates of 'exposure' (intensity of exposure and duration of exposure), and latent interval between first exposure and development of cancer or death.

1.5.6 Is the SMR significantly different from 100?

Whenever the SMR for a specific subgroup of the population has been calculated there is interest in determining whether it differs sufficiently from 100 for this to be unlikely to be a chance effect. The answer will be directly influenced by the number of deaths upon which the SMR is based; this seems intuitively plausible as, if based on relatively few deaths, one or two more or less might have occurred within the data period and would have an appreciable impact on the results. The actual play of chance can be fairly readily estimated by a simple calculation as follows:

$$\chi^2 \text{ (indicator of chance effect)} = \frac{(O-E)^2}{E}$$

where O is the number of observed deaths and E the number of expected deaths.

If, in a particular occupational group, the SMR for leukaemia was 150 and this was based upon 24 observed deaths, then

$$\chi^2 = \frac{(24-16)^2}{16} \quad E = \frac{O}{SMR} \times 100$$

$$= 4$$

but if this is based upon only 21 observed deaths, then

$$\chi^2 = \frac{(21-14)^2}{14}$$

$$= 3.5$$

The indicator being used is in fact χ^2, and it is technically known as being based on one degree of freedom in this comparison. The above fictitious

Table 1.3 Minimum number of deaths required for SMR to be significantly different from 100, at *P<0.05* or *P<0.01*

SMR	P<0.05	P<0.01
150	23	40
145	28	48
140	34	58
135	43	73
130	56	96
125	77	133
120	116	200
115	197	340
110	423	732
105	1614	2796
95	1460	2529
90	346	599
85	146	251
80	77	133
75	47	80
70	30	52
65	21	35

examples have been chosen for ease of calculation and also because they span an important value of χ^2, i.e. 3.84. This is the figure for one degree of freedom, which, if exceeded for the specific set of data, indicates that the difference between the observed and the expected values has a probability of less than 0.05. This is the level usually used to reject the suggestion that the results are chance findings, in which case they are referred to as 'statistically significant'.

To save calculation when scanning tables of SMRs or PMRs, a look-up table is provided (*Table 1.3*) which shows the minimum number of observed deaths required before specific values of the SMR are significantly different from 100. These are based on calculations which give a chi-squared value that is sufficiently large to be significant, either *P<0.05* or *P<0.01*.

1.5.7 Internal analyses in prospective studies

A very different approach is to use some form of internal analysis instead of calculating the expected mortality from national data. Oldham and Rossiter (1965) used a discriminant function to give a linear combination of 18 measurements made on a sample of men; their results facilitated interpretation of the data, and did not appear to be very dependent on the distributional assumptions that were involved. A discussion with a number of statisticians on the appropriate analysis of occupational-cohort studies (Liddell, 1975) distinguished (*a*) *a posteriori* analyses (relating effects to causal variates) in order to determine the best hypothesis, with probability statements adjusting for simultaneous inference; (*b*) *a priori* analyses (relating hypothesized causes to subsequent effects) to obtain mortality rates for defined subcohorts; (*c*) summarized data in life-table form comparing subcohorts. This approach was used in a major study of asbestos miners in Canada reported by Liddell, McDonald and Thomas (1977); they suggested that the conventional analysis was useful to place the cohort mortality rates in the appropriate demographic context. The regression analyses, which were more complex to perform, provided absolute risks when the complete data set was used. Further analyses by the same method (McDonald *et al.*, 1980) suggested that the *a posteriori* analyses had the advantages that interaction between several variables could be examined and it avoided the requirement for external rates. Darby and Reissland (1981) developed a test for trend which examined the distribution of observed and expected deaths in exposure categories across age/calendar-period/time-since-first-employment subgroups. The expected values were calculated assuming a no-dose effect. They had to exclude subgroups where there were no deaths or where all the person-years in any given category was the only entry. The authors also carried out a conventional analysis using national rates and obtained comparable results from both approaches.

Alderson, Rattan and Bidstrup (1981) were asked to see if control of the environmental exposure had reduced the risk of lung cancer in workers in the chromate-producing industry. However, because of the nature of the data available, those who had worked before the plant had been modified had, in general, a longer duration of work, and had been followed to older ages. There were thus confounding factors between duration of exposure, length of follow-up, and whether or not the individual had worked before the plant modification. In order to disentangle these confounding factors a multiple-regression analysis was carried out using death from lung cancer as the dependent variate. *Table 1.4* shows the main results for this analysis; duration of work and duration of follow-up were associated with appreciable variation in risk of lung cancer, though an independent contribution did come from calendar period of employment (i.e. distinguishing the influence of modification). This internal multivariate analysis thus confirmed the suggestion that the plant modification had had an effect on risk of lung cancer, although it also indicated that duration of employment and duration of follow-up were more important factors in determining risk of lung cancer.

Appendix: national publication of occupational incidence and mortality

The following notes indicate the main publications that are available for various countries; these are provided in alphabetical order. The most extensive material has been published for England and Wales; two tables indicate some of the results from the decennial publications, whilst a third table provides a limited comparison of the international publications.

A subset of the national material may be used to examine (*a*) the risk for a specific cancer in different occupations, or (*b*) the risk in a specific occupation of different cancers. Such *ad hoc* studies usually only cover a few sites of malignancy on a defined locality within a country. Many reports have been published of this nature; the method points discussed in 1.1 are relevant to such work. Though a review of all such work is not included here, key results on specific hazards stemming from such work are included in Chapters 2 and 3.

Australia

McMichael and Hartshorne (1982) used male deaths in the age range 30–64 in Australia in 1968–78 and census estimates by occupation to examine broad causes of mortality for 9 occupational groups. Direct age standardization was performed. This limited report presented the ratio of observed to expected deaths for 8 sites of malignancy for the 9 occupational groups.

In addition results for 5 specific occupations are given for lung, and mouth/pharynx/oesophageal cancer. The numbers of deaths upon which these results were based were not provided.

Table 1.4 Results of multivariate analysis, showing the independent contributions of various factors to risk of lung cancer in chromate workers

Factor	Category	Contribution to risk of lung cancer*
Duration of employment (years)	9	− 59
	10−	+ 2
	20+	+164
Duration of follow-up (years)	9	+118
	10−	+ 56
	20+	− 88
Period of employment	Pre-change	+ 73
	Pre-/post-change	+ 50
	Post-change	−112
Factory	Bolton	− 96
	Eaglescliffe	− 33
	Rutherglen	+ 62

Source: Alderson *et al.* (1981)
*The scores may be compared to indicate the relative contribution to the risk of cancer; they approximately indicate the percentage variation from average risk of lung cancer for all men in the study.

Appendix: national publication of occupational incidence and mortality 25

Canada

Records of occupations were available for a 10% sample of the Canadian labour force from 1965 to 1968. This file for 415 201 males was matched with the national mortality files for the period 1965–73. SMRs were calculated using (a) the Canadian population mortality rates, and (b) the entire study cohort rates to obtain the expected deaths. Howe and Lindsay (1983) presented preliminary results on cancer mortality for: (a) 12 occupation divisions, and (b) 11 industrial divisions for 13 sites of cancer. More specific occupations or industries were listed where the SMR for any given site was significant (P<0.05 on a one-tailed test) and O≥5.

Denmark

Introduction of a personal identification number in Denmark in 1968 and computerization of the central population index permitted linkage of data from the 1970 census to subsequent deaths. An analysis of occupational mortality has been published covering deaths in 1970–75 (Danmarks Statistiks, 1979). Due to the relatively small number of deaths, only one table relates cancer mortality to occupation; this is restricted to deaths from all cancers occurring in 93 occupational units (with results for some broader occupational groups). The total number of deaths is given and SMRs for males and females are given separately. These data, because of the broad cause

Table 1.5 Occupational units showing consistently raised SMRs for certain cancers in the period 1911–71, for males aged 15–64, England and Wales

Occupational unit	Oesophagus				Stomach						Lung				Leukaemia		
	1911	1921	1951	1971	1911	1921	1931	1951	1961	1971	1931	1951	1961	1971	1951	1961	1971
Farmer																	
Agricultural worker																	
Coal-face worker					138	118	121	167	260	171							
Coal-gas manufacturer											367	129	152	178			
Chemical worker	+	136	111	129													
Welder											..	118	122	151	114	121	115
Plumber											67	125	124	126			
Shoemaker																	
Cotton spinner					61	160	117	110	144	167							
Brewer																	
Tobacco worker																	
Paper manufacturer					..	105	178	141	136	136							
Compositor																	
Rubber worker																	
Bricklayer											104	113	136	147			
Mason																	
Painter/decorator											117	149	145	136			
Building labourer											153	175	124	97			
General labourer																	
Bus driver																	
Goods driver											110	118	135	145			
Postman																	
Bus conductor					..	112	114	102	120	139							
Railway porter	156	140	..	183	..	127	90	128	130	135							
Dock labourer					..	102	172	137	171	216	183	149	169	182			
Clerk																	
Commercial traveller																	
Police																	
Publican											146	144	142	153			
Barman											+	117	137	165			
Chimney sweep					..	+	133	143	+	127							
Hairdresser																	
Medical practitioner																	
Teacher																	
Clergy																	
Lawyers																	

Note: (1) Criteria for entry was that the RSMR was consistently raised and the SMR≥110 for the majority of the calendar periods for which data were available.
(2) The number of data-years around the census were: 1910–12; 1921–23; 1930–32; 1949–53; 1959–63; 1970–72.
(3) Symbols used: .. no data available; + too few deaths for calculation of SMR.
(4) Source: Logan (1982) Appendix Table E.

used, are unsuitable for comparison with the other national material.

Work is in progress to extend the mortality to 1970–80 and to add in cancer registrations for 1970–80 (Lynge, E., personal communication, 28/5/84).

England and Wales, 1911–71

Logan (1982) utilized the published series of decennial supplements for England and Wales for 1885–1971 to examine cancer mortality by occupation and social class. (Note: despite the title 1911–71, he made some use of the decennial supplements that had appeared since 1885.) Appendix *Table E* in the report presented SMRs for 36 occupations for 1911–71, for deaths from 11 cancer sites in males aged 15–64. Also a PMR, referred to as a relative standardized mortality ratio (RSMR), was calculated. Data have been abstracted from this where the RSMR was consistently raised, and the SMR was over 110 for the data-years available (not every occupation or site was tabulated in each of the 6 reports). The results in *Table 1.5* show the 4 sites for which at least one occupation has consistently

high SMRs. There was no such occupation for the other 7 sites: buccal cavity and pharynx; large intestine; rectum; pancreas; skin; prostate; bladder.

England and Wales, 1970–72

The decennial supplement for 1970–72 is the latest yet published in the series and provides extensive material in tables and microfiche (Registrar General, 1978). An abstraction of some of this material is included in *Table 1.6*; SMRs for men aged 15–64 in various occupational orders have been selected if significant ($P<0.01$) and where the $O \geqslant 20$. The data have also been examined for occupational units, using three different criteria to select jobs that are associated with increased SMRs: (*a*) using the same as for orders, i.e. SMR significant at $P<0.01$, with $O \geqslant 20$, and the actual SMR = 120; (*b*) PMR for those aged 65–74 significantly raised with $P<0.01$, and the SMR raised with $P<0.05$; (*c*) the PRR for registrations in 1966–67 or 1968–69 significantly raised with $P<0.01$ and the PMR for those aged 15–64 significantly raised, with at least $P<0.05$. These statistics are used for some of the international comparisons that follow and data are presented in

Table 1.6 Occupation orders with raised SMRs for deaths from cancer in males aged 15–64 in England and Wales

Occupation	Tongue		Hypoph.		Oesoph.		Stomach		Colon		Rectum	
	O	SMR	O	SMR	O	SMR	O	SMR	O	SMR	O	SMR
Farmer, forester, fisherman							320	171	207	120	107	150
Miners and quarrymen							320	171	207	120	107	150
Gas, coke, chemical							93	150				
Glass and ceramics												
Furnace, forge, foundry							115	144	117	131		
Electric and electronic												
Engineering and allied trades							1143	115			461	118
Woodworker												
Leather worker												
Textile worker							99	149				
Clothing worker												
Food, drink, tobacco						46	151					
Paper and printing												
Maker of other products												
Construction							382	142			131	126
Painter and decorator												
Driver stationery engine												
Labourer n.e.c.	32	218			190	134	872	150	354	115		
Transport and communication					194	128	752	124				
Warehousemen, storekeeper							371	117				
Clerical												
Sales	21	177										
Service, sport, recreation					154	128						
Admin. and managerial												
Professional, technical, artist												

Note: (1) Entry only if the SMR$\geqslant$110, $P<0.01$, and E$\geqslant$10.
   (2) The following sites did not have a single SMR eligible for entry: oropharynx, nasopharynx, bone, connective tissue, other skin, eye, CNS, thyroid, non-Hodgkin's lymphoma, Hodgkin's lymphoma, leukaemia, multiple myeloma.
n.e.c. = not elsewhere classified.

the chapters by individual site of malignancy and occupation.

Finland

Data from censuses held in 1970, 1975, and 1980 are accessible, in principle, by computer; this includes coded occupation. The 1970 census has been linked to deaths in 1971–75, and an analysis of cause of death and occupation published (Sauli, 1979). The current occupation was used for the economically active; conscripts and unemployed were classed by the last job held. There were 218 000 deaths in the period, which were linked to the census records for persons aged 15–64. There was a small proportion of mismatches (about 2%); there were also thought to be about 0.5% deaths in persons recorded at the census who died abroad. For males, data were presented for 72 different occupational groups; if numbers permitted, age-specific deaths, rates, and an SMR were provided for 5 broad sites of malignancy. However, due to the number of deaths available, results were only presented for: 28 occupations for alimentary tract; 3 for buccal cavity, pharynx, and larynx; 38 for lung; 4 for prostate; and

7 for leukaemia. Raised SMRs ($P<0.01$) were only found for lung cancer (for 10 occupations).

Extension of this work is linking the 1975 census to the original file and adding deaths and cancer registrations after 1975. No results are yet available for this later period.

France

The only data available are based on a special study (Desplanques, 1976). A sample of males aged 30–69 was selected from the index of the population in 1954. Information was collected on year of birth, marital status, region of residence, type of commune, qualifications, and social/professional status. For married subjects, information was collected from their wives. The final sample included 464 000 males and 328 000 females. Subsequent deaths were identified up until 1971; mortality rates by age were then calculated.

The study excluded those born outside France, such as immigrant workers, and the unemployed. The occupation used was that recorded in 1954, which may have changed over time—although restriction to persons over the age of 30 had reduced

Table 1.6 Continued

Liver		Gall bl.		Pancreas		Nose		Larynx		Lung		Melanoma		Testis		Bladder	
O	SMR	O	SMR	O	SMR	O	SMR	O	SMR	O	SMR	O	SMR	O	SMR	O	SMR
										315	123						
										515	155						
																63	141
										4894	119						
										802	113						
																73	145
		17	245							659	129						
										1595	144						
				95	135					847	139						
										796	113					66	152
53	156					29	205	92	186	3521	146						
								73	140	3225	128					224	127
										1517	115						
45	156							66	159	2437	120						
												72	142	103	145		

the likelihood of major job change. Using manual methods to identify deaths may have resulted in errors or omissions of differing degree for the 3 time periods of 1955–60, 1961–65, 1966–71.

The analyses by cause of death only provided a very limited examination of this topic, presenting statistics for 7 broad causes for 12 socio-economic groups, with mortality rates for the age groups 35–44, 45–54, and 55–64.

Italy

A cohort study has linked the 1981 census for the Turin population (about 1 million people) with deaths recorded in the local death index. A postal follow-up of those known from the city population register to have emigrated from the locality will be carried out in 1985. It is thought that the cohort size is too small for analyses by occupation and mortality of cancer sites (Costa, G., personal communication, 1984).

Northern Ireland

The Registrar General for Northern Ireland arranged for an analysis of occupational mortality for the years 1960–62, using the 1961 Census as denominator; no official report has been published. Age-standardized mortality ratios were calculated for males aged 15–64 for 27 occupation orders and social classes for all causes and 4 broad causes of death. Crude mortality rates were also shown for males and married women for 27 occupation orders. Park (1965–66) published these limited results, but emphasized that detailed tabulations were available upon request.

Norway

The information from the census in 1970 was linked to deaths occurring in 1970–73, which permitted analyses of mortality by occupation (Haldorsen and Glattre, 1976). This activity was then extended by

Table 1.7 Lung cancer SMRs for occupational units from 6 countries

Occupation	Canada	England & Wales	Finland	Norway	Scotland	US
Fishermen		250				
Orchardists						132
Forestry worker			153			
Mining and quarrying			225		125	
Furnacemen, coal/coke		178				
Chemical worker				158		
Glass formers		147		174*		
Smelter worker						171
Furnacemen—metal		155				
Moulders, coremakers					279	
Metal mill operators		184				
Electrical engineer		271			144	
Sheet metal worker		145			289	128
Steel erectors		197			298	127
Metal plate worker		151			200	
Welders, braziers		151	145	131	156	135
Turner					140	
Machine tool operator		164			208	
Tool maker		123				
Motor mechanic		133				124
Fitter n.e.c.					136	
Electroplater		171				
Plumber	168	126				130
Pipe fitter		133				
Metal making other		144				
Shipyard worker						119
Carpenter		120	135			
Leather worker					188	
Baker		128			159	
Butcher		119	190		140	
Food processor n.e.c.		129				
Printers		142			125	

Table 1.7 Continued

Occupation	Canada	England & Wales	Finland	Norway	Scotland	US
Rubber worker					195	
Bricklayer		147			176	
Mason		157			163	
Plasterer		160	190		277	154
Roofer						152
Builder		152				
Bricklayers' labourer		298				
Road construction worker						126
Construction worker		123				
Aerographer, paintsprayer		162				
Painter, decorator		136			149	121
Boiler fireman		159	143	152†		
Crane operator		138			145	
Foundry worker		195				
Other labourer		199	188	153‡	140	
Navy coastguard						135
Deck engine room rating	223			213§	192	154
Driver railway engine					158	
Railway guard	162					
Railway switchman						160
Driver bus/coach	125			152†		
Driver road goods vehicle	145		183		140	
Bus conductor	138					
Dock labourer	182				176	
Warehousemen	120					
Shop salesman					133	
Roundsman	143				219	
Garage proprietor	145					
Guards					165	
Publican	153					
Barman	165					
Cook					196	
Caretaker	124					
Launderer	157			174*		
Service sport recreation worker	132					
Civil/structural engineer					167	

*Glass, ceramics, laundry and dry cleaning, other production processes.
†Road transport and stationery engine driver.
‡Games supervisor, messenger, caretaker, cleaner, labourer.
§Ships crew.
All entries restricted to $O \geqslant 20$ and $P < 0.01$

Sources:	Canada	Howe and Lindsay, 1983.
	England and Wales	Registrar General, 1978.
	Finland	Sauli, 1979.
	Norway	Kristofersen, 1979.
	Scotland	Registrar General, Scotland, 1981.
	US	Milham, 1983.

n.e.c. = not elsewhere classified.

linking the 1960 Census information; this provided the opportunity to study 4 groups of subjects: (*a*) those economically active in 1970, plus non-active in 1970 but active in 1960; (*b*) active in 1960 but non-active in 1970; (*c*) active in 1960 and 1970 in the same occupational group; (*d*) active in 1960 and 1970 in different occupational groups (Kristofersen, 1979). The results are based on over 25 000 deaths in males amongst a workforce of over 1 million, and 4500 deaths in females in a workforce of nearly 0.5 million. Direct standardization was provided using the population for each of the 4 groups of subjects as standard. Despite these numbers, the material becomes of limited stability when examined by sex, occupational group, and cause of death.

A major extension of the analyses will utilize a file of the 1970 Census linked to all deaths in the period 1970–80.

Scotland

The Registrar General for Scotland has published data following each decennial census in Scotland, using exactly the same technique as in England and Wales. The same problems apply, plus the fact that Scotland only has a population of about 10% of that of England and Wales. The latest data (Registrar General, Scotland, 1981) have been used for the international comparison presented in *Table 1.7*.

Sweden

A linked file was obtained in Sweden from records of the 1960 census of population and housing, and cancer registrations in the period 1960–73 (National Board of Health and Welfare, 1980). After cross-checking information for persons not linked through their personal identification number, data were available for 376 015 matched records (98% of the total).

It was acknowledged that the rate of autopsies can influence the detection of cancers and if these cancers are also reported they can influence the regional registration rates (for example, there were higher rates in the Malmo area, where there is an autopsy on all deaths). Also the report draws attention to the change in occupation that can occur over time after the census, thus mixing and diluting the influence of specific occupations.

Tables were provided of the number of registrations by site and (*a*) industry and (*b*) occupation. However, no age-standardized statistics are provided and the populations by age within occupation are not included.

The deaths for 1961–70 were matched to the 1960 census records to provide a linked file of occupational data and subsequent deaths (Statistika Centralbyran, 1981). A second exercise linked the 1970 census to deaths in 1971–80; the intention is to combine this into one file linking the 1960 and 1970 Censuses and all deaths from 1960 onwards.

In order to respond to *ad hoc* requests, a system has been developed for quick and easy access to the linked files. The intention is that this will permit specific requests to be answered rapidly and relatively cheaply. In certain circumstances it is possible for *bona fide* research workers to be provided with a magnetic tape from the 'cancer-environment register', thus facilitating further detailed analyses. However, Axelson (1981) has suggested that record linkage was over-rated from the Swedish experience: 'I think it has taken away a lot of thinking and money from regular epidemiology, and in my view we have gained nothing so far.'

A further report (Malker and Weiner, 1984) provides examples of the use of the linked files. Brief descriptions and analyses are given for 33 occupational groups (some of which are subdivided into a number of different categories). For example, the final section presents data for 3 sites of cancer for 7 subgroups exposed to formaldehyde.

United States

Britten (1934) presented mortality rates by occupational class in the US based on deaths in 10 states in 1930 and census estimates of the populations in different occupations. No data were provided for specific cancers. More detailed analyses are provided by Whitney (1934), using the same material. These were the first publications of official data by cause and occupation for the US. One table showed death rates for 15–24, 25–44, and 45–64 age groups for all malignant tumours for 48 specific occupations and 14 broader groupings.

After a campaign to boost the recording of occupation at death registration, extensive special analyses were prepared of mortality for deaths in males aged 20–64 in the US in 1950 (Guralnick, 1962; 1963a and b). Census counts provided the denominators of population at risk. Analyses by occupation and industry were prepared for whites and non-whites for any occupation having at least 400 deaths in non-whites; the observed deaths were used to generate (*a*) SMRs based on the age and cause-specific death rates for all males, (*b*) PMRs based on the data for a given occupational or industrial group. The PMRs were used to overcome the census death registration biases in the material and highlight SMRs that warranted further consideration.

The most recent data from the US have been published by Milham (1983). This is based on 429 926 deaths in males aged 20 or more, resident in Washington State in 1950–79; proportional-mortality analysis was used to examine 217 occupations and 49 different malignant neoplasms. Data are also presented for 25 066 deaths in working women, excluding housewives. Three preliminary studies had suggested that the occupation recorded at death certification was of adequate validity. Industry was poorly recorded and inadequate to use. As less than 3% of the deaths were in non-whites, these were excluded from the tables.

This report was an extension of Milham(1976), which covered male deaths in Washington in 1950–71. Though only based on deaths in one state, the span of years results in nearly half a million deaths. Though the distribution of occupations may not represent the national profile, the value of material is tacitly acknowledged by the sponsorship of the publication by the National Institute for Occupational Safety and Health.

Rosenberg (1981) indicated that a study had been recently completed showing that the Bureau of Census coding procedures were compatible with the information on the death certificate. This was being extended to see if coding of occupation could become an integral part of the national mortality files in the US. Consideration was also being given to obtaining, in a survey, information about decedents' work history from informants.

International comparisons

The limited results where it is possible to compare SMRs for occupations of similar nature from the various national publications, are shown in *Table 1.7*.

Dubrow and Wegman (1983) have examined the results from 12 studies using mortality or cancer registration data plus occupations recorded at death or cancer registration, together with the Third National Cancer Survey in the US, and the patients' histories recorded at Roswell Park Institute. They discussed the problems of comparing the findings for these different 'surveillance' systems and suggest ways of probing the data to highlight possible occupational hazards.

Recommended reading

Epidemiology

ALDERSON, M.R. (1983) *An Introduction to Epidemiology*, 2nd edn. London: Macmillan

BARKER, D.J.P and ROSE, G. (1984) *Epidemiology in Medical Practice*, 3rd edn. Edinburgh: Churchill Livingstone

BOURKE, G.J. (1983) *The Epidemiology of Cancer*. London: Croom Helm

MORRIS, J.N. (1975) *Uses of Epidemiology*, 3rd edn. Edinburgh: Churchill Livingstone

MOSS, L. and GOLDSTEIN, H. (1979) *The Recall Method in Social Surveys*. London: University of London

SCHOTTENFELD, D. and FRAUMENI, J.F. (1982). *Cancer Epidemiology and Prevention*. Philadelphia: Saunders

Statistics

ARMITAGE, P. (1977) *Statistical Methods in Medical Research*. Oxford: Blackwell

BRESLOW, N.E. and DAY, N.E. (1980) *The Analysis of Case-control Studies*. Lyon: IARC

OSBORNE, J.F. (1979) *Statistical Exercises in Medical Research*. Oxford: Blackwell

ROTHMAN, K.J. and BOICE, J.D. (1983) *Epidemiologic Analysis with a Programmable Calculator*, 2nd edn. Massachusetts: Epidemiology Resources Inc.

Occupational health

McDONALD, J.C. (1981) *Recent Advances in Occupational Health*. Edinburgh: Churchill Livingstone

MONSON, R.R. (1980) *Occupational Epidemiology*. Florida: CRC Press

ROM, W.N. (1983) *Environmental and Occupational Medicine*. Boston: Little Brown

SAX, N.I. (1981) *Cancer-causing Chemicals*. New York: Reinhold

SCHILLING, R.S.F. (1981) *Occupational Health Practice*. London: Butterworths

2

Agents which cause occupationally induced cancers

This chapter reviews the known causes of occupationally induced cancers, when these are chemical or physical agents. Some studies have identified an increased incidence of mortality from cancer, without a particular agent being identified as (possibly) responsible; these studies are covered in the next chapter. It must be borne in mind that sometimes reports referring to workers exposed to a particular agent may indicate a spurious degree of precision, particularly if there has been job movement or exposure to multiple agents during the working lifetime of the subjects. The agents in this chapter are presented in alphabetical order; should a particular substance not be readily located, the index should be consulted.

In general, within any section, the comments are in the order of results from occupational mortality, case reports, case-control and prospective studies. This is then usually followed by a conclusion subsection. Sometimes the order of the material differs depending on particular aspects of the topic, including the fact that there may not be data from a particular type of study available. Case reports are only provided where they have played an appreciable part in defining the hazard involved, or there is a dearth of analytical studies in the literature. Laboratory studies are briefly referred to where human data on a particular hazard are either non-existent or very weak, and animal or short-term mutagenicity tests have helped to confirm the likelihood of risk to man. In some of the topics, studies of the hazard to the next generation have been reported, as these may play an important part in defining the overall hazard to the workforce and the community. Similarly studies of the distribution of cancer in the environment of a plant have been reported, where this is thought to add to knowledge of the potential hazard of a process or agent. Specific subsets of such studies are those involving the household of the workers. These have been included where they contribute to evaluation of the overall hazard from a process or agent.

Due to the large number of studies that have been reviewed for this chapter, space does not permit detailed description of each study. It has been the aim to identify the type of study and the key points: where it was carried out, when, the numbers of individuals involved, the source of comparison, the method of analysis, and any major problems with the particular study. In order to cover as many references as possible, tables are provided with collated material from all relevant reported studies for some of the topics. Sometimes the key facts of the study design are given in the tables, with very little discussion in the text. Where results are given in the text, these are usually in standard format, giving observed events (O), expected events (E), ratio of observed to expected (O/E), and the 95% confidence limits (95% CL). Both in the text and the tables, the data are usually presented in an order that considers reports country by country, and then either by year of publication or chronologically by data-years involved. This order may vary in certain circumstances, but is the usual pattern. One of the reasons for a high number of references is that many studies have produced a sequence of publications; great effort has been taken to try and identify the different publications that refer to the same plant or group of men. Sometimes this is not declared overtly in the different papers, and sometimes different research teams have published reports of the same or overlapping cohorts of subjects. Whether the multiple publications are a series of reports or examples of double publication of the same results it has been thought necessary to identify each of these—otherwise the actual number of positive results in the literature can be readily misjudged.

The points described in the method chapter should be borne in mind when interpreting the material presented in this chapter; the previous chapter indicated the basic requirements for a satisfactory study, and the relative weight that can be placed upon the different types of study.

For each major factor reviewed, a subsection provides a conclusion, which relies upon the judgement of the method points, including those on the issue of interpretation of data and drawing of inferences. The conclusions freely quote from the International Agency for Research in Cancer (IARC) evaluations where they have covered the topic in the series of monographs on the evaluation of carcinogenic risk of chemicals to man. The impact on this evaluation of results made available since the working group had prepared its report is noted.

One point to emphasize is that some of the agents identified in the chapter by a specific section heading refer to particular chemicals; this may be the case where there is no epidemiological data, and a chemical has been subject to appropriate laboratory investigation. At the other extreme are very general headings, such as herbicides; though laboratory data may relate to individual chemicals, the epidemiological material may not distinguish individual compounds, there may have been multiple exposure to different agents, or the summary of an article may have suggested the report was relevant to a particular compound when the text did not support this. In such circumstances, a more general heading is preferable.

2.1 Acrylonitrile

Prospective studies of workers with potential exposure to acrylonitrile in 4 different countries are briefly described, with the main results being collated in *Table 2.1*. Reference is also made to laboratory investigations of exposed workers.

2.1.1 Prospective studies

England and Wales

Werner and Carter (1981) followed 1111 workers at 6 factories in the UK over a 29-year period and suggested that there was a non-significant excess of cancers from a variety of sites. Examination of subsets of the data showed that significant excesses of lung cancer occurred in the males aged 15–44 for which no reason could be found, and stomach cancer in males aged 55–64. (The latter was possibly associated with the locality of the factory.) It was concluded that continued surveillance of these workers was required.

Germany: 1

Kiesselbach *et al.* (1979) identified 884 males exposed to acrylonitrile in 1950–77 at a German plant; 824 (93.2%) were followed to 1/8/77. Expected deaths were calculated from mortality rates for the region. There was a marked overall deficiency of deaths, a rather atypical result from a proportional-mortality analysis, and no evidence of a dose–response relationship; this made interpretation difficult.

Germany: 2

Twelve plants in a German chemical complex (BASF) used acrylonitrile in various manufacturing processes. Men working at least 6 months were followed up until 15/5/78; 98% of 1081 German workers, but only 56% of 388 foreigners could be traced. Expected deaths were based on national mortality rates. There was mixed exposure of the subjects but the authors concluded that the significant lung cancer excess was due to the acrylonitrile (Thiess *et al.*, 1980).

Netherlands

A study of workers on all plants producing acrylonitrile in the Netherlands was attempted

Table 2.1 Risk of various cancers in workers exposed to acrylonitrile

Study*	Stomach		Colon		Lung		Bladder		RES	
	O	E	O	E	O	E	O	E	O	E
England and Wales	5	1.9	2	1.1	9	7.6	1	0.5		
Germany: 1	4	3.0			6	6.7†				
Germany: 2	3	2.8	1	1.3	11	5.1	2	0.6	4	1.7
US: 1			3	0.5	6	1.5				
US: 2					8	4.4				
US: 3					9	5.9	2	0.5	4	1.8
Total O & E	12	7.7	6	2.9	49	31.2	5	1.6	8	3.5
O/E	1.56		2.07		1.57		3.12		2.29	
95% CL	0.8–2.7		0.8–4.5		1.2–2.1		1.0–7.3		1.0–4.5	

*See text for description of method.
†Respiratory tract.

(Association of Dutch Chemical Industry, 1980). There was great difficulty in obtaining data on workers who had left the industry. Nine cancer deaths were identified, but it was impossible to estimate an expected figure. Results from this study are not included in *Table 2.1*.

US: 1

Male employees first exposed to acrylonitrile at a US plant in 1950–52 were followed for over 20 years. Cancer incidence and mortality were compared with expected events based on (*a*) company statistics, (*b*) national mortality rates. There was an excess of lung cancer, but no data were available on smoking (US Department of Labour, 1978).

US: 2

Workers at Du Pont had been followed over a 26-year period and there was an excess incidence and mortality from cancer, when compared with company rates (O'Berg, 1980). In particular, there was a non-significant excess of lung cancer; examination of smoking data suggested that there was not sufficient discrepancy between the cohort of workers and the general public to explain the lung cancer findings. Examination of degree and duration of exposure suggested that there was a relationship between increased exposure and increased risk of cancer. The risk was highest in those who had worked in the early years of the plant operation.

US: 3

Delzell and Monson (1982a) followed, until 1/7/78, 327 men who had worked in 2 departments in a Goodrich rubber plant in Akron, Ohio and were potentially exposed for at least 2 years to acrylonitrile between 1940–71. Mortality was compared with that of the general population; the nominal roll was also checked against the cancer registries in the area and an internal comparison made against incidence in other workers. There had been some exposure to other chemicals on the plant. There was a non-significant excess of lung cancer.

US: 4

There was a suggestion that textile workers exposed to acrylonitrile had an excess of colorectal cancer (American Occupational Medical Association, 1977), but this has not been confirmed in other cohort studies of these workers.

2.1.2 Laboratory studies

Analysis of lymphocyte cultures for 18 workers exposed to acrylonitrile for about 15 years and 18 workers unexposed to known toxic agents showed no differences in the percentage of chromosome aberration (Thiess and Fleig, 1978).

2.1.3 Conclusions

The International Agency for Research in Cancer (IARC) (1979a), bearing in mind the evidence for mutagenicity and other experimental data, concluded that acrylonitrile should be regarded as if it were carcinogenic to humans. Since this was published further studies on workers have reported positive findings particularly for lung cancer, with an overall significant excess shown in *Table 2.1*. The increases for bladder and reticulo-endothelial system (RES) neoplasms are of borderline significance.

2.2 Alkyl sulphates

The alkyl sulphates (dimethyl sulphate, diethyl sulphate, diisopropyl sulphate etc.) are widely used as alkylating agents. The production of isopropyl alcohol may lead to all 3 alkyl sulphates appearing as byproducts and these may be the carcinogenic agent in that process (*see* 2.3.8).

2.3 4-Aminobiphenyl (xenylamine)

A number of reports have appeared on the risk of bladder cancer in a small group of workers exposed to 4-aminobiphenyl. Apparently, the initial paper was sufficient to prevent widespread use of the chemical.

Melick *et al.* (1955) reported 171 males who had been exposed to 4-aminobiphenyl in 1935–55; 19 had developed bladder cancer. The study was extended by Koss, Melamed and Kelly (1969) to 503 men exposed in 1935–55. By 1968, 35 had developed histologically confirmed bladder cancer, whilst a further 33 had cytological abnormalities in cells in their urine. Though no expected figures are provided, this is an extremely high incidence of bladder neoplasms in these workers, some of whom had limited exposure to the chemical. Other reports on these men have been published by Melamed *et al.* (1960), Koss *et al.* (1965), and Melick, Naryka and Kelly (1971).

2.3.1 Conclusion

IARC (1972) considered that bladder cancer was strongly associated with occupational exposure to 4-aminobiphenyl.

2.4 Anaesthetics

A number of studies have reported on the cancer incidence or mortality of operating theatre staff. Those relating to anaesthetic staff are discussed below, though no information is available about the specific exposures involved. Key results are given in *Table 2.2*. This is also one of the topics where many studies have been done on the outcome of pregnancy; key papers are briefly reviewed.

2.4.1 Cancer incidence and mortality of theatre staff

Using membership particulars from the American Society of Anesthesiologists, Bruce *et al.* (1968) calculated mortality rates for the period 1947–66 and compared these with rates for US males and also Metropolitan Life Insurance policy holders. It was suggested that there was a reduced risk of lung cancer but increased risk of neoplasms of lymphoid and reticulo-endothelial sites.

A questionnaire to 621 female nurse anaesthetists in Michigan produced an 84.5% response; this identified an excess of non-skin cancers in 1971, that was significantly raised when compared with age-adjusted incidence based on registry data: O = 7; E = 2.12; O/E = 3.30; 95% CL = 1.3–6.8 (Corbett *et al.*, 1973). It is not at all clear that the questionnaire answers will equate with registration incidence, e.g. those dying very soon after diagnosis or diagnosed at autopsy will not be identified in the questionnaire response.

A much more extensive postal survey of US operating room personnel obtained a 66.3% response in males and a 57.7% response in females, with an even lower response in the control groups of 41.3% and 43.5% (Cohen *et al.*, 1974). It suggested an increase in prevalence of cancer in female staff, the age-standardized rates for lymphoma/leukaemia

being the only site with a reported significant difference. The comparison groups were 2 other societies without operating room exposure, and the results are difficult to interpret. Subjects with cancer may have been particularly likely to be unable to respond.

Lew (1979) reported the mortality of the American Society of Anesthesiologists for 1954–76. It was stated that the proportion of deaths from all cancer was as expected; no details are given by site.

The prospective study of UK doctors in relation to their smoking provided the opportunity to examine the mortality of 547 anaesthetists followed for 20 years (Doll and Peto, 1977). There was no evidence of an excess of deaths from cancer (O = 29; E = 32; O/E = 0.91, 95% CL = 0.6–1.3), and there was a non-significant deficiency of deaths from lung, mouth and oesophageal cancer (O = 6, E = 10.5, O/E = 0.57, 95% CL = 0.2–1.2).

2.4.2 Hazard to the next generation

A high rate of miscarriage was observed among pregnant anaesthetists in Russia—in 18 of 31 pregnancies (Vaisman, 1967).

Questionnaires were sent to 578 nurses in anaesthetic departments and to 174 anaesthetists; 570 replies were adequate for analysis, with information on 212 pregnancies before and 392 during employment. The latter ended about twice as often in abortion or premature death, including pregnancies in unexposed wives of male anaesthetists. There was no evidence of difference in frequency of congenital malformations (Askrog and Harvald, 1970).

Questionnaires were sent to female anaesthetists in the UK and a sample of other women doctors; usable replies were obtained from 82% of the anaesthetists and 80% of the controls eligible for the study. Obstetric histories were obtained from 563

Table 2.2 Risk of various malignancies in persons exposed to anaesthetic gases*

Occupation	Country	Data–years	Sex	No. subj.	Site	O	E	O/E	Author
Nurse/ Anaesthetists	US	1971	F	621	All less skin	7	2.2	3.18	Corbett *et al.* (1973)
Anaesthesiologists	US	1947–66	M	5500	Lung	9	28.1	0.32	Bruce *et al.* (1968)
Anaesthesiologists	US	1947–66	M	5500	Leukaemia	6	6.2	0.97	Bruce *et al.* (1968)
Anaesthesiologists	US	1947–66	M	5500	RES less leukaemia	17	8.9	1.91	Bruce *et al.* (1968)
Operating room personnel	US	1963–72	F	49 585	RES	11	3.7	2.97	Cohen *et al.* (1974)
Anaesthetists	UK	1951–71	M	547	Lung, mouth, oesophagus	6	10.5	0.57	Doll and Peto (1977)

*See text for description of method.

married women anaesthetists and 828 women doctors, who acted as controls. The anaesthetists who worked during pregnancy had: twice the involuntary infertility of the controls; significantly greater frequency of spontaneous abortions than controls; significantly higher proportion of babies with congenital abnormalities than anaesthetists not at work, but a non-significant increase compared with the control doctors (Knill-Jones *et al.*, 1972).

This study was subsequently extended. A questionnaire was sent to anaesthetists in UK who qualified after 1931 and were thought to be in practice in 1972. This obtained usable replies from 5507 (69.3% of those receiving the form). There was a higher proportion of children of exposed fathers reported to have congenital malformation than in controls (3.09% versus 2.35% in controls), whilst maternal exposure appeared to double the proportion of abortions (Knill-Jones, Newman and Spence, 1975). A further questionnaire was completed by 5700 women doctors (72% of those sent this), who had qualified in England and Wales in 1950–75. Those who had worked in anaesthetic appointments had higher rates of stillbirth and congenital malformations of the cardiovascular system, but no difference in the spontaneous abortion rates in comparison with other doctors (Pharoah *et al.*, 1977).

A questionnaire to 621 female nurse anaesthetists in Michigan in 1971 obtained an 84.5% response. Those who had worked in pregnancy reported that 16.4% of their children had birth defects, compared with 5.6% if the mother had not worked in pregnancy. Two children (0.5%) whose mothers had worked in pregnancy had neoplasms, and 1 (0.4%) when the mother had not practised in pregnancy (Corbett *et al.*, 1974).

Tomlin (1979) reported on health problems of anaesthetists and their families; his methods were such that his results were quite unfounded. There was selective quoting of positive results from the literature, comparisons with other studies using quite different definitions, insufficient consideration of the bias in recall of the prevalence of congenital malformation, comparison of a cumulative lifetime figure with annual incidence, and incorrect statistical testing.

2.4.3 Conclusions

IARC (1976a) concluded that available studies indicated that working in operating theatres was associated with an increased risk of cancer, teratogenic effects, and possibly mutagenic effects. It was not possible to determine which particular factor was responsible.

Spence *et al.* (1977) and Spence and Knill-Jones (1978) concluded that there were effects on the fetus in female anaesthetists and wives of male anaesthetists. They found no adequate evidence for risk of cancer in those working in operating theatres. However, the results presented in *Table 2.2* are compatible with an increased risk of RES neoplasms.

2.5 Anthraquinones

Gardiner, Walker and Maclean (1982) identified 1975 men who had been employed in dyestuff manufacturing with potential exposure to anthraquinones for more than 6 months in 1956–65; the men were followed until June 1980. There was no evidence of an excess of cancer deaths in these workers.

2.6 Aromatic amines

2.6.1 Classic studies

Rehn (1895) observed that 3 of his patients with bladder tumours had been involved in a group of 45 men manufacturing fuchsin; one for 15, one for 20, and one for 29 years. (His original paper also refers to a fourth worker, who he had not examined.) Over the next 9 years he identified a further 20 patients who had been involved in the dye industry. Rehn felt that there might be a causal relationship. With the First World War, there was a major increase in the chemical industry and in particular in those countries that could not obtain products from Germany. Young *et al.* (1926) indicated, from an examination of mortality statistics, that workers involved in chemical manufacturing and textile dyers appeared to be at excess risk of bladder cancer. Subsequent work in England and Wales after the Second World War is now a classic of occupational epidemiology and is discussed in some detail below.

With the collaboration of the industry and 21 firms, Case *et al.* (1954) assembled a nominal roll of 2466 males exposed to 4 dyes for at least 6 months in 1921–50; this was checked against a file of death certificates mentioning bladder cancer. A comparison against expected figures was based on national rates allowing for age, sex, and calendar period. The risk of bladder cancer varied for the specific exposure:

Agent	O	E	O/E	95% CL
1-Naphthylamine	6	0.70	8.57	3.1–18.7
Benzidine	10	0.72	13.89	6.6–25.5
2-Naphthylamine	26	0.30	86.67	56.6–127.0
Mixed	81	1.48	54.73	43.5–68.0

An extension of this study identified 1555 men who had been exposed for at least 6 months to manufacture or processing of aniline, magenta, and/or auramine (Case and Pearson, 1954). Again the observed and expected mentions of bladder cancer on the death certificate were compared:

Agent	O	E	O/E	95% CL
Aniline	1	0.83	1.20	0.0–6.7
Auramine	3	0.13	23.08	4.6–67.4
Magenta	6	0.45	13.33	4.9–29.0
Auramine and magenta	0	0.2	0	—

During these studies an excess of bladder tumours was noted in a large county borough of England, in which there was a major plant processing rubber. Henry (1931) had pointed out that naphthylamine was used in antioxidants that had been introduced in some rubber producing firms in this country in 1927–28. A survey was therefore made of the death certificates mentioning bladder tumours and giving a rubber occupation; an approximate expected figure could be calculated from the estimated age structure of the workforce in the period 1921–51 (Case and Hosker, 1954). This showed:

Period	O	E	O/E	95% CL
1921–35	9	8.5	1.06	0.5–2.0
1935–51	26	15.9	1.64	1.1–2.4

Scott (1962) warned that the hazard might extend to cable manufacture, makers of pigments and paints, workers in the paper industry using auramine and magenta, and laboratory personnel handling benzidine.

A specific application of rubber, with the particularly hazardous antioxidant, was in the electric cable industry. Davies (1965) utilized the bladder cancer death certificates to identify that 65 mentioned work in the electric cable industry in 1945–64, but she was unable to calculate an expected value as the size of the potentially exposed workforce was not available. However, one factory in London identified 139 male employees who had worked in the rubber mill in the period 1935–49 and who were exposed to the antioxidant. Four bladder tumour deaths had occurred in this group, with only 0.2 expected (O/E = 20.0; 95% CL = 5.4–51.2).

Subsequent investigations in the rubber industry are reviewed in 3.30. These add no further information about hazards from specific aromatic amines.

2.6.2 Miscellaneous issues

Carcinogenic aromatic amines have been widely used in laboratories as reagents. However, because of the mixed nature of exposure and confounding factors, there has been no clear evidence of a hazard. Other risks with exposure to derivatives of the dyes have been: rat exterminators using the rodenticide 1-naphthylthiourea; manufacture of some paints and pigments; some textile printing; exposure to induline or nigrosine dyestuffs (Somerville *et al.*, 1980). The following notes indicate some specific points of concern from epidemiological data. Other related chemicals are dealt with in the sections on 4-aminobiphenyl and on anthraquinones (*see* 2.3 and 2.5).

2.6.2.1 Aniline

Goldblatt (1949) reported that 3 men exposed to aniline in 1934–47 in 2 chemical factories developed bladder papilloma, whilst those exposed to 2-naphthylamine and benzidine developed cancers. The number exposed and the possible contamination of the aniline was not discussed.

2.6.2.2 1-Naphthylthiourea (ANTU)

Davies, Thomas and Mason (1982) made special enquiries of the occupation of 28 men dying with bladder tumours mentioned on the death certificate where the job was given as pest control. No information was obtained for 10, but 4 of the remaining 18 had definitely been exposed to ANTU. Information from a variety of sources identified another 10 men who had developed bladder cancer after use of ANTU. The results are difficult to interpret in the absence of information about the size of the exposed population.

2.6.2.3 Benzidine

A review (IARC, 1982c) listed 14 different authors who had published case reports of the development of bladder tumours in workers exposed to benzidine.

Mancuso and El-Attar (1967a) followed 639 males employed in 1938–39 until 1965; some of the men had been exposed to benzidine and others to 2-naphthylamine. It was suggested that there was an excess of bladder cancer in those exposed only to benzidine compared to Ohio males, but the data provided do not permit calculation of RR. Preliminary results from this study had been published by Mancuso and El-Attar (1966).

A case-control study of 200 males with bladder cancer and controls with other bladder conditions showed an excess risk for work in the silk-dyeing industry (8.5% of cases, 1.4% of controls, RR = 6.8). A mixture of benzidine-based dyes had been used (Yoshida and Myakawa, 1972).

A small group of US workers manufacturing benzidine had a very high incidence of bladder cancer (13 out of 25 men). Some of the men had also been exposed to 2-naphthylamine and o-toluidine (Zavon, Hoegg and Bingham, 1973).

Tsuchiya, Okubo and Ishizu (1975) identified bladder cancer developing in 346 production workers and 669 users of benzidine in Japan in the period 1949–70: 72 developed bladder tumours, but no expected figure was provided. There had been mixed exposure to other dyes (2-naphthylamine and possibly others); absence of a person-years analysis makes interpretation difficult.

2.6.2.4 Dichlorobenzidine

This is one of the substances controlled under the British Carcinogenic Substances Regulations (1967). However, 3 negative reports have been published. Follow-up of 207 workers in the US potentially exposed to dichlorobenzidine for 17.0 years on average showed no death from bladder cancer (Gerarde and Gerarde, 1974). Though details of the person-years are not provided, or expected values based on these, it was considered that the results did not indicate a hazard. MacIntyre (1975) investigated 225 men who had been exposed in a UK plant in the previous 30 years of operations. There was no evidence of bladder cancer in any man and negative cytology in all providing 6-monthly urine specimens. No bladder tumour was found in a historical prospective study of 35 workers, who had predominantly been first exposed less than 20 years before (Gadian, 1975).

2.6.2.5 Double primaries

Moringa, Oshima and Hara (1982) identified 244 workers exposed to benzidine and 2-naphthylamine who had died from genito-urinary cancer. Of these, 11 had had second primaries elsewhere. Compared with control patients with bladder cancer, there was a statistically significant excess of hepatobiliary second primaries in the exposed workers. This was thought to indicate that these carcinogens could affect sites other than the bladder.

2.6.2.6 Dyeing and printing textiles

Proportional-mortality analyses of 1429 deaths occurring in 1957–68 in men who had worked for at least 12 months in Yorkshire prior to 1937 showed no evidence of increase in bladder cancer (Newhouse, 1978).

2.6.2.7 Gas workers

Henry, Kennaway and Kennaway (1931) had noted an excess of bladder cancer deaths in men with occupations recorded as gas workers in England and Wales in 1921–28. A Norwegian study indicated a possible excess of bladder cancer in gas workers (Brunsgaard, 1959). Follow-up of 2449 men aged 40–65 who had worked in coal carbonizing plants for at least 5 years in England in 1953–61 showed 5 dead from bladder cancer, with only 2.94 expected (Doll *et al.*, 1965). A test for trend against other groups of workers in the industry was nearly significant ($P = 0.06$). Extension of this follow-up for 4 years and addition of data for another group of 1176 carbonizing plant workers followed for 7–8 years was reported by Doll *et al.* (1972). This showed that the age-standardized mortality from bladder cancer was significantly greater than in the population; for those in the carbonizing plants: O = 12, E = 5.55, O/E 2.16, 95% CL = 1.1–3.8. It was suggested that this might be due to the naphthylamines present in the tar fumes to which the men were exposed.

2.6.2.8 Genetic variation in sensitivity

Study of bladder cancer patients who had been exposed to dyestuff intermediates showed that an excess had the slow phenotype for N-acetyltransferase. It was suggested that acetylator status identified susceptible individuals, who might be more likely to develop tumours when exposed to N-substituted aryl compounds or that they might develop more invasive lesions (Cartwright *et al.*, 1982).

2.6.2.9 o-Toluidine

A number of studies included workers exposed to o-toluidine, who were also exposed to other aromatic amines: the aniline workers in Case and Pearson (1954) and Case *et al.* (1954); a mixed group of dye workers in Germany (Gropp, 1958); workers exposed to 2-naphthylamine and benzidine (Viglianni and Barsotti, 1961); men exposed to fuchsin, safranine-T and other amines (Rubino *et al.*, 1979a). No results are available for risk of cancer in those exposed to o-toluidine without exposure to other known hazardous aromatic amines.

More specific studies on exposure to toluidine have been reported from USSR, but only limited details are available on person-years at risk, expected bladder tumours, or degree of mixed exposure (Khlebnikova *et al.*, 1970; Lipkin, 1972).

These results are insufficient to confirm a risk from exposure to o-toluidine.

2.6.2.10 Other dyes and pigments

It was considered that the use of finished dyestuffs was safe; however, doubts had now been raised and the matter is a current issue not resolved by present studies (Health and Safety at Work, 1980).

Follow-up of 342 workers producing aromatic amine-based dyes other than those discussed above (indigo, bromindigo, and acetanilide) in 1940–75 showed no deaths from bladder cancer, nor significant excess for other sites (Ott and Langner, 1983).

Records of 2589 workers employed in a pigments factory handling aromatic amines in Scotland, including results of screening over the period 1968–80, were analysed. There were 7 bladder tumours identified, including papilloma, with about 0.8 expected in males (Gillis, Boyle and MacIntyre, 1982).

2.6.3 Conclusions

The dyes are discussed in alphabetical order.

Aniline

IARC (1982a) considered that there was inadequate evidence of cancer risk to humans, only limited evidence from animal studies, and inadequate evidence from short-term tests (STT).

Auramine

On the basis of Case and Pearson (1954), IARC (1972) judged that there was sufficient evidence of carcinogenicity from the manufacture of auramine; IARC (1982d) concluded that there was insufficient evidence of a hazard from use of this agent.

Benzidine

IARC (1979c) considered there was sufficient evidence of a causal association of cancer with industrial exposure to benzidine, that was supported by animal tests and STT.

Magenta

IARC (1974a) accepted that one study had indicated a causal association of bladder cancer with manufacture of magenta, though animal tests and STT results were inadequate.

1-Naphthylamine

IARC (1974a) considered there was insufficient evidence of cancer hazard to man, due to the likely contamination of commercial 1-naphthylamine with 4–10% 2-naphthylamine in the study of Case *et al.* (1954). There was inadequate animal evidence, but STT had shown mutagenicity.

2-Naphthylamine

IARC (1979c) accepted that there was sufficient epidemiological evidence of a causal association of

exposure with subsequent bladder cancer. This was in agreement with results from animal tests and STT.

o-Toluidine

IARC (1982a) considered that the epidemiological studies were inadequate to assess the hazard, but both carcinogenicity in animals and activity in STT had been demonstrated.

2.7 Arsenic

There have been suggestions over the past century that occupational exposure to arsenic might lead to various cancers, particularly of the skin and lung. These historical reports are briefly noted and then the hazards from (*a*) mining, (*b*) copper smelting, (*c*) pesticide manufacture, and (*d*) pesticide use are reviewed. Key results are given in *Table 2.3*. The final section discusses risk of other malignancies.

2.7.1 History

A much-quoted early reference (Paris, 1825) drew attention to cancer of the scrotum in smelter workers in Cornwall. However, later review of this suggested that a clearcut causal relationship was by no means demonstrated. Pye-Smith (1913) reviewed 28 arsenic skin cancers of which 26 were from medicinal use of arsenic. He pointed out that the other 2 were due to employment in the sheep-dip industry. O'Donovan (1924) reported 6 further cancers of the skin known at the London Hospital, where all the men had been employed at a small local factory making sheep-dip.

In an extensive review of arsenical cancer, Neubauer (1947) indicated that some of the early suggestions of occupational risk had been disproved. For example, it was no longer thought that smelting workers in Cornwall or miners in Schneeberg and Joachimsthal had arsenical-induced cancer. However, he accepted some of the early reports that exposure to sheep-dip or arsenical insecticides could lead to skin and lung cancer.

In a clinical description of 31 patients with multiple cancers thought to be due to arsenic, Sommers and McManus (1953) suggested that 6 out of 31 were of varied occupational origins.

2.7.2 Mining

Osburn (1957) noted an excess of lung cancer in men who had worked in the Rhodesian gold mines where the ore contained arsenic. Further study showed that the miners with lung cancer had evidence of chronic arsenism (Osburn, 1969). The expected figures are based on comparison of crude lung cancer rates in blacks in Africa.

2.7.3 Copper smelters

2.7.3.1 Geographical studies

A preliminary assessment may come from geographical studies. Blot and Fraumeni (1975) showed that the average mortality rates for lung cancer in white males and females in the United States in 1950–69 were significantly increased in those counties with copper, lead, or zinc smelting and refining industries, in comparison with counties where non-ferrous ores were processed. There was no indication that this excess mortality could be attributed to geographical region, urbanization, socio-economic status, or other manufacturing process. It was suggested that community air pollution from industrial emissions containing inorganic arsenic was the likely factor.

Lyon, Fillmore and Klauber (1977) found that there was no evidence of excess lung cancer in males or females downwind of a copper smelter in Utah, in comparison with the distribution of lymphoma patients. The choice of control may have biased the results.

Mortality in 1961–74 in two parishes adjacent to a Swedish metallurgical smelter showed a significant excess of lung cancer. However, when the deaths in employees in the smelter were excluded, the excess of an SMR of 173 based on local rates was not significant (Pershagen, Elinder and Bolander, 1977).

2.7.3.2 Occupational studies

The following studies on workers in smelters are listed by country; there have been a number of reports from the US and these are given in chronological order.

Japan

Kuratsune et al. (1974) observed an excess of lung cancer in Saganoseki, Japan. The number of deaths was relatively small but they obtained details from the next of kin for 19 males who had died from lung cancer and a control matched for age at death. The only significant difference for the two groups was that 11 of the 19 with lung cancer had been employed as stokers in the local copper factory. Obviously, only limited weight can be placed on results based on occupational histories obtained for a limited number of deaths, and when the source of information was the next of kin. Further statistics from this smelter (Tokudome and Kuratsune, 1976) confirmed a markedly increased SMR for lung cancer, with evidence of a dose–response relationship to risk.

Sweden

Rather different was the case-control study of Axelson et al. (1978a) which was based on lung cancer deaths in the vicinity of a copper smelter in Rominskar, northern Sweden and control deaths in 1960–76. The exposure of each subject to arsenic was assessed from work histories and judgements of the hygiene standards in the factory departments. A prospective study was subsequently carried out of workers in this smelter in the period 1928–76. This confirmed the risk of lung cancer, which was particularly associated with work in the roasting and arsenic departments of the smelter (Wall, 1980).

US: 1

Snegireff and Lombard (1951) reported limited data from the metallurgical industry; there were few deaths and only a simple proportional-mortality analysis was carried out. There was no clear indication from this of an excess of cancer in the workers concerned. There were only 9 cancer deaths out of a total of 72 deaths from the plant for which they had data.

US: 2

Lee and Fraumeni (1969) examined the mortality experience of over 8000 white male smelter workers who had been exposed to arsenic in the period 1938–63. Again there was an excess overall mortality due mainly to malignant disease of the respiratory system and diseases of the heart. The three-fold excess respiratory cancer appeared to be related to duration of exposure and estimated intensity of arsenic exposure. Those workers with high exposure to arsenic had also been exposed to sulphur dioxide; the authors point out that chemical exposure other than the arsenic may be unidentified and specifically related to risk of lung cancer. Those who were alive in 1963 were then followed during the period 1964–77. A pilot study first determined the feasibility (Higgins et al., 1981); Lubin et al. (1981) reported on the mortality in the second period 1964–67. Then Lee-Feldstein (1983) analysed mortality for the whole period 1938–77. Again there was evidence of increased risk of lung cancer for higher levels of arsenic exposure; the SMRs were: light exposure = 231, medium = 446, heavy = 514. (This was exposure to trivalent arsenic.)

US: 3

A series of papers have appeared on the mortality of workers in a large smelter in Washington. Pinto and Bennett (1963) examined the mortality occurring in 1946–60. There were 18 deaths from lung cancer, but 15 of these had occurred in workers not thought to be specifically exposed to arsenic in the smelter.

Table 2.3 Risk of lung cancer in various occupational groups exposed to arsenic*

Occupation	Country	Data–years	Sex	No. subj.	O†	E†	O/E	Author
Mining	Rhodesia	1948–56	M		22	1.6	13.7	Osburn (1957)‡
	Rhodesia	1957–63	M		36	5.9	6.1	Osburn (1969)‡
Copper smelter	Japan	1967–69	M		11		7.3	Kuratsune *et al.* (1974)‡
	Japan	1949–71	M	839	29	2.4	11.9	Tokudome and Kuratsune (1976)
	Sweden	1960–76	M		29		4.3	Axelson *et al.* (1978a)
	Sweden	1928–76	M	3919	76	26.4	2.9	Wall (1980)
	US: 1	1925–49	M		7			Snegireff and Lombard (1951)
	US: 2	1938–63	M	8047	(147)	(44.7)	3.3	Lee and Fraumeni (1969)
	US: 2	1964–77	M	5403	(146)	(88.5)	1.6	Lubin *et al.* (1981)
	US: 2	1938–77	M	8045	302	106.0	2.8	Lee-Feldstein (1983)
	US: 3	1946–60	M		(18)	(8.6)	2.1	Pinto and Bennett (1963)
	US: 3	1950–71	M		(40)	(18.0)	2.2	Milham and Strong (1974)
	US: 3	1949–73	M	527	32	10.5	3.0	Pinto *et al.* (1977); Pinto, Henderson and Enterline (1978)
	US: 3	1940–76	M	2802	100		1.9	Enterline and Marsh (1982a)
	US: 4	1959–69	?	244	17	5.6	3.0	Rencher, Carter and McKee (1977)
Pesticide manufacture	Wales	1900–43	M		7	3.5	2.0	Hill, Lewis and Fanning (1948)§
	US: 1	1940–73		606	20	5.8	3.4	Ott, Holder and Gordon (1974)
	US: 2	1946–77	M	1050	23	13.5	1.7	Mabuchi, Lilienfeld and Snell (1979)
	US: 2				23	8.8	2.6	Mabuchi, Lilienfeld and Snell (1980)
	US: 2	1946–77	F	343	1	1.2	0.8	Mabuchi, Lilienfeld and Snell (1980)

*See text for description of method.
†Figures in parentheses are subsets of data included in other published results.
‡Case-control study.
§PMR.

Using a relatively crude proportional-mortality analysis they suggested there was no excess of cancer of specific sites in the workers. However, Milham and Strong (1974) obtained the causes of death for workers in the same plant in the period 1950–71. They identified 40 deaths due to respiratory cancer in refinery workers in the death records of the locality; using the population at risk in the smelter (published in the previous paper) and applying US mortality rates, only 18 deaths were expected (the excess being significant, $P<0.001$). Pinto *et al.* (1977) studied the mortality experience of 527 pensioners in the same copper smelter who were alive on 1/1/49. They showed a higher than expected mortality which was chiefly due to respiratory cancer. Analysis of estimated lifetime arsenic exposure in the smelter showed a linear relationship between exposure and respiratory cancer mortality. The authors point out that these workers would have been exposed to much higher levels of arsenic than existed when monitoring became available. A further paper (Pinto, Henderson and Enterline, 1978) contains the same results for lung cancer. Enterline and Marsh (1980a) traced 2776 male workers until 1976. The excess of lung cancer was evident in both smokers and non-smokers. Risk appeared to increase with duration of exposure, but not with latent interval. In a further analysis of the data, Enterline and Marsh (1982a) showed there was a gradient in risk of lung cancer in relation to time-weighted arsenic exposure.

More details than usual have been provided on the above because this series of papers indicates how, with improved quality of data and better techniques of analyses, rather different results can be obtained. It is not clear what the specific reason is for the negative in the first publication.

US: 4

Rencher, Carter and McKee (1977) analysed deaths in persons employed in a copper mine, smelter, and associated plant in 1950–69 in Utah, US. There was an excess of lung cancer in those who had worked in the smelter in comparison with (*a*) other parts of the plant, (*b*) the surrounding county. The paper uses an unconventional statistical analysis and does not state the sex of the subjects.

2.7.3.3 Laboratory studies

There was some evidence of differences in the proportion of well and poorly differentiated lung cancers in men who had worked in a copper smelter compared with miners and those living in the same locality as the US smelter (Newman *et al.*, 1976).

In investigating the health of smelter workers in northern Sweden, Beckman, Beckman and Nordson

(1977) examined cultured lymphocytes from 9 workers known to be exposed to arsenic. The proportion of chromosome aberrations in these workers was significantly raised compared to other subjects; again, the simultaneous exposure to other agents could not be assessed.

2.7.4 Pesticide manufacture

2.7.4.1 Geographical study

Rather different is the study by Matanoski *et al.* (1981). This examined the age-adjusted deaths in persons living within three-quarters of a mile of an arsenical pesticide plant in Baltimore in 1958–62 and 1966–74. In the later period there was an excess of deaths from lung cancer compared with men in control locations. The plant had been in existence for about 50 years, but had been rebuilt in 1952. It was not clear why the increase only occurred from the late 1960s and did not affect women.

2.7.4.2 Occupational studies

England and Wales

Hill and Lewis Fanning (1948) obtained the causes of death for all individuals who had worked in a factory manufacturing arsenical sheep-dip in Wales in the period 1910–43. They also used the causes of death for other residents in the same locality and carried out a proportional-mortality analysis. There was a significant excess of deaths from cancer in the workers, which was confined to those involved in the chemical processes rather than in the general operatives. Though the numbers were small, the data suggested that lung and skin cancer were particularly common. Perry *et al.* (1948) in a companion probe of the environment of the factory made no other suggestion to account for the excess cancer than arsenic exposure.

US: 1

Ott, Holder and Gordon (1974) compared the cause of death for 173 workers exposed to lead and calcium arsenate in pesticide production in a US factory who died in 1940 with 1809 decedents not so exposed. There was a significant excess of lung cancer in the exposed, which rose appreciably with estimated dose. A limited historical prospective study of 606 workers followed in 1940–73 showed a significant excess of lung cancer in comparison with national rates.

US: 2

Mabuchi, Lilienfeld and Snell (1979) followed 1393 persons employed in 1946–74 at a plant manufacturing arsenical pesticides; this included a 20% sample of those who had worked for less than 4 months. Using various company, state, and other methods for tracing, 901 were found to be alive, 240 had died and causes of death were obtained, whilst 252 (18%) could not be located; this latter group was considered to be alive at the end of the study (1977). Using Baltimore rates to calculate expected values, a significant excess of lung cancer was observed in males; the risk increased with intensity and duration of exposure. A case-control study suggested that evidence of arsenism was present before the lung cancers occurred. The data were taken as evidence of cancer risk from inorganic arsenic; no information was available on an effect of valency and there was not thought to be interaction with other chemical exposure. Very similar results were obtained by using national mortality rates for males, but there was no evidence of any hazard in a small group of females (Mabuchi *et al.*, 1980).

2.7.5 Pesticide use

Braun (1958) reviewed the case notes of 16 vineyard workers from the Palatinate with exposure to arsenic pesticides, who had been treated for various cancers in Heidelberg from 1952 to 1957. All showed keratoses; 9 had lung cancer, 2 with squamous cell skin cancer, and 2 with Bowen's disease; 1 had bile duct cancer; 1 a neoplasm of the lymph nodes; 1 a skin cancer; 1 Bowen's disease. The other 3 had no evidence of malignancy.

Roth (1959) reported 82 autopsies on vineyard workers in Germany: 61 showed deaths from cancer, of which 44 were respiratory tract. Often there were multiple tumours of the skin, though it is suggested that only 2 subjects died solely from skin cancer. There had been considerable use of an arsenic fungicide and insecticide in the period 1930–42. This was not restricted to the German vineyards; Galy *et al.* (1963) published case reports of 3 deaths from lung cancer in vineyard workers from the Beaujolais district, who had been exposed in the 1930s to antifungal arsenic solutions.

Nelson *et al.* (1973) followed up 1231 men who had been classified by exposure to lead arsenic insecticides used in orchards in 1938; by 1969 there were 452 deaths, but no evidence of increased mortality from all cancers in comparison with expected values based on state mortality rates. (Data were not presented for specific sites of malignancy.)

2.7.6 Other sites of malignancy

Ott, Holder and Gordon (1974), in a proportional-mortality analysis of 173 men who had worked in a pesticide factory and died in 1940–72, found an excess of Hodgkin's disease and other lymphoma. A prospective study of 606 workers in 1940–73 showed an excess. Using national rates to calculate the expected: O = 5; E = 1.3; O/E = 3.85; 95% CL = 1.2–9.0.

Mabuchi, Lilienfeld and Snell (1979; 1980) studied workers from a pesticide plant in Maryland. Initially there was evidence of a significant excess of lymphoma (Baetjer, Levin and Lilienfeld, 1975). However, analysis of data from 1050 male and 343 female employees traced over the period 1946–77 showed deaths from 4 such neoplasms, with 2.7 expected: O/E = 1.48, 95% CL = 0.4–3.8.

In a case-control study of persons dying from various diseases in the vicinity of a Swedish copper smelter in 1960–76, Axelson *et al.* (1978a) identified 6 deaths from leukaemia plus myeloma in former workers, when there was only one in the unexposed controls: O/E = 6.0, 95% CL = 0.9–38.5. It was not clear whether this was related to arsenic exposure.

Follow-up of 527 smelter workers in the period 1949–73 showed no excess risk of lymphoma: O = 2, E = 2.1, O/E = 0.95, 95% CL = 0.1–3.4 (Pinto *et al.*, 1977; Pinto, Henderson and Enterline, 1978). Extension of this to 2802 male smelter workers followed in 1940–77 showed no excess of lymphoma: O = 6, E = 6.67, O/E = 0.90, 95% CL = 0.2–2.0 (Enterline and Marsh, 1982a).

A register of 26 patients with angiosarcoma of the liver diagnosed in 1970–75 in New York was used for a case-control study. Two cases were exposed to arsenic, but the report does not confirm whether or not any controls were also exposed (Brady *et al.*, 1977).

2.7.7 Hazard to the next generation

To check on the observation that women living close to a smelter in Sweden had an increased risk of abortion, Beckman and Nordstrom (1982) investigated the spouses of male employees at the smelter from 1978, collecting information on pregnancies which were checked against hospital records. The fetal death rate was significantly increased after the husbands' employment, with no such change in control office workers and no difference in rate of induced abortion. The initial non-responders had a higher induced abortion rate, which made interpretation difficult.

2.7.8 Conclusions

A review by Blejer and Wagner (1976) stated that: (a) there was sound evidence of an excess of lung cancer from the various studies of smelter workers, and those making and using pesticides, (b) skin cancer had been confirmed as a risk in those workers manufacturing sheep-dip, and (c) there were 2 groups who produced arsenical pesticides in which

there was an excess risk of lymphatic system neoplasms. After consideration of the limited data on dose–response, it was suggested that the arsenic body-burden of workers should not be occupationally increased above that accumulated from the natural ambient level.

Sunderman (1976) concluded that occupational exposure to arsenic was responsible for cancers of: the respiratory tract (though he did not specify if this included the nose or larynx); skin; 'diverse' internal organs.

The working group convened in 1979 (IARC, 1980) concluded that there was sufficient evidence on humans that inorganic arsenic compounds were carcinogenic for skin and lung, but the data were inadequate for evaluation of a risk to other sites.

2.8 Benzene

Early warning of a hazard came from case reports. These are briefly reported and then some laboratory studies of chromosome abnormalities in exposed workers. Other evidence comes from case-control studies of patients with leukaemia. Historical prospective studies of workers exposed to benzene in (a) petroleum, (b) rubber, and (c) other industries are reviewed. Key results are given in *Table 2.4*.

Workers in both the petroleum and rubber industries are exposed to benzene and many other chemicals. General sections on the health of workers in these two industries should also be consulted when considering the issue of benzene (*see* 3.23 and 3.30).

2.8.1 Case reports

Suggestions of a hazard from benzene exposure in the early part of the twentieth century were supported by a report of a patient with leukaemia associated with benzene exposure in Italy (Delore and Borgamano, 1928).

Since then, many case reports of leukaemia associated with benzene have been reported from various parts of the world.

Goguel, Cavigneaux and Bernard (1967) reported 50 patients with leukaemia in 1950–65 treated in Paris, who had had solvent exposure to benzene. Other cases have been reported from the USSR (Tareef, Koutchalovskaya and Zorina, 1963). A variety of cytological forms were involved. Vigliani (1976) described 66 patients seen at a Milan clinic in 1942–76 with benzene 'haemopathy' of whom 11 developed leukaemia. The occupations were listed, but in the absence of population at risk the data are hard to interpret (*see also* Vigliani and Forni, 1976).

Aksoy, Erdem and Dincol (1974) reported 26 patients with acute leukaemia or pre-leukaemia amongst 28 500 shoeworkers in Turkey who were chronically exposed to high levels of benzene (used as a solvent by these workers). They estimated that the incidence was significantly greater than that of the general population. Many papers have been published by Aksoy and his colleagues, but these do not provide statistics of person-years or an event rate to enable a specific risk ratio to be calculated. Aksoy (1978) pointed out that from 1969 the use of benzene declined in shoemaking in Istanbul and the peak of occurrence of leukaemia was in 1973, followed by a rapid decline in patients reporting exposure.

2.8.2 Chromosome studies

Tough and Court Brown (1965) found chromosomal abnormalities in 2.5% of cells cultured from the peripheral blood of men who had been exposed to benzene. This was significantly greater than the figure for controls. However, extension of the study found an increase in the number of chromosome aberrations in exposed and non-exposed in a second location, whilst at a third location both exposed and non-exposed workers had no excess of aberrations compared with the general population (Tough *et al.*, 1970). The direct influence of benzene exposure was questionable. These results are difficult to interpret, but it was noted that factory 3 had the lowest benzene levels. The importance of adequate control data in such studies had been emphasized by Littlefield and Goh (1973). They pointed out that chromosomal breakage frequencies vary both within and between normal individuals at different times.

2.8.3 Case-control studies

In a study of 50 male patients treated in 1969–77 in Sweden for acute non-lymphocytic leukaemia and 3 categories of controls (patients with non-malignant disorders, allergic disorders, and chronic leukaemia) Brandt, Nilsson and Mitelman (1978) recorded excess occupations with exposure to petroleum products in those with acute leukaemia. However, only general information was available about the work involved, which meant it was not certain whether there had been specific exposure to benzene.

All deaths from lymphomas in New York State in 1950–69 in men who had worked in 14 occupations thought to be exposed to benzene were identified (Vianna and Polan, 1979). There appeared to be a significant excess of deaths in comparison with the State population, which was confined to those aged over 45 at death; however, absence of a denominator with occupation derived under the same conditions may have introduced bias. A similar study of all Hodgkin's and other lymphomas diagnosed in Tasmania in 1972–79 showed no increased risk for men with a work history of benzene exposure (Smith and Lickiss, 1980). However, these workers and also Linos *et al.* (1980) studying leukaemia patients diagnosed in Olmsted County Minnesota in 1955–74 found an increased risk with benzene exposure.

A case-control study of 42 patients with acute myeloid leukaemia treated in Linkoping in 1972–78 indicated a six-fold risk from exposure to various solvents, including petroleum products. It was suggested that there was a multiplicative effect with background radiation (Flodin *et al.*, 1981).

A case-control study of 255 children with leukaemia diagnosed in California in 1975–80 showed no difference in parental occupation (Shaw *et al.*, 1984). The material recorded at death registration had been used to assess potential exposure to benzene at the work of parents.

2.8.4 Prospective studies
2.8.4.1 Petroleum industry

See also 3.2.3. Monitoring the work environment of bulk petroleum loading installations and typical filling stations indicated that the airborne benzene concentrations were much less than the existing threshold limit value (TLV) ceiling value, which was 25 parts per million (ppm) at the time of the study (Parkinson, 1971).

A mortality study of workers in a variety of petroleum and petrochemical locations in Europe found no evidence of a benzene-associated mortality from leukaemia, in comparison with the expected mortality on national population rates (Thorpe, 1974).

A study of over 20 000 petroleum refinery workers in 17 refineries in the US (Tabershaw and Cooper, 1975) identified excess mortality from lymphomas but no excess of leukaemia. Review of occupational records of patients dying from lymphoma and leukaemia identified no excess of exposure to benzene in those individuals who had died from leukaemia.

A study of 8 UK oil refineries (Rushton and Alderson, 1981a) found 30 deaths from leukaemia with 31.96 expected. A case-control study was carried out for all deaths with mention of leukaemia on the certificate, assessing blind the potential benzene exposure from job records. Using 2 forms of analysis, a significant increase in risk from leukaemia was found for those potentially exposed to benzene when length of service was taken into account (Rushton and Alderson, 1981b). However, lack of an overall excess of leukaemia, and doubts over the validity of the assessment of benzene exposure, makes this result difficult to interpret.

Table 2.4 Risk of leukaemia in workers exposed to benzene*

Occupation	Exposure (ppm)	Country	Data years	Sex	No. subj.	O	E	O/E	Author
Patients	210–650	Turkey	1967–73	M/F		26	?		Aksoy, Erdem and Dincol (1974)
Patients	200–500	Italy	1942–74	M/F		24	?		Vigliani (1976)
Petroleum workers	<25	Europe	1962–78	M	38000	18	23.2	0.77	Thorpe (1974)
Rubber workers	?	US	1964–72	M	6678	8	1.86	4.3	McMichael, Spirtas and Kupper (1974)
Rubber workers	10–100	US	1940–75	M	748	7	1.5	4.76	Infante (1978)
Rubber workers	2–25	US	1940–73	M	594	3	0.8	3.75	Pagnotto *et al.* (1979)
Chemical workers	?	US	1940–77	M	259	3	0.9	3.23	Decoufle, Blattner and Blair (1983)
Total						39	28.29		
O/E						1.38			
95% CL						1.0–1.9			

See text for description of method.

Tsai *et al.* (1983) followed 454 males employed in 1952–78 in a Texas (Gulf) oil refinery, exposed to benzene at levels rarely above 1 ppm. There was no death from leukaemia, but this is based on too small a number of subjects to pick up a modest risk.

The above studies have each specifically probed for benzene exposure and related this to risk of RES neoplasms. More general studies have examined the mortality patterns of workers in oil refineries. Pooled data from 12 studies on petroleum workers (*see* 3.23) showed a significant excess of leukaemia (O = 161, E = 137.4, O/E = 1.17, 95% CL = 1.0–1.4).

In a rather different type of study, Ishimaru *et al.* (1971) interviewed 303 patients developing leukaemia in 1945–67 (or their relatives) and controls in Hiroshima and Nagasaki, in 1960–69. The risk of leukaemia was approximately 2.5 that expected amongst those with occupational exposure to benzene plus history of medical X-rays. Though this general conclusion was proposed, there were a large number of subgroups of occupation that were studied and some of those most closely associated with high benzene exposure showed no excess, whilst other occupations showed an excess when benzene exposure was unlikely.

2.8.4.2 Rubber industry

See also 3.30. McMichael, Spirtas and Kupper (1974) followed a cohort of 6678 male rubber workers in Akron for 9 years; they demonstrated that for men dying in the age range 40–64 there was a three-fold excess of leukaemia. This study did not separate the workers into categories with varying exposure to benzene (thus there may have been appreciable dilution in the risk of the exposed workers). Further work suggested an association between leukaemia and jobs entailing exposure to solvents, which would have included benzene in the

past (McMichael *et al.*, 1975). Investigation of workers involved in tyre repair, and association of this with solvent exposure that was heavy, medium, or light showed a six-fold difference in the relative risk of lymphatic leukaemia (predominantly of chronic type). A further study (McMichael, Andjelkovic and Tyroler, 1976) showed that there was a strong association with lymphatic leukaemia in those working in the synthetic plant, a location where there was no clear benzene exposure. There was no appreciable difference between results from mortality in active workers or retirees (Andjelkovic, Taulbee and Symmons, 1976). Monson and Nakano (1976a) followed up 13 571 white male rubber workers at Akron; they showed a significant excess of deaths from leukaemia in the processing division (O = 10; E = 4.2), and elevator/cleaning workers (O = 3; E = 0.4). Some excess was also seen in tyre workers, the chemical division, the 'shops', and 'industrial products' sections of the works; none of these reached the 5% level of significance. Tyroler *et al.* (1976) in a review of these studies emphasized the consistent excess deaths from leukaemia and lymphosarcoma linked particularly to solvent exposure.

Using a case-control approach for men in the industry developing lymphocytic leukaemia, Wolf *et al.* (1981) again found some evidence of a risk from exposure to solvents, but suggested that this was lower than indicated from earlier studies. (O/E = 3.2, P = 0.07 for lymphatic leukaemia in men with high exposure in one company, but only O/E = 1.6 for 4 companies combined.) A case-control study showed 15 lymphocytic leukaemia subjects in the rubber industry were 4.5 times as likely to have direct exposure to benzene and other solvents than controls in the industry. The effect appeared to be with coal-tar-based benzene and xylene, rather than petroleum-derived solvents (Arp, Wolf and Checkoway, 1983).

Infante (1978) reported a study of men working in an Ohio plant, in which rubber and benzene were mixed in a tank, to produce rubber film. Those working from 1/1/40 to 31/12/49 were followed to 30/6/75. Of 748 men, 75% were traced and the remainder were assumed to be alive. Person-years by age and calendar period were calculated; expected deaths were calculated from US national rates and also data on mortality amongst glass-fibre construction workers in the same state as the plant. There were 140 deaths observed and 187 expected; it is suggested that the deficit was due to incomplete follow-up. For leukaemia O = 7, E = 1.38 from national rates and 1.47 from the glass-fibre workers. There was a greater excess for acute myeloid leukaemia. There were no firm data on levels of benzene exposure, but it is suggested that it was 100 ppm in 1941 and 10 ppm in 1971. These are substantially the same results as reported by Infante *et al.* (1977), but the estimates of levels of exposure were revised following the query by Tabershaw and Lamm (1977). These results have also been published by Rinsky, Young and Smith (1981). It was not clear whether the workers had been exposed to other hazardous chemicals.

Pagnotto, Elkins and Brugsh (1979) followed up 594 workers exposed for at least a month to benzene in a Dow rubber-coating plant in the US in the period 1940–73. In those with a low or very low level exposure [10 ppm time-weighted average (TWA)] there was a significant excess of mortality from leukaemia (O = 3, E = 0.8, O/E = 3.75). Follow-up of 38 workers exposed to benzene for 1–24 years at concentrations of 5–50 ppm (with some levels of 90–140 ppm) had not identified a single patient with leukaemia within 13 years after ceasing exposure. This report relates to the same group of men studied by Ott *et al.* (1978), Townsend, Ott and Fishbeck (1978), Fishbeck, Townsend and Swank (1978), and is an extension of the limited follow-up reported by Pagnotto *et al.* (1961).

2.8.4.3 Other industries

Two hundred and fifty-nine males employed in 1947–60 and potentially exposed to benzene were followed until the end of 1977. There were 3 deaths from leukaemia and 1 of multiple myeloma (E = 1.06). One of the workers dying from leukaemia had previously had myeloma. There was no information on exposure other than that there had been benzene exposure from the process (Decoufle, Blattner and Blair, 1983).

Proportional-mortality analysis of 347 deaths of male employees in a printing plant in Washington in 1948–77 suggested a subgroup who had worked in the bindery with some benzene exposure had an increased risk of leukaemia (Greene *et al.*, 1979).

A cohort of 4602 men who had worked at 7 chemical plants in the US for at least 6 months and had been exposed to benzene in 1946–75, were followed until 1977. Expected deaths were obtained from (*a*) 3074 workers in the same or related plants not exposed to benzene, and (*b*) US national mortality rates. There was a non-significant increase in mortality from leukaemia, non-Hodgkin's lymphoma, and other lymphopoietic neoplasms. The leukaemia risk showed a significant association with estimated benzene exposure, though there were no deaths from acute myelogenous leukaemia (Cox, 1983).

2.8.4.4 Other compounds

Girard *et al.* (1969) reported 7 patients with severe 'haemopathies' including 4 with leukaemia, who had occupational histories of exposure to compounds of chlorinated benzenes (especially *o*-dichlorobenzene). These case reports were not accompanied by any estimate of risk.

2.8.5 Conclusions

IARC (1982c) concluded that there was sufficient evidence that benzene was carcinogenic to man, and that it led to the development of acute myelogenous leukaemia. Most of the earlier reports referred to acute myelocytic or lymphocytic types, but more recent studies have also indicated risk of chronic forms of leukaemia. In a review, Infante and White (1983) suggested epidemiological studies were too insensitive to determine risk from specific cell types where the RR<5.0.

The main difficulty has been to determine a safe exposure level. The clear evidence of leukaemogenesis may have been based on very high levels of exposure in the past. The Health and Safety Executive (1982a) indicated that the hazard in the shoe workers involved exposure to 100–600 ppm; there were only limited data on workers exposed to around 100 ppm, and no adequate evidence of risk at 10 ppm.

2.9 Benzotrichloride

Mortality was examined for 953 workers in an organic chemical plant employed in 1961–70 and followed to 1976. There was an increased SMR for cancers, especially in the earlier entry group of workers. Using a regression model in a life-table analysis, it was suggested there was a cancer hazard in a subgroup of workers exposed to chlorinated toluenes, of which benzotrichloride was thought to be the possible hazard (Sorahan *et al.*, 1983).

Table 2.5 Risk of lung cancer in various occupational groups exposed to beryllium*

Occupation	Country	Data–years	Sex	No. subj.	O	E	O/E	Author
Beryllium register	US: 1	1952–66	?	535	3	—	—	Hardy, Rabe and Lorch (1967)
Beryllium register	US: 1	1952–75	M	357	7	3.3	2.1	Infante, Wagoner and Sprince (1980)
Beryllium side-effects	US: 2	1944–69	M/F	60	0			Stroeckle, Hardy and Weber (1969)˙
Beryllium plants	US: 3	1937–66	M	3685	34			Mancuso and El-Attar (1969)
Beryllium plants	US: 3	1942–75	M	3266	65	41.6	1.6	Mancuso (1980)
Beryllium plants	US: 3	1937–76	M	3685	80	57.1	1.4	Mancuso (1980)
Beryllium plants	US: 4	1942–75	M	3055	47	34.3	1.4	Wagoner, Infante and Bayliss (1980)
Total					134	94.7		
O/E							1.41	
95% CL							1.2–1.7	

*See text for description of method.

2.9.1 Conclusion

IARC (1982c) could not make an evaluation from the available information.

2.10 Benzoyl chloride

In a small plant in Japan manufacturing benzoyl chloride, 3 lung cancers occurred in the workforce of about 20 (Sakabe, Matsushita and Koshi, 1976). Based on a staff of about 20, it was estimated that E = 0.06 in the period 1953–73. Sakabe and Fukuda (1977) reported 2 other patients with lung cancer from a second small plant producing benzoyl chloride. No expected figure was available. Both groups of workers were potentially exposed to a range of precursor chemicals.

2.10.1 Conclusion

IARC (1982c) decided that no evaluation was possible of the hazard to man.

2.11 Beryllium

The following notes discuss 4 studies that have been carried out on workers exposed to beryllium in the United States. *Table 2.5* presents the results. There have been no other definitive studies from other countries that contribute to assessing the cancer hazard to workers exposed to this substance.

2.11.1 Prospective studies

US: 1

A review of the US beryllium case register for the period 1952–66 noted that 3 patients had developed bone cancer with less than 0.1 expected. Apart from this, there was no evidence of excess cancer. The sex

of the subjects was not recorded. Attention was directed to the incomplete ascertainment of those with effects of beryllium and it was acknowledged that those registered may be a biased subgroup of all with marked exposure (Hardy, Rabe and Lorch, 1967).

A more extensive follow-up of 357 men alive in 1952–75 when entered on the register identified 139 who had died. There was a non-significant excess of lung cancer, compared with an expected value based on national rates. As before, there was an appreciable excess of deaths from non-respiratory disease (Infante, Wagoner and Sprince, 1980).

US: 2

Stroeckle, Hardy and Weber (1969) followed up 60 patients who suffered various effects from beryllium exposure in 1944–66. By 1969 there had been 17 deaths, but none from cancer (the mortality seemed to be raised for complications of respiratory disease).

US: 3

Mancuso and El-Attar (1969) followed up 3685 white male workers employed in 2 plants handling beryllium in Ohio and Pennsylvania in 1937–48 until 1966. Comparison was made with a cohort of rubber workers. It was appreciated that the number of deaths from lung cancer was slightly higher than in the control group, but no value for this was given.

An examination of those with respiratory disease following exposure (a subset of the subjects from the previous report) was thought to indicate an enhanced risk of lung cancer (Mancuso, 1970). This work was extended (Mancuso, 1980), including deaths up until 1976; the expected values were based on national rates. The excess of lung cancer was more marked in the Ohio plant, and in the workers who had (*a*) worked less than 5 years, and (*b*) been first employed at least 15 years prior to death. A comparison was also made with lung cancer in viscose rayon workers (Mancuso, 1980); again a significant excess of lung cancer showed in the beryllium workers. A more limited analysis of these data appeared in Mancuso (1979).

US: 4

The 3055 workers at the Pennsylvania plant involved in the above studies were also studied by Wagoner, Infante and Bayliss (1980), who followed those who had worked in 1942–68 until 1975. An expected value was obtained using national mortality rates. The excess of lung cancer was most marked in those who had worked for less than 5 years (and who may have had higher acute levels of exposure). The same results were presented by Infante, Wagoner and Sprince (1979). An earlier version of this work (Baylis and Lainhart, 1972) had been criticized by Eisenbud *et al.* (1978). It was argued that smoking and geographical location had not been adequately considered, and mortality rates for 1965–67 were used to estimate expected deaths in 1968–75, thus providing a low expected figure. In response, it was pointed out that more non-smokers occurred in the beryllium workers, also more were heavy smokers— which could only have led to a 14% excess in deaths. Use of national rates actually overestimated the local expected by 19% (Wagoner, Infante and Mancuso, 1978). There had apparently been 'internal' doubts about the Baylis and Lainhart (1972) report—one of the authors had written to the director of the organization in which the work was done, pointing out defects in the study (evidence for this was quoted by Smith, 1981).

2.11.2 Conclusion

Particular caution is required in interpreting the above 4 studies, as it is not clear to what extent there is overlap in the individuals included in each of the studies. It is conceivable that the same man could be represented in each of the 4 studies. In the monograph (IARC, 1980), it was concluded that the epidemiological evidence that occupational exposure to beryllium may lead to an increased lung cancer risk is limited. However, in conjunction with the laboratory data it was thought that beryllium should be suspected of being a human carcinogen. In a brief review, Kuschner (1981) concluded that the epidemiological studies were strongly suggestive that beryllium was carcinogenic in man.

2.12 Brominated chemicals

There is one study involving a mixture of a number of chemicals. Because of the non-specific nature of this report, it is located under this general title, rather than under a more specific chemical. (*See also* Polychlorinated biphenyls—2.49.)

Wong (1981) identified 3579 workers who had been employed at 3 manufacturing plants and one research location in the US in 1935–76 and were potentially exposed to a range of brominated chemicals (1,2-dibromo-3-chloropropane, 2,3-dibromopropyl phosphate, polybrominated biphenyls, DDT, and other agents). The subjects were virtually all white males, and 95% were successfully followed up; national rates were used to calculate expected deaths. There were no significant excesses of any cancer site in the whole group; examination by duration of employment showed no site with an SMR that increased with longer duration of work. In a further analysis of the results (Wong *et al.*, 1984), in a subgroup exposed to organic brominated compounds such as methyl bromide, there was a significant excess of testicular cancer: O = 2, E = 0.11, O/E = 17.99, 95% CL = 2.0–64.9.

2.12.1 Conclusion

IARC (1979b) found sufficient evidence of carcinogenicity in rats and mice that, in the absence of adequate human data, it was concluded that 1,2-dibromo-3-chloropropane should be considered a carcinogenic risk to humans. As far as polybrominated biphenyls were concerned, IARC (1978b) could not make an evaluation.

2.13 Cadmium

The initial report of a cancer hazard implicated risk for prostate cancer. The series of papers that have studied this issue are dealt with first; prospective studies of 5 groups of workers are briefly reviewed, and then reports based on geographical distribution of prostate cancer, and a case-control study. This is followed by comments on the risks of other cancer sites. The results of the prospective studies are given in *Table 2.6*.

2.13.1 Prospective studies

England and Wales: 1

Potts (1965) reported that a small group of cadmium battery workers had an excess mortality from cancer; this was based on 3 prostate cancers in 8 deaths. Kipling and Waterhouse (1967) then reported a significant excess of 248 nickel–cadmium workers had developed prostate cancer: O = 4, E = 0.6, O/E = 6.67, 95% CL = 1.8–17.1. However, of the 4 patients, 3 had already been included in the report by Potts. Further follow-up of the same workers then failed to confirm a significant excess mortality from this site (Sorahan and Waterhouse, 1983). The overall risk was 1.21; 95% CL = 0.5–8.4 (O = 8, E = 6.6), with no gradient in relation to degree of exposure.

US

A US study examined workers who had been in post in the period 1940–69 for at least 2 years in a smelter involved in the production of cadmium metal and cadmium compounds. Standard techniques were used which showed that there was a significantly increased overall malignancy risk, and excesses in particular from lung cancer and prostate cancer; lung O = 12, E = 5.11, O/E = 2.35, 95% CL = 1.2–4.1; prostate O = 4, E = 1.15, O/E = 3.48, 95% CL = 0.9–8.9 (Lemen *et al.*, 1976).

Sweden

A small group of battery workers and alloy workers in Sweden were followed from 1940 to 1975; there was a non-significant excess of prostate cancer (Kjellstrom, Friberg and Rahnster, 1979).

until the end of 1979 showed no excess of prostate cancer and a non-significant increase in lung cancer (Armstrong and Kazantzis, 1983).

The results from the 5 historical prospective studies are presented in *Table 2.6*. The overall excess of prostate cancer is of borderline significance (one more reported death would have made the result significant). The largest study dominates the results and this did not show any increased risk in prostate cancer.

2.13.2 Case-control study

A rather different study involved histories obtained from patients admitted to Roswell Park hospital in the US. For 176 men with prostate cancer, there was a non-significant risk from reported exposure to cadmium, in comparison with other cancer patients: RR = 1.6, $P < 0.20$ (Kolonel and Winkelstein, 1977).

2.13.3 Geographical study

An investigation of geographical clustering of prostate cancer in south-east Alberta has appeared

Table 2.6 Risk of prostate cancer in 5 historical prospective studies of workers exposed to cadmium*

Occupation	Country	Data–years	Sex	No. subj.	O	E	O/E	Author
Smelter workers	US	1940–69	M	272	4	1.1	3.5	Lemen *et al.* (1976)
Battery and alloy workers	Sweden	1940–75	M	363	6	3.9	1.5	Kjellstrom, Friberg and Rahnster (1979)
Cadmium vicinity	England	1921–78	M	624	8	3.0	2.7	Holden (1980)
Battery workers	England	1946–81	M	3025	8	6.6	1.2	Sorahan and Waterhouse (1983)
Cadmium industries	England	1942–79	M	6995	23	23.3	1.0	Armstrong and Kazantzis (1983)
Total					49	37.9	1.29	
95% CL							1.0–1.7	

*See text for description of method.

England and Wales: 2

Holden (1980) contrasted the mortality of (*a*) 347 men who had worked for at least 1 year manufacturing cadmium–copper alloys, (*b*) 624 men employed at the same building as those in group (*a*), but not directly employed in handling the cadmium–copper alloy, and (*c*) 537 men in a control group employed in iron and brass foundries. The 'vicinity' workers had a significant excess of prostate cancer, but not the smaller group of highly exposed workers. Holden (1969) had previously reported a death from prostate cancer in 42 men exposed to cadmium fumes, but no expected figure was provided.

England and Wales: 3

Follow-up of nearly 7000 men exposed to cadmium who had worked for at least 1 year from 1942–70,

to implicate environmental exposure to cadmium (Johnstone, 1981). Bako *et al.* (1982) subsequently reported that census divisions of Alberta with high incidence of prostate cancer in 1969–73 had high levels of cadmium in water, soil, and crops.

2.13.4 Other cancers

Incidence data for patients in Los Angeles in 1972–75 did not show an increased risk for occupations associated with cadmium exposure.

Men employed in photography, painting, welding, and metal plating had a combined SRR = 0.87 (Ross *et al.*, 1979).

Lung cancer

Three studies already mentioned have shown evidence of an increased risk of lung cancer; Lemen *et al.* (1976), O = 12, E = 5.1; Holden (1980), O = 36, E = 26.1; Sorahan and Waterhouse (1983), O = 89, E = 70.2. The pooled results show a significant excess of lung cancer: O = 137, E = 101.4, O/E = 1.35; 95% CL = 1.1–1.6.

Renal cancer

Kolonel (1976) in a case-control study of renal cancer found a significant association of this with previous exposure to cadmium. There was also an increase in nasopharyngeal cancer in the Swedish workers (O = 2, E = 0.2, O/E = 10, 95% CL = 1.1–3.6), but there had also been exposure to high levels of nickel (Kjellstrom, Friberg and Rahnster, 1979). There is no support from the other studies for these findings.

2.13.5 Conclusion

IARC (1976a) considered that available studies indicated that occupational exposure to cadmium in some form increases the risk of prostate cancer in man. One study suggested an increased risk of respiratory tract cancer.

The Health and Safety Executive (1983) concluded that there was clear evidence that exposure to high concentrations of cadmium (i.e. several mg/m^3) was associated with increased mortality from respiratory cancer. They noted that the positive associations with prostate cancer were based on small groups of workers; since then, a large study in England has shown no such association (Armstrong and Kazantzis, 1983). The pooled data in *Table 2.6* shows O/E = 1.29, which is just significant at the 5% level.

2.14 Carbon disulphide

Follow-up of 343 viscose rayon workers exposed to carbon disulphide and a comparison group of paper mill workers over a 15-year period in Finland identified a lower mortality from lung cancer in the rayon workers (Nurminen and Hernberg, 1984). Though the difference was not significant (4 per 4685 person-years and 9 per 4830 person-years), the results are of interest as a higher proportion of the rayon workers smoked (55% versus 49%).

2.14.1 Conclusion

As there was increased smoking in the rayon workers, the results are not readily explained. They require replication before analytical studies are instituted to search for any factors reducing the risk of lung cancer.

2.15 Carbon tetrachloride

There has been no epidemiological study reported on workers exposed to carbon tetrachloride, but 2 case reports need to be considered.

A fireman who was acutely intoxicated by carbon tetrachloride developed cirrhosis and subsequently an 'epithelioma' of the liver 4 years after the original exposure (Simler, Maurer and Mandard, 1964).

A man developed acute poisoning when exposed to carbon tetrachloride for a few days, which had been used to clean his rug. Seven years later a hepatocellular carcinoma was diagnosed (Tracey and Sherlock, 1968).

2.15.1 Conclusion

IARC (1979b) noted that there was sufficient evidence of carcinogenicity in animals; there were also the case reports above. It was concluded that carbon tetrachloride should be considered as a carcinogen to man.

2.16 Chloroform

There is limited production and use of chloroform as an intermediate in various chemical processes. No study of workers specifically exposed to chloroform has been reported.

2.16.1 Conclusion

IARC (1979b) concluded that chloroform was carcinogenic to mice and rats, and should be regarded as a carcinogenic risk to humans.

2.17 Chloromethyl ethers

A number of studies have been carried out on workers exposed to chloromethyl methyl ether (CMME). In its synthesis it may be contaminated by 1–7% of bischloromethyl ether (BCME), and laboratory evidence suggests it is the BCME that is the carcinogen involved. This section has the more general heading chloromethyl ethers (CME), though the studies are more correctly classified as potential exposure to CMME contaminated with BCME.

The most extensive series of papers stem from studies on one plant in the US; these studies are described first, followed by brief notes on studies from 3 other countries.

2.17.1 Prospective studies

US: 1

Figueroa, Raszkowski and Weiss (1973) followed 125 men potentially exposed to CMME at one plant in Philadelphia from December 1962, after excess lung cancer had been reported in the workers. It was known that the CMME was contaminated with BCME. Over the next 5 years, 4 men developed lung cancer; compared with other non-exposed workers this was thought to be an eight-fold excess. Further reports extended the period of follow-up, examined the dose–response, relationship of risk to smoking, and reported on the histology of the neoplasms (Weiss and Boucot, 1975; Weiss, 1976; Weiss and Figueroa, 1976; Weiss, 1977a; Weiss, 1980). The study was extended to other workers at the plant (De Fonso and Kelton, 1976; Weiss, Moser and Auerbach, 1979). Of 91 men definitely exposed to CME in 1948–71, 14 had developed lung cancer by 1979; 13 of these were small cell cancers, occurring at a relatively young age with higher risk in non-smokers. The early results from this study were also quoted by Lemen *et al.* (1976).

US: 2

Records from 6 of the 7 producers of CME in the US identified 1827 exposed workers and 8870 non-exposed control workers employed in 1948–72 (Pasternack, Shore and Albert, 1977). It was estimated that follow-up to 1972 was 89.8% complete, but only about 1% of the deaths were lost. Expected deaths were based on national rates. There was an increased risk of lung cancer only at the firm involved in the previous study, where it was known that exposure levels had been high; a clear dose–response relationship was found at this firm. In the other 5 plants there was a slight deficiency of lung cancer (O = 3; E = 4.5). Preliminary results from this study were reported by Albert, Pasternak and Shore (1975).

England and Wales

McCallum, Wooley and Petrie (1983) studied a factory in South Wales with 276 men exposed to CME in 1948–80 and a factory in the north-east of England with 394 exposed workers. Expected mortality was based on urban rates in the vicinity of the factories. Estimates of exposure levels over time were made. In the South Wales plant there was a significant excess of lung cancer, which was more clearly related to the degree of exposure than the duration. The plant was modified in 1972 and there was no evidence of a hazard after this time. There was no excess of lung cancer over the whole period studied in the plant in north-east England.

Germany

Thiess, Hey and Zeller (1973) reported 8 lung cancers, 2 of which were in 50 process workers and 6 in 18 laboratory staff exposed to CME. These had developed in 1964–71, after 8–16 years from first exposure. No expected figures were provided. The minimum exposure had been 6 years.

Japan

Sakabe (1973) reported the occurrence of 5 lung cancers amongst 32 workers exposed to CME in 1955–71 from one plant in Japan. Only 0.02 were expected on national rates. There had not been any other lung cancer amongst the factory personnel in this period, who had not worked on the CME plant.

2.17.2 Conclusions

IARC (1974a) accepted the initial study in the US and suggested there was an increased risk of lung cancer in the workers potentially exposed to CME. This review did not indicate whether the risk was most likely to be due to BCME impurities.

Since the IARC evaluation, many further papers have appeared on the first US plant studied, with positive results from 3 other countries. It appears that the hazard is restricted to lung cancer, occurs in those who do and do not smoke, and has been controlled by plant engineering.

2.18 Chloroprene

Two authors have reported studies on workers exposed to chloroprene. However, because of the difficulty in interpreting the results from these studies, brief reference is also made to case reports, laboratory studies, and investigations of hazard to the next generation.

2.18.1 Case reports

Infante (1977) reported a worker, exposed to chloroprene but neither thorotrast nor vinyl chloride, who developed an angiosarcoma of the liver.

2.18.2 Prospective studies

USSR

Khachatryan (1972a) reported 87 patients with lung cancer in workers exposed to chloroprene; it was suggested this was higher than expected from other patients treated in the oncology clinic. Khachatryan (1972b) indicated increased prevalence of skin cancer in 2 groups exposed to chloroprene compared with 3 groups of workers with other chemical or no chemical exposures. It was pointed out (IARC, 1979a) that these studies had a number of method faults: failure to adjust for age and sex, variable case ascertainment, lack of information about confounding factors, and lack of histology.

US

Company records identified 1576 male employees potentially exposed to chloroprene in a Louisville plant in 1957; 98.8% were followed until 1974 (Pell, 1978). A second plant using chloroprene to produce synthetic rubber in New Jersey did not have adequate records, but discussion with known workers identified 234 males first employed in 1931–46 on the plant. Again 98.8% were followed until 1974. Expected figures for both groups were calculated (a) from Du Pont company and (b) national mortality rates. Excess cancer deaths occurred for 4 sites: digestive organs, respiratory system, urinary organs, RES. However, all were based on small numbers and only that for urinary tract was of borderline significance (RR = 2.12; 95% CL = 0.8–4.4).

2.18.3 Laboratory studies

IARC (1979a) quoted 4 reports of increased chromosome aberrations in workers exposed to chloroprene.

2.18.4 Hazard to the next generation

Davtyan, Fomenko and Andreyere (1973) quoted cases of children born with physical and mental defects to female workers in a polymerization area of a chloroprene rubber factory.

Disturbance of spermatogenesis in workers and increased spontaneous abortion rates in workers' wives have been reported by Sanotskii (1976).

2.18.5 Conclusion

IARC (1979a) stated that it was not possible to evaluate the carcinogenic hazard from chloroprene. No adequate study has been reported since that date to revise that opinion.

2.19 Chromium

There were a number of reports of lung cancer developing in workers in the chromate-producing industry in Germany in the 1930s (for a review *see* Baetjer, 1950a). It was not until after the Second World War that epidemiological studies provided confirmatory statistics on the extent of the hazard.

The following notes cover the studies on lung cancer in workers exposed to chromium in (a) production, (b) pigment manufacture, (c) plating, and (d) the ferrochromium industry. Brief comments are then made about the risk of cancer at other sites. *Table 2.7* summarizes the published material.

2.19.1 Chromate producing

The following provide brief descriptions of the studies carried out in different countries. The countries are arranged in alphabetical order, the studies chronologically. A number of the studies have been carried out on the same group of workers; the sequence of such studies is identified in the text, whilst *Table 2.7* has results in parenthesis where there is possibly repeat publication.

England and Wales

Bidstrup (1951) reported the prevalence of lung cancer in 724 workmen employed in the 3 chromate-producing locations in Great Britain. Follow-up was then carried out until 1955, when a three-fold increase in lung cancer was noted (Bidstrup and Case, 1956). A more extensive follow-up was then performed, including tracing those who had left the industry prior to retirement. There was evidence that plant modification carried out in the 1950s had led to a reduction in risk of lung cancer, after taking into account age and duration of employment (Alderson, Rattan and Bidstrup, 1981).

Germany

Zober (1979) reviewed the number of lung cancers developing in workers in 7 chromate factories. Again no person-years at risk nor expected number of cancers are provided.

Japan: 1

Tsuchiya (1965) obtained numbers of deaths and numbers of employees by questionnaire from 200 large employers in 1957–59. There was an excess of lung cancer, compared with the expected based on national rates, for exposure to chrome and nickel, but the 2 metals were not separated in the results.

Japan: 2

Watanabe and Fukuchi (1975), in an abstract, reported an excess of lung cancer in chromate-producing workers in Hokkaido observed in 1960–73. Ohsaki *et al.* (1978) discussed the lung cancers developing in a small group of workers in 1972–76, but gave no indication if the same or a different factory was involved. A conventional person-years analysis was not presented.

US: 1

Machle and Gregorius (1948) studied the mortality in the 7 chromate-producing plants in the US. Multiple and overlapping studies have subsequently been carried out on these workers; the numbers in post in 1937 were:

Location	Employees	Study 1	2	3	4	5
Glen Falls NY	50	+			+	
Jersey City NJ	350	+			+	+
Jersey City NJ	150	+			+	
Baltimore Md	450	+	+		+	+
Kearney NJ	135	+			+	
Newark NJ	100	+			+	
Painesville Ohio	210	+		+	+	+

The first study compared the mortality with that in a control group of industries.

US: 2

Baetjer (1950b) examined the records of lung cancer patients and controls treated at 2 Baltimore hospitals in the period 1925–48. There was a chromate-producing plant in the locality and the percentage of lung cancer patients employed there was higher than in controls. (This plant included about 31% of the workforce in studies (1) and (4).) Hayes, Lilienfeld and Snell (1979) followed over 200 men employed at the Baltimore plant in 1954–74 until 1977. A conventional analysis suggested a two-fold excess risk of lung cancer, with increased risk from long duration of employment or work at the 'wet' end of the plant (rather than in the 'mill' and 'roast' departments). An unconventional analysis of preliminary data from the same plant (Hill and Ferguson, 1979) does not contribute any additional guidance.

US: 3

Mancuso and Hueper (1951) compared the proportion of lung cancer in all deaths in workers from an Ohio plant with that in the local male population. (This plant had about 14.5% of the workforce included in studies (1) and (4).) Subsequent follow-up of the workers at this plant identified 41 lung cancer deaths in 1931–74 (Mancuso, 1975). An attempt was made to analyse these data by type of chromium and duration of exposure, but the result was not conclusive.

US: 4

Brinton, Frasier and Koven (1952) studied workers from the same 7 plants extracting chromates in the US as studied by Machle and Gregorius. In the age range 15–74 there were 32 deaths from lung cancer,

with only 7.2 expected, based on national mortality rates. (The same results were published by Gafafer, 1953.)

US: 5

Taylor (1966) identified over 1000 men employed in 3 chromate plants in the US in 1937–40, who were followed until 1960. It was stated that in 1937 these men included about 70% of the total number of such workers in the US. Enterline (1974) re-analysed the data for the same men. No further follow-up was presented, but it appeared that the risk of lung cancer was greatest shortly after the cohort was identified as being actively employed in the industry. It is not clear if this is due to a short latent interval, or a reflection of the entry criteria for the cohort (they may have been employed before the records of deaths were available).

2.19.2 Chrome pigments

Case reports from Germany described lung cancer in workers at several plants exposed to lead and zinc chromate pigments (Gross and Kolsch, 1943; Letterer, Neidhardt and Klett, 1944). These early studies have been followed by epidemiological investigations in a number of countries.

England and Wales

Davies (1978) followed 646 men who had worked at 3 factories making chrome pigments in the UK; all had worked for at least 3 months prior to 1967 and were followed until 1977. Those with high or medium exposure in 2 factories had a significant excess of lung cancer (O = 25, E = 9.6, O/E = 2.6, 95% CL = 1.7–3.8). These 2 locations had handled lead and zinc chromate, whilst only lead pigment was used at the location which failed to generate excess deaths. In an extension of this study, Davies (1984a) followed 897 male workers exposed to lead and zinc chromate pigments in the period 1933–81 and 255 exposed only to lead chromate pigments. Expected figures were based on national rates. All had worked for at least 1 year by 1975 in one of the 3 factories in England; office staff were excluded. There was no evidence of a hazard from handling lead chromate, whilst that from zinc chromate increased with degree and duration of exposure.

France

Haguender *et al.* (1981) followed up 251 male workers employed for at least 6 months in a chrome pigment factory in France in 1958–77. Expected figures were based on mortality for the appropriate department. For lung cancer, O = 11, E = 2.38,

Table 2.7 Studies of lung cancer in men with various categories of chromate exposure*

Occupation	Country	Data–years	Sex	No. subj.	O	E	O/E	Author
Chromate producing	Great Britain	1949–55	M	723	(12)	(3.3)		Bidstrup and Case (1956)
	Great Britain	1948–77	M	2836	116	48.0	2.4	Alderson, Rattan and Bidstrup (1981)
	Japan	1960–73	M	136	8	0.3	24.2	Watanabe and Fukuchi (1975)†
	Japan	1972–76	M	554	14	0.3	49.5	Ohsaki *et al.* (1978)†
	US: 1	1933–47	M	1445	(42)		16	Machle and Gregorius (1948)†
	US: 2	1925–48	M		(10)	(0)		Baetjer (1950b)‡
	US: 2	1945–79	M	2101	(59)	(29.2)	2.0	Hayes, Lilienfeld and Snell (1979)
	US: 3	1931–49	M		(6)	(1.0)	5.8	Mancuso and Hueper (1951)
	US: 3	1931–74	M		(41)			Mancuso (1975)
	US: 4	1940–50	M	977	(16)	(0.2)	80.0	Brinton, Frasier and Koven (1952)
	US: 5	1937–60	M	1212	(71)	(8.3)	8.5	Taylor (1966)
	US: 5	1937–60	M	1200	(69)	(7.3)	9.4	Enterline (1974)
Chrome pigments	England and Wales: 2	1969–72	M	1238	17	10	1.7	Royle (1975)‡
	England and Wales: 2	1967–77	M	1646	(25)	(9.6)		Davies (1978)
	England and Wales: 2	1963–81	M	897	52	30.1	1.7	Davies (1984a)§
	England and Wales: 2	1947–81	M	255	7	6.4	1.1	Davies (1984a)‖
	Norway	1948–72	M	133	(3)	(0.08)		Langard and Norseth (1975)
	Norway	1948–80	M	133	7	0.13	53.8	Langard and Vigander (1983)
	Netherlands & W. Germany	1965–81	M	1396	19	9.3	2.0	Frentzel-Beyme (1983)
Chrome plating	England and Wales	1946–74	M	4167	49	34.9	1.4	Waterhouse (1975)
	Japan	1970–76	M	5170	5	7.1	0.7	Okubo and Tsuchya (1977)
	US	1959–77	M	48				Dalager *et al.* (1980)
	US	1959–77	M	202				Dalager *et al.* (1980)¶
Ferrochromium	Sweden	1951–75	M	1932	5	7.2	0.7	Axelsson, Rylander and Schmidt (1980)
	Norway	1953–77	M	976	7	1.8	3.9	Langard, Anderson and Gylseth (1980)

Figures in parentheses are subsets of data included in other published results.
*See text for description of method.
†No conventional person-years at risk analysis.
‡Case-control study.
§Zinc chromate exposure.
‖Lead chromate exposure.
¶Zinc chromate spray painters.

O/E = 4.61, 95% CL = 2.3–8.3. This excess was not accounted for by the smoking habits of the workers. Though there were 50 deaths in the group, cause was only available for 30 men.

Netherlands and West Germany

Follow-up of 1921 employees in 5 factories in the Netherlands and West Germany who had been exposed to lead chromate pigment dust (and also zinc chromate) showed an increase in lung cancer (Frentzel-Beyme and Claud, 1980). Further details on what appears to be the same study were reported by Frentzel-Beyme (1983); 1396 men were followed for 8–16 years; there were 19 lung cancers observed but only 9.34 expected.

Norway

All 133 workers employed in a small chromate pigment producing factory for at least 3 years in 1948–72 in Bergen, Norway were traced (Langard and Norseth, 1975). All workers had been mainly exposed to zinc chromate dust. There were 3 who had developed lung cancer, with only 0.079 expected. The men were subsequently followed to 1980 (Langard and Vigander, 1983). Six of 7 patients with lung cancer occurred in the 18 workers exposed for more than 5 years (E = 0.1, O/E = 60, 95% CL = 21.9–130.6).

US

Male workers in a chrome pigment plant (potentially exposed to lead and zinc chromate) in Newark were followed in the period 1940–69 and expected deaths calculated from US mortality rates (Sheffet *et al.*, 1982). There were 321 deaths in 1296 white and 650 non-white men. There was an increase in lung cancer that was non-significant, but was related to length of employment: O = 31, E = 23.0, O/E = 1.35, 95% CL = 0.9–1.9.

2.19.3 Chrome platers

Two cases of lung cancer in men working in a chrome-plating plant in Besancon, France were reported (Michel-Briand and Simonin, 1977). No expected figure was provided.

England and Wales: 1

Tracing of 1238 chromium platers in Yorkshire and 1284 control workers matched for age and sex in 1969–72 identified variation in the cause of deaths. There were 17 deaths from lung cancer in the male platers but only 10 in the male controls, which was not statistically significant (Royle, 1975). Though there were differences in the other jobs held by both cases and controls, these were not thought to account for the findings. Smoking histories taken from a sample of cases and controls showed no appreciable differences.

England and Wales: 2

Using company records for one factory, Waterhouse (1975) traced about 83% of 5000 men who had worked on chrome plating from 1946. There was a significant excess of lung cancers: O = 49, E = 34.88, O/E = 1.4, 95% CL = 1.0–1.9.

Japan

Okubo and Tsuchya (1977) identified from union records 3395 males and 1775 females who had worked in Tokyo in chrome plating in 1970–76. Compared with general Tokyo population, there was a slight deficiency of lung cancer.

US

Deaths in 1959–77 amongst men who had worked (*a*) as spray painters exposed to zinc chromate primer paints, and (*b*) electroplaters exposed to chromic acid were analysed by Dalager *et al.* (1980). The 48 electroplaters showed no abnormal cancer pattern, but the proportion of cancer deaths in the 202 spray painters was significantly raised. There was an excess of respiratory cancer in those who had worked at least 20 years prior to death, which increased with duration of work and length of follow-up.

2.19.4 Ferrochromium

USSR

Male and female workers producing chromium ferro-alloys in 1955–69 in the USSR were studied by Pokrovskaya and Shabynina (1973). Compared with local mortality rates, there was an increase in risk of lung cancer in the males (RR = 4.4 in those aged 30–39, increasing to 6.6 in those aged 50–59).

Sweden

Using company records Axelsson, Rylander and Schmidt (1980) identified men who had worked for at least a year in a Swedish ferrochromium plant at Trollhattan in 1951–75. Deaths were compared with the expected based on national rates for this period; cancer registrations were studied for 1958–75, being compared with national and county rates. There was no evidence of a risk for lung cancer.

Norway

Langard, Anderson and Gylseth (1980) identified all men employed for at least a year in a Norwegian plant producing ferrochromium and ferrosilicon in 1953–77. Deaths and registrations were identified and compared with expected figures based on national rates, with subsequent allowance for the rural location of the plant. An excess of lung cancer was of borderline significance.

2.19.5 Other cancers

Nose

Newman (1890) reported a workman, exposed to chrome pigments, who developed perforation of the nasal septum and then an adenocarcinoma of the left inferior turbinate.

A study of 1200 male employees in 3 chromate-producing plants in the US identified 2 deaths from maxillary sinus cancer in 1941–60. This was described as 'greatly in excess of expected' (Enterline, 1974).

In a study of chrome pigment workers in a small plant in Norway, mortality in 1948–72 was examined (Langard and Norseth, 1975). One worker developed nasal cancer, but he had only been employed for 3 months, 3 years before his cancer was diagnosed. No expected figure was given.

In a study of 2915 men who had worked for at least 1 year at the 3 chromate-producing factories in Britain between 1948 and 1977, there were 2 deaths from nasal cancer: E = 0.28, O/E = 7.1, 95% CL = 0.8–25.8 (Alderson, Rattan and Bidstrup, 1981).

A case-control study of patients with nasal cancer in Scandinavia (Hernberg *et al.*, 1983a) also found an increased risk of those exposed to chromium (O/E = 2.7; 95% CL = 1.1–6.6) and to welding of chrome and nickel (O/E = 3.3; 95% CL = 1.1–9.4).

Larynx

In a case-control study, 43 male residents treated in the Toronto General Hospital for squamous carcinoma of the larynx in 1974 and matched controls were interviewed, mostly at home (Shettigara and Morgan, 1975). It was stated that there was no evidence of risk from chromium exposure, but the specific results were not provided and this was based on very small numbers.

A case-control study in Denmark of laryngeal cancer patients in 1979–82, showed no evidence of risk from chromium exposure: RR = 1.1, 95% CL = 0.8–1.5 (Olsen and Sabroe, 1984).

Gastrointestinal

The workers studied by Langard and Norseth (*see* section above on nasal cancer) also appeared to have an excess of gastrointestinal cancers by 1975; O = 3; E = 0.47; O/E = 6.38; 95% CL = 1.3–18.6 (Langard and Norseth, 1975).

2.19.6 Conclusions

Sunderman (1976) suggested that hexavalent chromium compounds were causative of lung cancer.

The monograph by IARC (1980) stated that there was sufficient evidence of respiratory carcinogenicity in men occupationally exposed during chromate production, whilst there was insufficient evidence (*a*) from other occupations, or (*b*) for other sites. The more recent studies appear to confirm a lung cancer hazard in pigment workers and a risk of nasal cancer. In a review, Norseth (1981) concluded that there was no epidemiological evidence of carcinogenicity from trivalent chromium, but that the slightly soluble hexavalent salts appeared to be the most potent carcinogens. He emphasized that there was difficulty in interpretation of results as workers tend to have mixed exposure.

2.20 Dichlorodiphenyl-trichloroethane (DDT)

A number of the studies reviewed in the section on herbicides etc. (*see* 2.37) included references to potential exposure to DDT. However, all the individuals involved had multiple exposure to other suspect agents. The only other approach to studying this problem has been to estimate the tissue levels of DDT in cancer patients and controls.

Hoffman *et al.* (1967) found a tissue level of DDT of 9.6 ppm in 292 patients dying from cancer, and of 9.4 ppm in 396 with other disease. A smaller study of 38 patients showed a non-significantly higher prevalence of cancer in those patients with higher tissue levels of organochlorine: RR = 1.78, 95% CL = 0.2–17.2 (Casarett *et al.*, 1968). Radowski, Deichmann and Clizer (1968) also reported higher tissue levels of DDT in 50 patients with cancer than 42 controls, but marked variation occurred in the levels for individuals. These 3 studies show inconsistent results, with appreciable subject-to-subject differences in detected DDT.

2.20.1 Conclusion

IARC (1974b) had, at that time, insufficient epidemiological data to evaluate the carcinogenicity of DDT to humans. IARC (1982d) considered that there was sufficient information to designate this substance as carcinogenic to animals, but still insufficient information about the hazard to humans.

2.21 Dibromochloropropane (DBCP)

As there are no adequate epidemiological studies, laboratory investigations are briefly reviewed. DBCP is used as a pesticide; the section on herbicides and pesticides should be consulted (*see* 2.37).

2.21.1 Laboratory studies

Sperm counts were lower in 107 men exposed to DBCP compared to those in 35 men who had never been exposed—46 million/ml compared with 79 million/ml (Whorton *et al.*, 1979). There had also been potential exposure to a wide range of other chemicals. Two other studies were quoted by IARC (1979b) which had reported reduced sperm counts and sperm activity (Biava, Smuckler and Whorton, 1978; Glass *et al.*, 1979).

In another study, sperm counts in men exposed and unexposed to DBCP were similar. However, histories of reproduction showed differences in those who had been exposed, with most marked reduction in fertility after about 3.5 years of exposure, and a return to normal about 2 years after cessation of exposure (Levine *et al.*, 1983a).

2.21.2 Prospective study

A historical prospective study of 3579 white male workers exposed to various brominated chemicals in

1935–76 showed a lower all-cause SMR and no specific cancer with a significant increased risk in the total group (Wong, 1981).

2.21.3 Conclusion

IARC (1979b), in the absence of human case reports or epidemiological studies, judged DBCP a carcinogenic risk to humans on the basis of animal studies. The more recent studies mentioned above do not alter this conclusion.

2.22 3,3'-Dimethoxybenzidine

A Russian report noted that not a single bladder tumour had been identified in those exposed solely to 3,3'-dimethoxybenzidine (Genin, 1974). However, it has been pointed out that this chemical had been prepared on plants also used to produce benzidine, and the 3,3'-dimethoxybenzidine may be the agent involved in risk of bladder cancer.

2.22.1 Conclusion

IARC (1982d) considered that the above epidemiological data were inadequate, but there was sufficient evidence of carcinogenicity to animals and limited evidence of activity in short-term tests.

2.23 Dimethylcarbamoyl

Due to lack of epidemiological data, laboratory studies are briefly mentioned in the following notes.

A study of 39 production workers, 26 processing workers, 42 exworkers all aged 17–65 and exposed to dimethylcarbamoyl from 6 months to 12 years identified 6 deaths—none of which were from cancer. There was no evidence of lung cancer on X-ray of the men (von Hey, Thiess and Zeller, 1974).

Chromosome studies were carried out on 10 employees exposed to dimethyl- or diethylcarbamoyl for 4–17 years and a control group with no such exposure. The subjects were screened for other exposure that might cause chromosome damage. There was no significant difference in the parameters of chromosomal aberration investigated (Fleig and Theiss, 1978a).

2.23.1 Conclusion

IARC (1976b) considered the information then available inadequate to base a judgement upon. No further epidemiological results have appeared since that time.

2.24 Dimethyl sulphate

Having provided evidence of dimethyl sulphate being a direct carcinogen in rats, Druckrey *et al.* (1966) reported a 47-year-old man dying of lung cancer following exposure to dimethyl sulphate 11 years previously. Of 10 other workers also exposed, another 3 had died from bronchial cancer. It was suggested that occupational carcinogenesis from dimethyl sulphate should be recognized as a hazard.

2.24.1 Conclusion

IARC (1974a), on the basis of laboratory studies and the case report, decided that there was evidence of suspicion of a carcinogenic hazard to man.

2.25 Dusts

The majority of studies that have identified dusts as carcinogens have been associated with exposure to particular dusts, even if it is not confirmed whether a specific chemical is responsible. For example, sections cover the hazard from various organic dusts (flour—3.3; leather—3.20; peat—2.47; textiles—3.35; wood—3.38), and inorganic dusts (silica—2.51; fibres—2.32–2.34). This section covers a few studies where there has been reference to exposure to 'dusts', without qualification of the type involved.

2.25.1 Prospective studies

Vorwald and Karr (1938) assembled X-ray reports for 15 587 males exposed to inhaled dusts at work. Only 0.019% identified a lung cancer. Autopsies of 3739 exposed males identified 30 with such a cancer. It was suggested there was no evidence of increased risk of lung cancer in these workers.

Neuberger *et al.* (1982) followed 1630 male workers exposed to silicogenic or inert dusts in Vienna from the 1950s until 1980, together with 1630 matched controls. There was an excess of lung cancer (O = 175; E = 130, O/E = 1.35; 95% CL = 1.1–1.6).

2.25.2 Case-control studies

Nose and nasopharynx

In a study in Los Angeles in 1972–76, Preston-Martin, Henderson and Pike (1982) found that inhalation of dust, fumes, and vapour was associated with risk of nose, nasal sinus, and nasopharynx cancers.

Larynx

A case-control study of laryngeal cancer patients in Denmark treated in 1980–82 showed a raised risk in those exposed to dusts: $RR = 1.6$; 95% $CL = 1.2–2$ (Olsen and Sabroe, 1984).

2.25.3 Conclusion

The above studies are insufficient to evaluate the rather nebulous concept of a cancer hazard from dusts. There is hard evidence of specific risks for cancer from the organic dusts, inorganic dusts, and asbestos fibres mentioned in the opening paragraph of this section.

2.26 Epichlorohydrin

The only epidemiological reports are on workers exposed in Shell plants in the US. Brief reports (Enterline, 1982) on (*a*) 474 males potentially exposed for at least 3 months in 1948–65 and followed to 1978 and (*b*) 389 males exposed for at least 3 months in 1955–65 and followed to 1978 showed a non-significant excess of lung cancer. Pooling the results: $O= 10$, $E = 7.28$, $O/E = 1.37$, 95% $CL = 0.7–2.5$. However, it was pointed out that some of the workers on plant (*a*) had also worked on an isopropyl alcohol plant and the excess lung cancers occurred in this group with multiple exposures.

2.26.1 Conclusion

IARC (1982d) considered the above evidence inadequate for carcinogenicity in men, but there was sufficient evidence of carcinogenicity to animals and in short-term tests.

2.27 Ethylene dibromide (EDB)

Men who had worked at 2 ethylene dibromide plants (*a*) opened in the 1920s in Michigan, and (*b*) opened in 1947 in Texas were identified from lists showing those in post in January of each year. Of 161 men, all but 1 were followed to 1976 (99.4%). Expected deaths were based on US white male mortality rates. There was no clear excess of deaths from neoplasms: plant (*a*) $O = 2$, $E = 3.6$; plant (*b*) $O = 5$, $E = 2.2$; overall $O/E = 1.21$, 95% $CL = 0.5–2.5$. Ott, Scharnweber and Langner (1980) accepted that the results cannot rule out EDB as a human carcinogen.

2.27.1 Conclusions

IARC (1977b) had no case reports or epidemiological data available at the time of their review. The above study is inadequate as a basis for an evaluation.

2.28 Ethylene oxide

Laboratory studies of exposed men have suggested that there may be a hazard to man. The epidemiology reports are limited, though this is one of the agents for which studies of fetal loss are available.

2.28.1 Laboratory studies

Levinson (1981) referred to a US study of 75 workers in which chromosome abnormalities had been detected: no specific details are given. He also referred to a group of 31 workers exposed to as little as 1 ppm for an average of 15 years; no subject developed lymphatic leukaemia. Examination of levels of sister chromatid exchange in lymphocyte cultures showed no difference for 14 staff operating ethylene oxide sterilizers and matched controls in a US hospital (Hansen *et al.*, 1984).

2.28.2 Cross-sectional study

Joyner (1964) studied the health of 37 men employed on ethylene oxide production over an average of 10 years. Age-matched controls working on other production units were also reviewed. Previous medical history whilst on the plant, present health and results from examination and laboratory investigations were reviewed. There was no evidence of adverse health effects in the 37 operators, though because of small numbers interpretation as a 'negative' has to be qualified. No chromosome or sperm tests were performed on the men.

2.28.3 Prospective studies

The following studies are discussed in chronological order.

Sweden: 1

Between 1972 and 1977, 3 cases of 'leukaemia' (1 was of Waldenstrom's macroglobulinaemia) were diagnosed in a Swedish factory where 50% ethylene oxide and 50% methyl formate were used to sterilize hospital equipment.

The treated boxes of equipment were subsequently stored in a 'hall' where up to 30 women worked; apparently the boxes leaked and thus individuals working in or passing through this hall were exposed to a time-weighted average ethylene oxide concentration of 20 ± 10 ppm. Estimated person-years at risk indicated that 0.2 cases of leukaemia were expected (Hogstedt *et al.*, 1979).

Sweden: 2

Men working in a plant manufacturing ethylene oxide in 1961 have been followed until the end of 1977 (Hogstedt, Malmqvist and Wadman, 1979). No men were lost on follow-up of the 241 men employed for more than a year; expected deaths or incidence of cancer were calculated from national data. The men were divided into those not working in the production of ethylene oxide, exposed intermittently, or daily. Those exposed daily had a significant excess of deaths from tumours, especially stomach and leukaemia; there was no appreciable variation in the mortality for those intermittently or not exposed. It was pointed out that the workers had been potentially exposed to a number of different compounds associated with the process. Results from this study were also published by Hogstedt *et al.* (1979).

US

Personnel records identified 767 males who had worked for at least 5 years on a Texaco plant producing ethylene oxide in the period 1955–77. More than 95% were traced; expected mortality was based on US national rates (Morgan *et al.*, 1981). Overall there was a deficiency of neoplasms and no site showed a significant excess.

Germany

Theiss *et al.* (1982) followed 602 workers potentially exposed to alkylene oxides (such as ethylene oxide) and other agents in the period 1928–80. In comparison with another group of workers with styrene exposure, there were 14 deaths from neoplasms, with 16.7 expected; no site-specific data were provided.

2.28.4 Hazard to the next generation

Studies on the hazard to pregnant women are of interest because of the limited nature of the information about risk of cancer in exposed workers. Information on spontaneous abortion was obtained by (*a*) questionnaire, and (*b*) hospital discharge registers for all staff in Finnish hospitals employed in chemical sterilizing of equipment in 1980. Overall there was an increased abortion rate compared with nursing auxiliaries, which was particularly marked for pregnancies during which

sterilizing work was carried out—16.7% of these compared with 5.6% of 'non-exposed' pregnancies. Adjustment for confounding factors did not affect the results and it was concluded that ethylene oxide might be the factor involved (Hemminki *et al.*, 1982). Queries were raised about: bias in the exposure data, the validity of abortion recall over a long time period, the method of analysis for confounding factors, and the levels of exposure. Hemminki, Mutanen and Niemi (1983) emphasized that the recording of exposure by supervising staff was separated by 6 months from contact with individuals asking about work done during each pregnancy (the place of work being linked to the supervisors record of exposure). The information about abortions was obtained (*a*) from the respondents, (*b*) from hospital discharge records; there was good agreement between the 2 sources. Further data were provided comparing abortion rates (adjusted for age distribution) for exposed staff and nursing auxiliaries in the same hospitals who were not exposed. There was a significantly greater rate of abortion in the exposed staff. It was emphasized that these results related to pregnancies chiefly before environmental measurements of ethylene oxide levels had been made.

2.28.5 Conclusions

When ethylene oxide was reviewed by IARC (1976a), there was no published prospective study of workers for evaluation. Though there have been 2 reports from Sweden of excess of leukaemia in exposed workers, these have not been replicated in the studies from Germany and the US. It is not clear whether there is a definitive carcinogenic risk, let alone the levels of exposure that might be responsible.

2.29 Ethylene thiourea

Innes and his colleagues (1969) reported that ethylene thiourea caused thyroid cancer in rats. Smith (1976) used a nominal roll of persons in the rubber industry to cross-check against thyroid cancer registrations in the Birmingham region in 1957–71. Though there were records available for 1929 workers, no thyroid cancers were found; no expected figure was given, but it is very low. There was no information on the level of exposure to ethylene thiourea.

2.29.1 Hazard to the next generation

Smith (1976) checked a nominal roll of women who had worked in rubber manufacture in 1963–71 and were potentially exposed to ethylene thiourea, against birth records in Birmingham. Of 699 women, 255 were identified in the birth records as mothers to 420 children; 59 women had been at work in early pregnancy. There was no evidence of higher prevalence of congenital malformations compared with that in the locality.

2.29.2 Conclusions

IARC (1974a) had no case reports or epidemiological data upon which to base an evaluation. The above report does not alter the situation materially.

2.30 Fertilizers

One study on this general exposure is briefly described in this section. A more specific entry is that of nitrate fertilizer manufacture (2.45); also, farmers will be exposed to fertilizers, amongst other factors (*see* 3.14).

In a matched case-control study of 111 patients with prostate cancer treated in Chicago and Los Angeles, Rotkin (1977) observed an increased risk from exposure to fertilizers (RR = 2.57; 95% CL = 1.1–5.9). Interpretation is difficult because of the limited information provided and the inadequate statistical examination of the results.

2.30.1 Conclusion

The above report is an inadequate base to consider that those exposed to fertilizers have an increased risk of cancer.

2.31 Fibre (1): asbestos

This section indicates the background to concern about the cancer risk from exposure to asbestos and provides brief notes of the sources of exposure, types of fibres, and some of the problems specific to epidemiological studies of this hazard. Results of a number of studies are presented for: miners and millers, employees in various factories, insulators, and shipyard workers. The results from these studies for 5 sites of malignancy are given in *Tables 2.8–2.12*. Some case-control studies have focused on risk from asbestos for specific sites of malignancy, whilst there is a particular hazard for mesothelioma; sections cover these issues. Asbestos is one of the agents where there is clear evidence that 'industrial' processes can lead to exposure of persons in the workers' households and residents in the neighbourhood of installations. Some of the key papers on this are described. Specific issues of concern to planning preventive measures are the need to clarify the risk

from different types of fibre, and to confirm the relative contributions that asbestos makes to smokers' risk of lung cancer.

Because of the voluminous literature on this subject, the large number of individuals who have been exposed to asbestos, and the widespread concern about the hazard that such exposure generates, this section provides a more detailed exposition than other sections in this chapter.

2.31.1 Background

Case reports of lung cancer in patients with asbestosis came from the US (Lynch and Smith, 1935) and then the UK (Gloyne, 1933). Gilson (1966) emphasized how these case reports had been supported by the steadily rising proportion of lung cancer in persons dying from asbestosis in England and Wales noted in the reports of the Ministry of Labour.

Using certificates of death from lung cancer occurring in England and Wales in 1921–38, Kennaway and Kennaway (1947) suggested there was an increasing risk of lung cancer in those exposed to asbestos, but no ratio for this risk could be calculated due to the inability to estimate the number of exposed workers from the 1931 census.

Merewether (1949) provided a brief note of cancer of the lung in relation to asbestos; he referred to 235 deaths with asbestosis as a diagnosis, which had been reported to the Chief Inspector of Factories in the period 1924–46. Cancer of the lung or pleura was present in 31 (13.2%). When analysed by sex, 17.2% of the 128 male deaths and only 8.4% of the female deaths were affected by lung cancer. A tabulation was provided of the mean duration of exposure to asbestos dust: this was 16.5 years for those developing lung cancer in comparison with 13.4 years for those dying with no evidence of such cancer. It had been found impossible to classify the dustiness of the occupation, due to the frequency with which individuals were moved in their work. In comparison, subjects dying from silicosis only had cancer of the lung in 1.3%. No specific comment was made that this frequency of lung cancer in subjects with asbestos was of aetiological significance.

The problems of the validity of death certificates are particularly important in studies of asbestos workers, where some of the specific causes of death (pleural and peritoneal mesothelioma) may be misdiagnosed as other neoplasms. In the follow-up study of insulation workers in the US (Selikoff and Seidman, 1981), 49 death certificates gave cancer of the pancreas as the cause of death, with only 17.5 expected. Review of case notes indicated that only 23 deaths should have been so certified (including one originally given as myocardial infarction); there were, in addition, 16 peritoneal mesothelioma, 4 lung cancers, 2 colon cancers, and carcinomatosis with unidentified site in 5. Because of this difficulty, a number of authors have argued that it is important to check the diagnosis for all deaths in prospective studies of asbestos workers. However, Enterline (1976a) has suggested that this artificially raises the risk from asbestos exposure. It is not self-evident that this inflation always occurs, as review of the records may reduce or increase the number of deaths ascribed to a particular cancer. Where reports give results based on review of the diagnosis, these have been used in the tables in this section.

As with many other occupational hazards, there are problems of studying mobile workers with exposure in different industries. This is compounded by the difficulty of assessing past levels of exposure; even where there have been measurements of the fibre levels, the techniques have varied. Gold and Cuthbert (1966) emphasized the difficulty of confirming exposure in some occupations—for example a joiner may periodically use asbestos boards, or work in a confined space on ships alongside laggers.

This appears to be a topic where there have been overlapping studies on some groups of workers—often without clear specification in the papers that this is so. This is complicated by the multiple publication of results by the same authors of findings from a particular study (again without always acknowledging this).

The latent interval may also be very long. For example, Selikoff *et al.* (1967) reported that the interval from first exposure to asbestos until death from lung cancer varied from 22 to 54 years, with a mean of 32 years. Because of the need to consider year of first exposure, duration of exposure, and latent interval from first exposure, many papers provide a range of results from subsets of the data. This can lead to secondary quotation of different results from the same piece of work. The estimates of risk can differ appreciably if the analysis is restricted to those followed a minimum of 1, 10, or 20 years after first exposure. This has been further confused by erroneous abstraction or transcription of results that has apparently occurred in 2 major reviews on the subject.

When interpreting results, particularly in relation to type of fibre and exposure levels, it is important to appreciate the nature of asbestos fibres and the levels produced by various processes. Asbestos is a naturally occurring silicate fibre, which can be classified:

Different mines handle different types of fibre (*see* 2.31.2). (Actinolite and tremolite are not covered in the present review, because inadequate human studies have been reported.) Historically, the main fibre handled has been chrysotile, with increasing use of all 4 main types of fibre until the 1970s. As far as exposure levels are concerned, many of the papers reviewed have provided subjective or objective assessments of the work conditions. The issue of a 'safe' level is discussed in the chapter on prevention.

2.31.2 Mining and milling

The following notes cover 5 studies carried out on asbestos miners. They are listed in chronological order of the data-years involved.

Salary lists were used to identify 1092 employees at 2 Finnish anthophyllite mines, who had worked in 1936–67 for at least 3 months; 95.3% were traced until 1969. Expected deaths were based on national mortality rates in 1958. A questionnaire was sent to miners and population controls in 1967 to assess smoking habits (Meurman, Kiviluoto and Hakama, 1974).

Males mining crocidolite in Western Australia in 1943–66 were identified from company records and followed until 1977. Expected deaths were calculated from state mortality rates. No detail on exposure levels was given (Hobbs *et al.*, 1980).

Rubino *et al.* (1979b) studied over 900 chrysotile miners from Italy; they had first worked in 1930–65 for at least 1 month and their mortality was observed in 1946–75. Expected deaths were based on national mortality rates. An earlier report covered men employed in the period up to 1970 (Ghezzi, Aresini and Vigliani, 1972).

McDonald *et al.* (1971) traced, up to 1966, 88.4% of 11 788 persons born from 1891 to 1920, who had worked in the Quebec chrysotile mines and mills for at least 1 month. This study was subsequently extended to (*a*) 1969 (McDonald *et al.*, 1973; 1974); (*b*) 1973 (Liddell, McDonald and Thomas, 1977); (*c*) 1975 (McDonald *et al.*, 1980). The results from the latter paper are included in *Tables 2.8–2.10, 2.12* covering deaths in 1951–75. During the course of this work a number of method papers were produced: (*a*) examining the use of internal or external comparison, (*b*) handling the analysis in an *a priori* or *a posteriori* fashion, and (*c*) placing emphasis on a case-control analysis within the data.

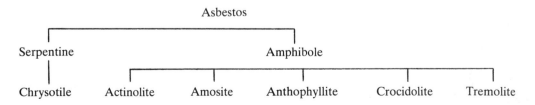

These issues are discussed in 1.2.6, 1.4.4 and 1.5.7. Dust measurements from the mines were used to examine the dose–response, whilst smoking histories permitted examination of the effect of asbestos and smoking on risk of lung cancer (*see* 2.31.12).

Union lists identified 544 men employed as miners and millers in Thetford mines, Quebec in 1960 for at least 20 years. They were followed to 1977; for 130 of 179 deaths clinic records were used to confirm the cause of death. Expected values were based on national mortality rates (Nicholson *et al.*, 1979). It is not clear whether these miners were included in the larger study mounted by McDonald and his colleagues.

2.31.3 Manufacture

These notes cover studies from Canada, Denmark, England and Wales, and the US. Within each country, the studies are in chronological order of the data-years involved.

Canada: 1

McDonald and McDonald (1978) identified 3 groups of workers who had been exposed to crocidolite in the manufacture of military gas masks in Canada: (*a*) 112 of 113 producing filter pads in Quebec in 1939–41 were traced until 1975; (*b*) 23 of 32 workers producing filter pads in 1940–41 in Montreal were traced in 1976; (*c*) 54 who had been exposed in Ottawa in 1939–42 during assembly of the masks: 41 were traced until 1975. The overall trace rate was 84%. The observed lung cancer deaths were compared with miners and millers from Quebec, by proportional analysis.

Canada: 2

Finkelstein (1983) identified 186 male production workers hired by 1960, at an Ontario asbestos cement factory, who had worked for at least 9 years; 97.3% were traced to 1980. Expected deaths were based on Ontario mortality rates.

Table 2.8 Risk of gastrointestinal cancer in various groups of asbestos workers*

Occupation	Fibre	Country	Data–years	Sex	No. subj.	O	E	O/E	Author
Mining/ milling	Anth	Finland	1936–69	M/F	1041	7	14.9	0.47	Meurmann, Kiviluoto and Hakama (1974)
	Chr	Italy	1946–75	M	933	19	19.3	0.98	Rubino *et al.* (1979b)
	Chr	Canada	1951–75	M	10939	209	203.7	1.03	McDonald *et al.* (1980)
	Chr	Canada	1961–77	M	544	20	9.5	1.05	Nicholson *et al.* (1979)
Manuf. cement	*Chr*, Cro	Canada: 2	1960–80	M	186	3	1.4	2.14	Finkelstein (1983)
Manuf. cement	Mixed	Denmark	1944–76	M	16089	45	39.1	1.15	Clemmensen and Jensen (1983)
Manuf. textiles	*Chr*, Cro	England: 1	1916–74	P	1369	16	15.7	1.02	Peto *et al.* (1977)
Manuf. mixed	Cro, Amo, Chr	England: 2	1933–75	M	3467	58	34.0	1.71	Newhouse and Berry (1979)
Manuf. mixed	Cro, Amo, Chr	England: 2	1936–75	F	922	26	10.2	2.55	Newhouse and Berry (1979)
Manuf. cement	*Chr*, Cro	England: 3	1936–77	M	1592	18	19.6	0.92	Thomas, H.F. *et al.* (1982)
Manuf. gas masks	Cro, Chr	England: 4	1940–78	F	578	10	12.3	0.81	Jones *et al.* (1980)
Manuf. gas masks	Cro	England: 5	1951–77	F	500	7	10.7	0.65	Wignall and Fox (1982)
Manuf. frict. prod.	*Chr*, Cro	England: 6	1941–79	M	7474	103	107.2	0.96	Berry and Newhouse (1983)
Manuf. frict. prod.	*Chr*, Cro	England: 6	1941–79	F	3708	29	27.4	1.06	Berry and Newhouse (1983)
Manuf. insul. prod.	Amo, Chr	England: 7	1947–78	M	4820	17	15.1	1.13	Acheson *et al.* (1984a)
Manuf. mixed	*Chr*, Amo, Cro	US: 1	1940–75	M	2666	50	41.4	1.21	Robinson, Lemen and Wagon (1979)
Manuf. mixed	*Chr*, Amo, Cro	US: 1	1940–75	F	537	8	6.0	1.33	Robinson, Lemen and Wagon (1979)

Table 2.8 Continued

Occupation	Fibre	Country	Data–years	Sex	No. subj.	O	E	O/E	Author
Manuf. mixed	Mixed	US: 2	1941–73	M	1075	55†	39.9	1.38	Henderson and Enterline (1979)
Manuf. cement	Chr, Amo, Cro	US: 3	1942–76	M	5645	25	50.1	0.50	Hughes and Weill (1980)
Manuf. paper board	Chr	US: 4	1945–74	M	264	4	3.8	1.05	Weiss (1977b)
Manuf. mixed	?	US: 5	1948–63	M	21 755	83†	78.3	1.06	Enterline and Kendrick (1967)
Manuf. textile	Chr	US: 6a	1959–77	M	2543	25†	17.1	1.46	McDonald et al. (1983a)
Manuf. mixed	Chr, Amo, Cro	US: 6b	1959–77	M	4137	50†	47.9	1.04	McDonald et al. (1983b)
Manuf. frict. prod.	Chr	US: 6c	1959–77	M	3641	59	51.6	1.14	McDonald et al. (1984)
Manuf. insul. prod.	Amo	US: 7	1961–77	M	582	15	7.2	2.08	Selikoff, Seidman and Hammond (1980)
Insulators	Mixed	England	1933–75	M	1368	3	4.3	0.70	Newhouse and Berry (1979)
	Mixed	N. Ireland	1940–75	M	162	13	0.7	18.57	Elmes and Simpson (1977)
	Chr, Amo	US	1943–76	M	632	43	15.1	2.85	Selikoff, Hammond and Seidman (1979)
	Chr, Amo	US	1943–76	M	833	3	1.5	2.00	Selikoff, Hammond and Seidman (1979)
	?	US	1945–65	M	152	4	1.8	2.22‡	Kleinfeld, Messite and Kooyman (1967)
	Chr, Amo	US/Canada	1967–76	M	17 800	99	59.4	1.67	Selikoff, Hammond and Seidman (1979)
Shipyards	Mixed	England	1947–78	M	6076	63	83.3	0.76	Rossiter and Coles (1980)
	?	Italy	1960–75	M	2190	78	58.6	1.26	Putoni et al. (1979)
(Insulators)	?	US	1967–76	M	440	3	3.1	0.97	Selikoff, Hammond and Seidman (1979)
Shipyards	Mixed	England	1960–69	M		416	408.5	1.02‡	Lumley (1976)

*See text for description of method.
†Based on ICD 150–156 (remainder are 150–154).
‡Proportional Registration Ratio.

Denmark

Company records were used to identify all males who had worked at an asbestos cement factory in 1944–76. This roll was matched against the national cancer register; expected cancers were based on national rates (Clemmesen and Hjalgrim-Jensen, 1981).

England and Wales: 1

Peto et al. (1977) traced 1106 persons (822 men) who had worked for at least 10 years in a textile factory in England by 1972; 96.8% were followed until 1974. This included 69 men with more than 10 years and 74 with less than 10 years exposure prior to 1933 when the hygiene standards were changed. Chrysotile was used predominantly, but also small amounts of crocidolite. Expected deaths were based on

national rates. Previous reports were: Doll, 1955; Knox, Doll and Hill, 1965; Hill, Doll and Knox, 1966; Knox et al., 1968.

England and Wales: 2

Newhouse and Berry (1979) followed 4835 male workers first employed in 1933–64 and 922 women employed first in 1936–42 at a factory in London making textiles, insulation and some other products until 1975. The trace rate was 94.8% for men and 77% for women. The main fibre used was crocidolite with some amosite and chrysotile. Of the men, 1368 had been employed as laggers, usually working on contract outside the factory; their results are presented separately. Expected deaths were based on national mortality rates. Previous publications were: Newhouse, 1969, 1973; Newhouse et al., 1972.

England and Wales: 3

Thomas *et al.* (1982a) traced 1592 men who had worked for at least 6 months at any time from 1936, until 1977 in an asbestos factory in South Wales. For the first year some crocidolite was used, but after that only chrysotile. Expected deaths were based on national rates; those for 1966–70 were used for the period 1966–77. Preliminary results were published by Elwood *et al.* (1964).

England and Wales: 4

Out of a workforce of 1600, 951 women who had worked on gas mask manufacture in Nottingham in 1940–45 were followed until 1978. Only 60.8% were traced. Some women had been exposed to chrysotile for a maximum of 5 months, whilst the majority were exposed to crocidolite for up to 5 years with a small number exposed to both fibres (Jones *et al.*, 1980). Expected values were based on national rates, applied to the original sample of 951, rather than the 575 who were traced.

England and Wales: 5

Wignall and Fox (1982) identified 535 women who had worked on military gas mask production in 1939–44 and been exposed to crocidolite in one room of the Nottingham plant (about one-third of the workforce of the previous study). Five hundred (93%) were traced until 1977; of these, 133 worked for less than 6 months. The source of expected deaths is not given.

England and Wales: 6

Berry and Newhouse (1983) identified 9113 men and 4347 women who had been employed at a factory producing friction materials in Chapel-en-le-frith, England in 1941 or at any subsequent date. Over 99% were traced to the end of 1979. Chrysotile was used almost exclusively, with crocidolite being used on one product in 1929–44. Expected deaths were based on national rates. Identical results were published by Newhouse, Berry and Skidmore (1982), though this is not pointed out in the paper.

England and Wales: 7

An Uxbridge, London factory, manufacturing asbestos board from 1947, used amosite with chrysotile being added up to 3% until 1973. Of the 6032 men ever employed in 1945–78, 5871 (97%) were traced until 1980; 4882 had been exposed to

Table 2.9 Risk of laryngeal cancer in various groups of asbestos workers*

Occupation	Fibre	Country	Data-years	Sex	No. subj.	O	E	O/E	Author
Mining/ milling	Chr	Italy	1946–75	M	933	6	1.9	3.16	Rubino *et al.* (1979b)
	Chr	Canada	1951–75	M	10939	16	14.9	1.07	McDonald *et al.* (1980)
Manuf. cement	Mixed	Denmark	1944–76	M	16089	6	2.9	2.07	Clemmesen and Jensen (1983)
Manuf. mixed	*Cro*, Amo, Chr	England: 2	1933–69	M	3467	2	0.4	5.00	Newhouse and Berry (1973)
Manuf. gas masks	*Cro*	England: 5	1951–77	F	500	1	0.1	10.00	Wignall and Fox (1982)
Manuf. frict. prod.	*Chr*, Cro	England: 6	1941–79	M	7474	2	3.6	0.56	Berry and Newhouse (1983)
Manuf. textiles	*Chr*	US: 6a	1959–77	M	2543	3	0.1	50.00	McDonald *et al.* (1983a)
Manuf. mixed	*Chr*, Amo, Cro	US: 6b	1959–77	M	4137	0	0.03	0	McDonald *et al.* (1983b)
Manuf. frict. prod.	Chr	US: 6c	1959–77	M	3641	4	0.04	100.00	McDonald *et al.* (1984)
Insulators	Chr, Amo	US	1943–76	M	632	6†	2.8	2.14	Selikoff, Hammond and Seidman (1979)
	Chr, Amo	US	1943–76	M	833	2†	0.5	4.00	Selikoff, Hammond and Seidman (1979)
	Chr, Amo	US/Canada	1967–76	M	17800	11	4.7	2.34	Selikoff, Hammond and Seidman (1979)
Shipyards	?	Italy	1960–75	M	2190	15	7.7	1.95	Putoni *et al.* (1979)
	Mixed	England	1960–69	M		20	18.5	1.08‡	Lumley (1976)

*See text for description of method.
†Larynx, pharynx, buccal cavity.
‡Proportional Registration Ratio.

asbestos, but only about 700 prior to 1960. Results for mesothelioma have been published (Acheson *et al.*, 1981), and cancers (Acheson *et al.*, 1984a). The number of the exposed are slightly different in the second paper; expected figures were based on national rates.

England and Wales: 8

Acheson *et al.* (1982) followed 1327 women employed in 1939 on gas mask assembly; 570 had been exposed to chrysotile in a factory in Blackburn, and 757 to crocidolite and chrysotile in a factory at Leyland. They were all traced to mid-1980.

National rates were used to calculate expected figures for 1951–80, with correction for local mortality for 1968–78.

US: 1

Robinson, Lemen and Wagoner (1979) followed 3276 workers employed for at least 1 year in 1940–67 at a plant producing textile, friction and packing materials in the US until 1975; 97% were traced. Chrysotile was the predominant fibre, with about 1% of amosite and less crocidolite. Expected deaths were based on national rates.

US: 2

One thousand and seventy-five men who had retired in 1941–67 from a US company and reached the age of 65 were traced until 1973; work had involved a variety of products, with different groups of men having exposure to amosite and/or chrysotile and/or crocidolite. Expected values were based on national white mortality rates (Henderson and Enterline, 1979). Previous papers had included 273 Canadian employees of the company (Enterline, 1970; Enterline, Decoufle and Henderson, 1972; Enterline and Henderson, 1973; Enterline and Weill, 1973).

US: 3

Hughes and Weill (1980) identified 5645 men employed for at least 1 month in 2 plants producing cement products in New Orleans from the early 1940s. The men were traced to 1974, but only contributed to the analysis from 20 years after first exposure. Chrysotile had been the predominant fibre, but crocidolite had also been used in both plants and amosite in one. Expected deaths were based on national rates for 1950, 1960, and 1970. Previous results appeared in Weill, Hughes and Waggenspack (1979).

US: 4

A US plant produced paper and millboard from

1896, until 1960 when working methods were changed. Company records identified 254 men recruited in the period 1935–45 and alive at the end of 1945; 94% were followed until 1974. Though all had worked for a minimum of 1 year, 56% had only worked for less than 5 years. Expected mortality was calculated from national rates (Weiss, 1977b).

US: 5

Enterline and Kendrick (1967) identified 21 755 white male employees in 1948–51 from asbestos production plants in the US, who were followed until 1963. This involved 9 textile plants, 11 friction plants, and 15 building product plants. Comparisons were made against mortality in cotton textile workers, and expected deaths were based on national rates. The type of fibre was not specified. Preliminary results were published by Enterline (1965).

US: 6(a,b,c)

A coordinated study in 3 US manufacturing plants aimed to compare the hazard from chrysotile use with that found in mining and to determine the risk of mesothelioma from this fibre. The studies involved plants in South Carolina (McDonald *et al.*, 1983a), Pennsylvania (McDonald *et al.*, 1983b), and Connecticut (McDonald *et al.*, 1984).

In the South Carolina plant 2543 men who had worked for at least a month in 1938–58 were followed until 1977. The trace rate is not quoted, though of the 863 found to be dead, certificates were found for 827 (95%). Only chrysotile had been used for the manufacture of textiles. The Pennsylvania plant also produced textiles with some friction materials and packings; it used mainly chrysotile with some amosite and crocidolite. Of 4137 who had worked for at least 1 month in 1938–59, 97% were traced until 1977. The third plant in Connecticut used chrysotile for friction products and packings. Of 3641 men employed for 1 month or more in 1938–58, 96.5% were traced until 1977. Only deaths occurring after 20 years from first exposure were included.

Preliminary results for all 3 plants were published by McDonald and Fry (1982). More detailed results were provided for the South Carolina plant by Dement *et al.* (1982, 1983), and for the Pennsylvania plant by Mancuso and El-Attar (1967b) and Robinson, Lemen and Wagoner (1979).

US: 7

A factory making insulation materials for ships from amosite was established in New Jersey in 1941, which closed in 1954. Selikoff, Seidman and Hammond (1980) identified 933 men who had begun

66

Table 2.10 Risk of lung cancer in various groups of asbestos workers*

Occupation	Fibre	Country	Data–years	Sex	No. subj.	O	E	O/E	Author
Mining/ milling	Anth	Finland	1936–69	M/F	1041	21	12.6	1.67	Meurmann, Kiviluoto and Hakama (1974)
	Cro	Australia	1943–77	M	6200	60	38.2	1.57	Hobbs *et al.* (1980)
	Chr	Italy	1946–75	M	933	11	10.4	1.06	Rubino *et al.* (1979b)
	Chr	Canada	1951–75	M	10939	230	184.0	1.25	McDonald *et al.* (1980)
	Chr	Canada	1951–75	F	440	1	1.2	0.83	McDonald *et al.* (1980)
	Chr	Canada	1961–77	M	544	28	11.1	2.52	Nicholson *et al.* (1979)
Manuf. cement	*Chr*, Cro	Canada	1960–80	M	186	17	2.0	8.50	Finkelstein (1983)
Manuf. cement	Mixed	Denmark	1944–76	M	16089	44	27.3	1.61	Clemmesen and Jensen (1983)
Manuf. textiles	*Chr*, Cro	England: 1	1916–74	M	143	20	4.5	4.44	Peto *et al.* (1977)
Manuf. textiles	*Chr*, Cro	England: 1	1934–74	M	942	29	18.4	1.58	Peto *et al.* (1977)
Manuf. textiles	*Chr*, Cro	England: 1	1934–74	F	284	2	0.9	2.22	Peto *et al.* (1977)
Manuf. mixed	*Cro, Amo,* Chr	England: 2	1933–75	M	3467	103	43.2	2.38	Newhouse and Berry (1979)
Manuf. mixed	*Cro, Amo,* Chr	England: 2	1936–75	F	922	27	3.2	8.44	Newhouse and Berry (1979)
Manuf. cement	*Chr*, Cro	England: 3	1936–77	M	1592	28	33.0	0.85	Thomas, H.F. *et al.* (1982)
Manuf. gas mask	*Cro*, Chr	England: 4	1940–78	F	578	12	3.8	3.16	Jones *et al.* (1980)
Manuf. gas mask	*Cro*	England: 5	1951–77	F	500	10	3.7	2.70	Wignall and Fox (1982)
Manuf. frict. prod.	*Chr*, Cro	England: 6	1941–79	M	7474	143	139.5	1.03	Berry and Newhouse (1983)
Manuf. frict. prod.	*Chr*, Cro	England: 6	1941–79	F	3708	6	11.3	0.53	Berry and Newhouse (1983)
Manuf. insul. prod.	*Amo*, Chr	England: 7	1947–78	M	4820	57	29.1	1.96	Acheson *et al.* (1984a)
Manuf. gas mask	*Chr*	England: 8	1951–80	F	570	6	4.8	1.25	Acheson *et al.* (1982)
Manuf. gas mask	*Cro*, Chr	England: 8	1951–80	F	757	13	6.2	2.10	Acheson *et al.* (1982)
Manuf. mixed	*Chr, Amo,* Cro	US: 1	1940–75	M	2666	49	36.1	1.36	Robinson *et al.* (1979)
Manuf. mixed	*Chr, Amo,* Cro	US: 1	1940–75	F	537	14	1.7	8.24	Robinson *et al.* (1979)
Manuf. mixed	Mixed	US: 2	1941–73	M	1075	63	23.3	2.70	Henderson and Enterline (1979)
Manuf. cement	*Chr, Amo,* Cro	US: 3	1942–74	M	5645	51	49.1	1.04	Hughes and Weill (1980)
Manuf. paper board	*Chr*	US: 4	1945–74	M	264	4	4.3	0.93	Weiss (1977b)
Manuf. mixed	?	US: 5	1942–63	M	21755	92†	67.3	1.37	Enterline and Kendrick (1967)
Manuf. textile	*Chr*	US: 6a	1959–77	M	2543	59†	29.6	1.99	McDonald *et al.* (1983a)
Manuf. mixed	*Chr, Amo,* Cro	US: 6b	1959–77	M	4137	43†	50.4	0.86	McDonald *et al.* (1983b)
Manuf. frict. prod.	*Chr*	US: 6c	1959–77	M	3641	73†	49.1	1.49	McDonald *et al.* (1984)
Manuf. insul. prod.	*Amo*	US: 7	1961–77	M	582	60	10.1	5.94	Selikoff, Seidman and Hammond (1980)

Table 2.10 Continued

Occupation	Fibre	Country	Data–years	Sex	No. subj.	O	E	O/E	Author
Insulators	Mixed	England	1933–75	M	1368	21	5.6	3.75	Newhouse and Berry (1979)
	Mixed	N. Ireland	1940–75	M	162	32	4.7	6.81	Elmes and Simpson (1977)
	Chr, Amo	US	1943–76	M	632	93	13.3	6.99	Selikoff, Hammond and Seidman (1979)
	Chr, Amo	US	1943–76	M	833	10	2.9	3.45	Selikoff, Hammond and Seidman (1979)
	?	US	1945–65	M	152	10	1.4	7.14‡	Klienfeld, Messite and Kooyman (1967)
	?	Sweden	1967–74	M	1699	6	1.9	3.20	Englund (1980)
	Chr, Amo	US/Canada	1967–76	M	17800	486	105.6	4.60	Selikoff, Hammond and Seidman (1979)
Shipyards	Mixed	Hawaii	1950–73	M	4779	35	32.5	1.08	Kolonel *et al.* (1980)
	Mixed	England	1947–78	M	6076	84	119.7	0.70	Rossiter and Coles (1980)
	Mixed	England	1960–69	M		363	338.0	1.07‡	Lumley (1976)
	?	Italy	1960–75	M	2190	123	54.9	2.24	Putoni *et al.* (1979)
	?	England	1964–?	M	429	19	4.0	4.75§	Edge (1979)
(Insulators)	?	US	1967–76	M	440	21	5.7	3.68	Selikoff, Hammond and Seidman (1979)

*See text for description of method.
†ICD 160–164.
‡Proportional Mortality/Registration Ratio.
§Case-control study.

work in 1941–45; 39 had worked with asbestos elsewhere. Two-hundred and seventy died within 20 years of first exposure, and 42 were lost-to-follow-up. One-third of the men had worked for less than 4 months in the factory. The 582 were traced to 1977 and observed mortality compared with the expected based on (*a*) state mortality rates, (*b*) results from the American Cancer Society prospective study. Only deaths occurring at least 20 years after first exposure were included. The cause of death was reviewed for those who died. Earlier results were published by: Selikoff, Hammond and Churg, 1972; Selikoff and Hammond, 1975; Siedman, Lilis and Selikoff, 1976; Seidman, Selikoff and Hammond, 1979.

2.31.4 Insulators

The following notes describe 5 studies of groups of insulators; a sixth formed a subset of the manufacturing study already discussed (England and Wales: 2).

Northern Ireland

Elmes and Simpson (1977) followed 162 Belfast insulators initially employed in 1940 until 1975. The cause of death was based on review of all available information, though the difficulty of distinguishing lung cancer from mesothelioma is emphasized. (The 11 undetermined deaths have been split between

bronchus and mesothelioma in the ratio of specified neoplasms in these two sites.) Expected deaths were based on national rates. The results are presented in histogram form in the paper, making retrieval of O and E difficult. Earlier results were presented by Elmes and Simpson (1971).

US: 1

Union records identified workers employed in the New York–New Jersey area who had worked prior to 1943 and were followed initially until 1962 (Selikoff, Churg and Hammond, 1964). They were subsequently followed until 1976 (Selikoff, Hammond and Seidman, 1979). Expected mortality was based on US white mortality rates for 1949–76, with extrapolation back to cover the period 1943–48. The 833 men joining the union in 1943–62 were also followed to 1976. Results for deaths in the period 1943–76 are shown in *Tables 2.8–2.10, 2.12*. Other reports on this group include: Hammond, Selikoff and Churg, 1965; Selikoff, Churg and Hammond, 1965; Selikoff and Hammond, 1975.

US: 2

Klienfeld, Messite and Kooyman (1967) identified from Union records 152 New York insulators who had had 15 years exposure by some date in the period 1945–65. A proportional-mortality analysis used expected figures based on national rates in 1948.

Sweden

Englund (1980) used employee certification to identify 1699 insulators in Sweden in 1967, who were followed to 1974. Expected deaths were calculated from national rates. The significant excess of respiratory cancer deaths was supported by an analysis from the national Cancer Environment files linking the 1960 census with cancer registrations up until 1973 (*see* Chapter 1, Appendix: Sweden).

US: 3, Canada

All 17 800 men on the insulation workers union rolls in US and Canada on 1/1/67 were entered into a further study. (This included men from the New York–New Jersey studies, US: 1 above.) The men have been followed to 1976 (Selikoff, Hammond and Seidman, 1979). For those who have died, the cause of death was reviewed and analysed by 'corrected' cause. Expected deaths were based on US rates. Other reports on this group of workers include those by Selikoff, Hammond and Seidman, 1973 and Selikoff and Hammond, 1975.

2.31.5 Shipyards

Prospective studies of men working in shipyards in Hawaii, UK, Italy, and the US are described. Then follow brief notes of (*a*) case reports of hazard from mesothelioma in France and the Netherlands, and (*b*) case-control studies of lung cancer in the US, which have included patients from shipyards.

Hawaii

All men employed in the naval shipyard in Hawaii in 1960 were identified, together with any recruited until 1969; all were followed until 1973. Men exposed to radiation, sandblasting, and rubber work were excluded. Other jobs were classified into those with likely or unlikely/minimal asbestos exposure; there had been little improvement in dust control

until the 1970s. Expected mortality was based on national rates, adjusting for race (Kolonel *et al.*, 1980).

England and Wales: 1

Workers in Devonport naval dockyard aged 15–36 in 1947 were followed until 1978. Expected deaths were based on national rates. Analyses of all-cause mortality were provided by trade. Though no information was given on the types of fibre, it was stated that exposure had been heaviest in the 1950s (Rossiter and Coles, 1980). A more limited study used cancer registrations in males for the Plymouth locality in 1960–69. Proportional analysis was carried out on those who had worked in the dockyard (Lumley, 1976).

Italy

Personnel records were used to identify men employed in the Genoa shipyard in 1960, who had retired but were alive at that time. Those who had retired or left the industry in the period 1960–75 were identified and deaths in the cohort identified. Expected deaths were based on mortality of either the male population of Genoa, or the male staff of a local hospital (Putoni *et al.*, 1979). The initial cohort was 2190; some analyses were carried out for 20 different occupational categories within the shipyard workers. Though there were important differences in the work of the different groups, many of these analyses were based on small numbers of events.

England and Wales: 2

Fletcher (1972) followed up male shipyard workers from Barrow, who had pleural plaques on routine X-ray in 1960–70; 16 developed cancer of the lung with 6.7 expected, whilst 3 mesotheliomas were also diagnosed. In a further study on these workers,

Table 2.11 Risk of ovarian cancer in various groups of female asbestos workers*

Occupation	Fibre	Country	Data years	No. subj.	O	E	O/E	Author
Manuf. mixed	*Cro*, Amo, Chr	England: 2	1936–75	595	3	0.7	4.29	Newhouse and Berry (1979)
Manuf. gas mask	*Cro*	England: 5	1951–77	500	5	2.8	1.79	Wignall and Fox (1982)
Manuf. frict. prod.	*Chr*, Cro	England: 6	1941–79	3708	8	8.1	0.99	Berry and Newhouse (1983)
Manuf. gas mask	*Chr*	England: 8	1951–80	570	5	3.4	1.47	Acheson *et al.* (1982)
Manuf. gas mask	*Cro*, Chr	England: 8	1951–80	757	12	4.4	2.73	Acheson *et al.* (1982)

*See text for description of method.

Edge (1979) identified 429 who had radiological evidence of pleural plaques in 1964–71. Follow-up mortality was compared with that in a matched sample of residents of Carlisle having had a normal X-ray. There appeared to be an excess risk of bronchial cancer; although a person-years analysis was performed, conventional expected values were not presented. The last year of follow-up was not stated.

US: 1

Selikoff, Lilis and Nicholson (1979) analysed the subset of 440 of their US insulation workers (*see* 2.31.4), who had exclusively worked in shipyards. These men were followed in the period 1967–76. Limited numbers only permitted examination of lung cancer and mesothelioma deaths; expected deaths were based on national rates.

France

Case reports have examined the risk of mesothelioma in shipyard workers. A clinical series of 70 patients with pleural mesothelioma treated in Nantes hospital in 1956–78 had occupational histories of asbestos exposure in 51. Of these, 44 had worked in the shipyards, with a range of trades—the minority of whom regularly handled asbestos, such as laggers (de Lajartre and de Lajartre, 1979).

Netherlands

There were 25 patients with mesothelioma diagnosed in the Walchren Islands in 1962–68, and a further 32 in 1969–78. All but 12 had been workers at the local shipyard, and 7 of the others had occupational exposure to asbestos elsewhere (Strumphius, 1979). (Though an estimate of the size of the workforce is given it is not possible to calculate an expected value.)

US: 2

Two case-control studies of the aetiology of lung cancer have specifically focused on the influence of work in shipyards. To explore the high lung cancer mortality in north-east Florida, a case-control study was carried out with 323 male patients with lung cancer and 434 controls. Increased risk was found for work with ship building, construction, and lumber/wood industries. There was no evidence of diagnostic reporting of migration factors influencing the mortality rates (Blot *et al.*, 1982).

US: 3

To follow-up the evidence of high lung cancer mortality in the south-east Atlantic coast of the US,

patients with lung cancer treated in 4 hospitals in 1970–76, or identified from death certificates, were matched with controls (excluding lung or bladder cancer, or chronic lung disease). Interviews were carried out with patients or next of kin, and results were available for 458 cases (89% of those initially identified). Those ever working in shipyards in the Second World War had RR = 1.6, 95% CL = 1.1–2.3, after adjustment for smoking and other occupations held. There was a multiplicative effect with smoking and it was suggested that asbestos was the relevant shipyard exposure (Blot *et al.*, 1978).

2.31.6 Other workers

Some of the studies on mesothelioma have indicated a wide range of occupations with potential exposure to asbestos. This is confirmed in the studies of shipyard workers, which indicate a hazard to many trades. An analogous example is a study of 'machinists' on a US railroad; these men were maintenance staff working on locomotives after laggers had removed and then replaced the insulation round the boilers. A cohort, alive in 1954 who had been employed for a number of years were followed until 1982; 47 (23.9%) could not be traced. Out of 132 deaths, 9 were from mesothelioma; observed but no expected figures were provided for other cancers (Mancuso, 1983). Case reports were also provided of 'machinists' in other industries who had developed mesothelioma.

3.31.7 Laryngeal cancer

The results on the risk of cancer of the larynx from prospective studies of various occupational groups have already been presented; unfortunately many of the reports have not separately distinguished this site of malignancy. In addition, a number of case-control studies have probed the association with asbestos exposure and these are described below. The results from 7 of these studies are given in *Table 2.13*.

In a case-control study of 100 male patients in Liverpool (Stell and McGill, 1973) a highly significant excess had been exposed to asbestos.

A matched-pairs analysis for 47 patients with laryngeal cancer treated in Washington State showed a non-significant increased risk from asbestos exposure (Hinds, Thomas and O'Reilly, 1979).

In a case-control study of lung cancer and cancer of the larynx in Virginia (Blot *et al.*, 1980), an increased risk was found for shipyard workers for lung but not laryngeal cancer.

A case-control study of male patients treated in London hospitals compared asbestos exposure in 83 patients with laryngeal neoplasms, 42 with cysts and polyps, 67 with inflammatory lesions, and 113 with

Table 2.12 Proportion of deaths from mesothelioma in various groups of asbestos workers*

Occupation	Fibre	Country	Data–years	Sex	No. subj.	No. mesothelioma			Author
						Pl.	Perit.	Percentage deaths	
Mining/ milling	Anth	Finland	1936–69	M/F	1041	0	0	0	Meurmann, Kiviluoto and Hakama (1974)
	Cro	Australia	1943–77	M	6200	17	0	3.2	Hobbs et al. (1980)
	Chr	Italy	1946–75	M	933	0	0	0	Rubino et al. (1979)
	Chr	Canada	1951–75	M	10939	10	0	0.2	McDonald et al. (1980)
	Chr	Canada	1951–75	F	440	1	0	1.2	McDonald et al. (1980)
	Chr	Canada	1961–77	M	544	1	0	0.6	Nicholson et al. (1979)
Manuf. gas masks	Cro	Canada: 1	1939–76	F	176	3	6	16.1	McDonald and McDonald (1978)
Manuf. cement	Chr, Cro	Canada: 2	1960–80	M	186	5	5	17.2	Finkelstein (1983)
Manuf. cement	Mixed	Denmark	1944–76	M	16089	3	0		Clemmensen and Hjalgrim-Jensen (1981)
Manuf. textiles	Chr, Cro	England: 1	1916–74	M	1085	9	0	3.1	Peto et al. (1977)
Manuf. textiles	Chr, Cro	England: 1	1934–74	F	284	1	0	4.2	Peto et al. (1977)
Manuf. mixed	Cro, Amo, Chr	England: 2	1933–75	M	3467	19	27	8.4	Newhouse and Berry (1979)
Manuf. mixed	Cro, Amo, Chr	England: 2	1936–75	F	922	12	6	9.0	Newhouse and Berry (1979)
Manuf. cement	Chr, Cro	England: 3	1936–77	M	1592	2	0	0.6	Thomas, H.F. et al. (1982)
Manuf. gas masks	Cro, Chr	England: 4	1940–78	F	578	17	12	17.5	Jones et al. (1980)
Manuf. gas masks	Cro	England: 5	1951–77	F	500	12	1	9.8	Wignall and Fox (1982)
Manuf. frict. prod.	Chr, Cro	England: 6	1941–79	M	7474	8	0	0.6	Berry and Newhouse (1983)
Manuf. frict. prod.	Chr, Cro	England: 6	1941–79	F	3708	2	0	0.7	Berry and Newhouse (1983)
Manuf. insul. prod.	Amo, Chr	England: 7	1947–78	M	4882	4	1	4.6	Acheson et al. (1981)
Manuf. gas masks	Chr	England: 8	1951–80	F	570	1	0	0.6	Acheson et al. (1982)
Manuf. gas masks	Cro	England: 8	1951–80	F	757	3	2	2.3	Acheson et al. (1982)
Manuf. mixed	Chr, Amo, Cro	US: 1	1940–75	M	2666	13		1.4	Robinson et al. (1979)
Manuf. mixed	Chr, Amo, Cro	US: 1	1940–75	F	537	4		3.1	Robinson et al. (1979)
Manuf. mixed	Mixed	US: 2	1941–73	M	1075	4		0.5	Henderson and Enterline (1979)
Manuf. textile	Chr	US: 6a	1959–77	M	2543	0	1	0.2	McDonald et al. (1983a)
Manuf. mixed	Chr, Amo, Cro	US: 6b	1959–77	M	4137	10	4	1.6	McDonald et al. (1983b)
Manuf. frict. prod.	Chr	US: 6c	1959–77	M	3641	0	0	0	McDonald et al. (1984)
Manuf. insul. prod.	Amo	US: 7	1961–77	M	582	7	7	4.6	Selikoff, Seidman and Hammond (1980)

Table 2.12 Continued

Occupation	Fibre	Country	Data–years	Sex	No. subj.	No. mesothelioma			Author
						Pl.	Perit.	Percentage deaths	
Insulators	Mixed	England	1931–75	M	1368	4	5	10.8	Newhouse and Berry (1979)
	Mixed	N. Ireland	1940–75	M	162	11	5	13.1	Elmes and Simpson (1977)
	Chr, Amo	US	1943–76	M	632	11	27	7.9	Selikoff, Hammond and Seidman (1979)
	Chr, Amo	US	1943–76	M	833	2	1	4.8	Selikoff, Hammond and Seidman (1979)
	?	US	1945–65	M	152	1	2	6.5	Klienfeld *et al.* (1967)
	Chr, Amo	US/Canada	1967–76	M	17800	104		4.6	Selikoff, Hammond and Seidman (1979)
Shipyard wks	Mixed	England	1947–78	M	6076	29	2	3.0	Rossiter and Coles (1980)
	Mixed	Hawaii	1950–73	M	4779	0	0	0	Kolonel *et al.* (1980)
	?	England	1964–?	M	429	23		18.1	Edge (1979)
(Insulators)	?	US	1967–76	M	440	3	5	10.1	Selikoff, Hammond and Seidman (1979)
Railway wks	?	US	1954–82	M	150	9	0	6.8	Mancuso (1983)

*See text for description of method.

Table 2.13 Results of 7 case-control studies of laryngeal cancer showing relative risks for asbestos exposure*

Author	Country	n†	RR	95% CL
Stell and McGill (1973)	England and Wales	100	14.5	5.2–40.9
Hinds, Thomas and O'Reilly (1979)	US	47	1.7	0.7–4.1
Blot *et al.* (1980)	US	63	0.9	0.1–7.1
Newhouse, Gregory and Shannon (1980)	England and Wales	83	0.4	0.2–1.2
Shettigara and Morgan (1975)	Canada	43	∞	n.a.
Burch *et al.* (1981)	Canada	204	1.4	0.8–2.4
Olsen and Sabroe (1984)	Denmark	326	1.8	1.0–3.4

*See text for description of method.
†Number of patients with laryngeal cancer in each study.
n.a. = cannot be calculated.

no disease on endoscopy (Newhouse, Gregory and Shannon, 1980). There was no evidence of excess risk from asbestos—a smaller proportion with cancer reported exposure either <15 years or >15 years prior to diagnosis.

A case-control study of 43 males and matched controls treated in Toronto in 1974 obtained information by trained interviewers, mostly visiting the patients in their own homes (Shettigara and Morgan, 1975). A more extensive study was then carried out on 204 patients diagnosed in 1977–79 and drawn from Ontario. Controls were individually matched with neighbourhood controls (Burch *et al.*, 1981).

Data were collected from patients diagnosed with laryngeal cancer in Denmark in 1980–82 and population controls matched on age and locality of residence (Olsen and Sabroe, 1984). In males, there was a significantly increased risk for exposure to asbestos.

As can be seen from the results of these 7 studies shown in *Table 2.13*, the first reported study showed a high and significant relative risk. Though the RR was over 1.0 for 3 of the other studies, it is only of borderline significance in one of these. This pattern of results suggests that the initial excess noted in Liverpool may have been an extreme finding, whilst the others approximate to the actual risk for this site of malignancy.

2.31.8 Lymphoma

Though this site has not usually been identified in the prospective studies of occupational groups, 2 case-control studies are relevant. A study of 28 men with lymphoma of the alimentary tract treated in Los Angeles in 1977–81 showed 12 had asbestos exposure at work compared with one control: RR = 12; 95% CL = 2.4–59.2 (Ross *et al.*, 1982).

Olsson and Brandt (1983), in a case-control study of 169 men in southern Sweden with non-Hodgkin's lymphoma, found no evidence to support the suggestion that asbestos exposure was a risk factor.

2.31.9 Mesothelioma

The background to the recognition of the hazard for mesothelioma from asbestos exposure is briefly described and then various case reports and case-control studies. The contribution from examination of the geographical distribution of mesothelioma deaths is then mentioned. The section ends with 2 important aspects of the problem of (*a*) assessment of the different fibres' risks, and (*b*) the use of models to quantify the extent of the hazard.

2.31.9.1 Background

Isolated case reports had noted the occurrence of mesothelioma in subjects with asbestosis (Weiss, 1953; Leicher, 1954). In the period 1956–59, a series of pleural tumours were referred for treatment from the North Western Cape Province in South Africa. Investigations showed that all but one of the 33 patients with histologically proven pleural mesothelioma had exposure to crocidolite asbestos (Wagner, Sleggs and Marchand, 1960). The authors emphasized that this tumour was very rarely seen elsewhere in South Africa. This was followed by a case report from Western Australia of a patient with mesothelioma having prior exposure to crocidolite (McNulty, 1962).

Investigation of a series of patients having coroners' autopsies in East London for asbestosis showed that 10 had primary mesothelioma of the peritoneum, with the same diagnosis being made in another patient with asbestosis in the period 1958–63. All had worked at the same asbestos factory and 52 autopsies had been carried out in this period on the patients. Histologically the lesions were difficult to define and Enticknap and Smither (1964) suggested they be called 'peritoneal tumours of asbestosis'.

2.31.9.2 Further studies on mesothelioma

Selikoff, Churg and Hammond (1965) contrasted the high proportional deaths from mesothelioma in insulation workers (3.3%) compared with the extreme rarity amongst the deaths in over a million subjects in the American Cancer Society prospective study (0.009% of all deaths).

In 55 patients with histologically confirmed asbestosis in Pennsylvania, 5 (9%) had mesothelioma (O'Donnell, Mann and Grosh, 1966). As the majority of the diagnoses of asbestosis were made at autopsy, it is not a suitable sample to assess the proportion who developed mesothelioma.

As part of the survey of the health of workers at Plymouth dockyard, Sheers and Templeton (1968) reported that 10 patients had been diagnosed with pleural mesothelioma in the previous 3 years. This was extended by Lumley (1976) who compared cancer registrations for dockyard workers in 1960–69 with those occurring in the male population in the locality.

On review of 32 cases of mesothelioma in Victoria, Australia there was evidence of exposure to crocidolite alone in 5, but the majority had mixed fibre exposure (Milne, 1976a).

Decoufle (1980) reported 3 deaths from mesothelioma in 3806 persons employed in the shoe industry, which he suggested might be due to asbestos used as a filler in rubber soles and heels.

A recent case-control study of 480 patients dying from malignant mesothelioma investigated occupational histories (the sample represented about 80% of the patients dying in Canada from this condition in 1960–75 and in the US in 1972). Asbestos exposure was found in 50% of males, but only 5% of females; the risk was greatest for insulation workers (RR = 46.0), but was also high for manufacture of asbestos products (RR = 6.1), and in the heating trade (RR = 4.4). There was no evidence of an increased risk in those exposed at work to man-made mineral fibres, living near zeolite deposits or from smoking (McDonald and McDonald, 1980).

Langer and McCaughey (1982) provided a report of a 55-year-old patient with mesothelioma who had worked on car repairs since the age of 19, including the replacement of brake linings. This was the sole known exposure to chrysotile.

Mancuso (1983) followed 197 machinists in the railroad industry for 1935–82. Out of 132 deaths, there were 9 from mesothelioma and 1 from endothelioma of the pleura.

Investigation of all cases of mesothelioma in the Connecticut cancer register in 1955–77 indicated a relative risk of 2.25 for carpenters, 3.87 for plumbers and pipefitters, and 5.08 for those ever employed in the rubber industry. For all 201 cases of mesothelioma occupational exposure to asbestos was indicated in 85% (Teta *et al.*, 1983).

Review of job histories for 321 mesothelioma patients diagnosed in 1972–79 in Los Angeles suggested that 42% had been exposed to asbestos (Wright *et al.*, 1984).

2.31.9.3 Geographical distribution of mesothelioma

An early clue came from a report of excess pleural malignancies in seaside towns in Denmark and

Germany compared with inland urban areas (Glatzel, 1943). A number of authors have subsequently used maps (Greenberg and Lloyd Davies, 1974; Whitwell, Scott and Grimshaw, 1977). The latter authors related the environmental sources of asbestos in Merseyside to the localities of deaths from mesothelioma subdivided according to the lung fibre counts of asbestos fibres.

As part of an analysis of mortality by area in England and Wales, Gardner, Winter and Acheson (1982) identified local authorities with raised mortality from mesothelioma in 1968–78. In men, the high mortality areas are mainly concentrated in ports with ship building, whilst women showed high rates where gas masks had been made. Both showed high mortality in the east of London, where various asbestos factories were located. They conclude that most, if not all, the localities identified as having raised mortality were known to have major use of asbestos.

The neighbourhood risk of mesothelioma has been studied by a number of authors—*see* 2.31.11.

2.31.9.4 Models

Using accumulated data on mesothelioma deaths amongst male and female workers followed from the 1930s from an East London textile factory, Newhouse and Berry (1976) predicted there would be ultimately 7–11% overall mortality from mesothelioma in males and perhaps a higher proportion in females. *Table 2.14* shows the death rates in the UK in 1968–73. These are based on the data obtained from the register of mesothelioma patients assembled by the Health and Safety Executive (HSE).

Peto, Seidman and Selikoff (1982) estimated that the incidence of mesothelioma was related to the third power of the interval since exposure first began. They suggested that the hazard could be ordered: North American insulators > New Jersey amosite workers in a factory > Barking factory handling amphiboles.

2.31.10 Type of fibre

It is important to consider whether one type of fibre is more hazardous than another. However, many of the groups of workers studied have had mixed exposure; the dose and duration may be important confounding factors, but poorly documented; variation of age at first exposure and length of follow-up also affect the results obtained in individual studies. *Tables 2.8–2.12* indicate the specific fibre involved in different studies, where this is recorded.

In a review of the topic, Gloag (1981a) accepted that there was a gradient in risk for both lung cancer and mesothelioma from low risk in those exposed to chrysotile, through amosite, to high risk from crocidolite. The data were not inconsistent with a linear dose–response relationship, with risks of both cancers being roughly proportional to the 'dose of fibres'. Gloag (1981b) also pointed out that crocidolite differed in structure between that obtained in the Cape and Transvaal mines, and this was associated with variation in risk of mesothelioma. Various sources of other hazardous fibres causing mesothelioma have been reported: mineral deposits in rural Turkey, zeolite used for building, and material containing tremolite with very little chrysotile which is used for stucco and whitewash.

McCullagh (1980) challenged the view that amosite was more hazardous than chrysotile. He suggested that the Advisory Committee on Asbestos had placed too great a reliance on the study of the Paterson, New Jersey workers employed in 1941–45 (*see* US: 7). McCullagh considered that: (*a*) the relative risk had been inflated about 15% by reviewing the cause of death, and (*b*) previous exposure to other forms of asbestos in jobs earlier had been grossly underestimated. However, Acheson and Gardner (1983) considered amosite was probably more dangerous than crocidolite. Using data on fibre counts in lung tissue from patients with mesothelioma and controls, Acheson and Gardner (1979) suggested that there was synergism between chrysotile and amphiboles. However, using further data derived from a refined technique for assessing fibre counts in lungs of 86 mesothelioma cases and 56 controls, Acheson and Gardner (1980) found no evidence for such synergism.

Acheson *et al.* (1981) reported 5 deaths from mesothelioma in 5871 men who had worked in a London factory which had manufactured insulation board from 1947 to 1978, using amosite predomi-

Table 2.14 Mesothelioma death rates per million persons by age, 1968–83, UK

Year	Age groups						
	0–24	25–34	35–44	45–54	55–64	65–74	75–84
1968–70	0.05	0.28	1.82	4.55	11.3	10.9	7.58
1971–75	0.03	0.49	1.44	6.55	13.5	16.6	10.5
1976–80	0.04	0.37	2.69	10.5	21.1	28.8	23.2
1981–83	0.06	0.24	3.64	10.8	28.3	33.7	31.0

Source: Deaths from HSE register (*see* text).

nantly, and as the only fibre since 1973. (Less than 3% of chrysotile had been used from 1947 to 1973, with crocidolite used only on an experimental basis for 5 days.)

To explore the possible effect of different fibres, Wagner, Berry and Pooley (1982) examined the lungs of men who had died of mesothelioma and a matched set dying of other causes. The lungs of those with mesothelioma did not differ in their content of either chrysotile or crocidolite from that of the controls; it was not possible to implicate a particular fibre from this study.

The reported fibre exposure for 38 studies is shown in *Table 2.12*. Though chrysotile is identified as the only or major exposure in half of these, the relative risk cannot be distinguished by fibre without detail on levels of exposure.

2.31.11 Household and neighbourhood risks

There have been many studies which have considered the extent to which members of a household where there is an asbestos worker, or residents in the vicinity of plants, are exposed to risk. The first definitive report on the hazard of mesothelioma in miners noted that some patients had only environmental exposure (Wagner, Sleggs and Marchand, 1960). In a review, Anderson *et al.* (1976) listed 17 studies which have reported excess mesothelioma risk to household members. Some of these are briefly discussed below.

Full occupational and residential histories were obtained for 76 patients treated at the London hospital for proven mesothelioma in the period 1917–64 (Newhouse and Thompson, 1965). Forty patients either had occupational (41% of total) or domestic (12% of total) exposure, whilst there was evidence of a neighbourhood effect in 11 (14%). This left only 25 of the original 76 for whom no source of asbestos was found (33%).

Lieben and Pistawka (1967) investigated 42 patients in Pennsylvania, diagnosed in 152 hospitals in 1958–63. Where necessary, employers were questioned. They found that: 10 worked in asbestos plants, 3 had family members in such plants, there was possible exposure in another 10, but no evidence of exposure in 11.

Bohlig *et al.* (1970) reported a striking concentration of mesothelioma patients in one part of Hamburg, near a large asbestos processing factory. Following review of the histories of the subjects, attention was drawn to the family hazard of the subjects from dusty clothes brought home, and also the risk from dismantling old insulations.

Investigation of 52 females developing mesothelioma and matched controls in New York in 1967–77 showed that 10 patients had indirect exposure through their husbands' and/or fathers' occupations,

but only 1 of the controls (Vianna and Polan, 1978). In addition, 3 cases lived within 3.6 km of asbestos factories, whilst there were no controls within 8 km.

In a follow-up of over 3000 household contacts of men exposed to amosite, 5 deaths from pleural mesothelioma were identified in about 510 deaths (Anderson *et al.*, 1979). These results are an extension of Anderson *et al.* (1976); the statistics are not presented in a clear fashion for ready interpretation.

The *British Medical Journal* (1978) concluded that 'the community at large seems most unlikely to be exposed to a perceptible risk'.

A related issue to household risk, is whether there is genetic predisposition to response to asbestos exposure. Evans, Lewinsohn and Evans (1977) reported that there was an excess of asbestos workers with advanced pulmonary fibrosis who had excess of a particular histocompatibility antigen (HLA-B12), but not HLA-B27 as reported by others. Burrell (1974) concluded that the immunological evidence at that time was scanty and unimpressive in relation to asbestos. He quoted some unpublished laboratory evidence suggesting immunological specificity for mesothelioma. There was a higher proportion of HLA-B27 in 92 subjects with asbestosis in comparison with (*a*) control workers exposed to asbestos without respiratory disease, and (*b*) blood donors (Turner Warwick, 1977).

In their study of women with mesothelioma, Vianna and Polan (1978) noted a significant excess of cancer reported in parents; they suggested this might be from genetic predisposition.

A family of 2 parents and 12 children in whom 5 members developed mesothelioma was reported from Sweden. There appeared to be direct occupational exposure in 4 of the 5 members. Though Risberg, Nickels and Wagermark (1980) suggested that a genetic risk factor may have played a part, there seems no need to invoke this on the basis of such data.

Liddell and Miller (1983) emphasized the importance of assessing whether there is appreciable variation in individual susceptibility to carcinogens. Discussing asbestos hazard, they advocated that cases of lung cancer with assessed asbestos exposure should be compared with controls of equal degrees of exposure, to determine what other factors were associated with development of the cancer.

2.31.12 Smoking and asbestos exposure

Selikoff, Hammond and Churg (1968) emphasized how important it was to determine the combined effect of asbestos exposure and smoking upon risk of lung cancer. In an analytical study, they obtained details of smoking habits of the New York insulators under follow-up. Deaths were available in the period 1963–67 for 370 men who had worked for at least 20 years. Amongst 87 non-smokers, none died of lung cancer; amongst 283 regular smokers 24 had died, when only 3 were expected from their level of smoking. This led the authors to suggest that asbestos workers who smoked should stop.

Smoking histories were obtained for the 180 male and 98 female deaths in 1960–70 amongst workers from the Barking asbestos factory. On balance the results for the males were not sufficiently clearcut to distinguish additive from multiplicative effects, but the women showed evidence of a multiplicative increase in risk for smokers who had been heavily exposed to asbestos (Berry, Newhouse and Turok, 1972).

Meurman, Kiviluoto and Hakama (1979) presented data on lung cancer and smoking habits of Finnish anthophyllite miners. The data could not distinguish a multiplicative effect from an additive effect of asbestos.

Utilizing results from the study of 17 800 US and Canadian insulators followed in 1967–76, Hammond, Selikoff and Seidman (1979) concluded that there was a very strong synergistic effect between asbestos exposure and smoking, in respect of lung cancer.

A further study of 933 men manufacturing amosite asbestos products followed from 1941 to 1977 suggested that smoking and asbestos exposure increased the risk of lung cancer 80-fold (Selikoff, Seidman and Hammond, 1980).

In the study of Canadian miners and millers (McDonald *et al.*, 1980) there was a clear linear dose–response to asbestos exposure, but there was insufficient material to distinguish an additive from a multiplicative effect with smoking.

A case-control study of 200 men with lung cancer suggested that 58 had some occupational exposure to asbestos compared to 29 controls. Martischnig *et al.* (1977) emphasized the additional risk from smoking and the number of occupations to which incidental exposure to asbestos occurred.

In a method paper, Berry (1980) found a better fit for an additive model of asbestos plus smoking, but limitation in the data may have concealed a multiplicative effect.

In discussing interaction with smoking, Acheson and Gardner (1983) point out that the weight of evidence supports a 'smaller than multiplicative interactive term'. This would increase the slope of the dose–response curve, which would also be shifted upwards if the workers smoked more than the comparison population.

McMillan, Pethybridge and Sheers (1980) noted that smoking also influenced the prevalence of other lung pathology independently of the degree of asbestos exposure, whilst Saracci (1981) suggested that over 90% of the excess of lung cancer could be prevented if exposed workers did not smoke.

2.31.13 Conclusions

There is no argument that exposure to asbestos in the past had led to increase in deaths from lung cancer and mesothelioma in various groups of exposed workers. *Tables 2.8, 2.9* and *2.11* also indicate an excess of gastrointestinal, larynx and ovarian cancer. Enterline (1976a) noted the variation in risk of lung cancer ranged from 1.2 to 9.2 in 11 studies. In 6 of these he attempted to correct for (*a*) inclusion of those only recently exposed, (*b*) use of an inappropriate population to calculate expected deaths, (*c*) adjustment of cause of death in the study deaths, not in the 'expected' deaths. This removed much of the variation in the results, even though there may have been appreciable differences in the level and duration of exposure.

The important issues of the variation in the hazard for different fibres, and the influence of smoking have already been discussed. A related issue is the assessment of the dose–response curve. Using data for Canadian miners and millers, McDonald *et al.* (1980) indicated a fairly steady increase in risk of lung cancer with increase in asbestos exposure:

Dose	O	E	O/E
30	91	97.6	0.93
30–	43	36.7	1.17
100–	38	31.8	1.19
300–	29	16.6	1.75
600+	41	14.6	2.81

where dose is 10^6 particles/foot^3 per year, for exposure over 20 years since start of work.

In addition to the Canadian miners and millers, a linear relationship appears to hold for factory workers in the UK and US, and the insulators in the US. Acheson and Gardner (1983) concluded that the range in estimated slopes of dose–response curves had widened in recent years. This varied from a steep slope in textile manufacture in North Carolina, to a questionable effect in a cohort manufacturing brake linings. The evidence pointed to a linear relationship.

It is usually considered that the fibres exert a direct physical effect at the site of the body they reach. However, Goldsmith (1982) reviewed 11 studies and examined the excess cancers for (*a*) the gastrointestinal tract, (*b*) other non-pulmonary sites, (*c*) all non-pulmonary sites. He suggested there was a generalized increase in cancers and that this was due to a systemic effect of asbestos rather than a site-specific effect. This was compatible with an effect on 'cancer defense mechanisms'.

An important issue is the extent to which the 'removal' of individuals from exposure is followed by reduction in relative risk. Walker (1984) reviewed published data and emphasized that long-term follow-up of workers showed a decline in risk of lung cancer following cessation of exposure to asbestos. He suggested that the relative risk began to decline 'sometime after exposure to asbestos'. This was not as marked as the effect of giving up smoking, and was not clearly due to the removal of high risk subjects through death.

Nicholson, Perkel and Selikoff (1982) attempted to quantify the number of workers exposed to asbestos in the US in 1940–79. Bearing in mind the latent interval, they estimated that the annual deaths from cancer due to this exposure would rise to the year 2000, and only decrease after that time.

In 1966 a central register of mesothelioma deaths was established for England and Wales. Information was collated from: death registration; cancer registration; claims for benefit from mesothelioma handled by the Pneumoconiosis Medical Panels; informal registration by clinicians, pathologists, and coroners. The material for 1967–68 was reviewed and it was suggested that there was considerable under-reporting (Greenberg and Lloyd Davies, 1974). *Table 2.14* shows the latest available rates for England and Wales; as yet there is still evidence of increasing rates, especially at the older age groups.

IARC (1977a) concluded that it was not possible to assess whether there is a level of exposure in humans below which an increased risk of cancer would not occur.

2.32 Fibre (2): man-made mineral fibres

Because of some of the physical similarities of asbestos fibres to those that are man made, concern has been expressed about the potential hazard to health from production and use of such material. The following notes cover the historical prospective studies on various groups of workers; results are given in *Table 2.15*.

Canada: 1

A glass wool plant in Ontario, Canada opened in 1948 and used steam blowing until changing to centrifugal formed fibres in 1961. All 2576 men working at least 90 days from 1955 onwards were studied; 97.2% were traced until 1977. Expected deaths were based on Ontario mortality rates (Shannon *et al.*, 1984).

Canada: 2

As part of a study of asbestos-cement workers, Finkelstein (1983) followed 87 men who were employed on rock wool or glass fibre production, with no or minimal exposure to asbestos. The men had been hired prior to 1960 and worked a minimum of 9 years; 94.3% were traced to 1980. Mortality was compared with that in Ontario males.

Denmark

All 5543 workers employed in the Danish mineral wool industry were matched against the national cancer registry for 1944–79 (Olsen and Jensen, 1983). Expected figures were based on national incidence (with and without correction for locality of residence). The data for those first employed more than 20 years before, indicated a non-significant excess of bladder cancer: O = 4, E = 1.6, O/E = 2.5; 95% CL = 0.7–6.4; skin cancer: O = 5, E = 2.4, O/E = 2.1, 95% CL = 0.7–4.9.

Table 2.15 Lung cancer mortality in studies of man-made mineral fibre workers*

Exposure	Country	Data–years	Sex	No. subj.	O	E	O/E	Author
Glass wool	Canada: 1	1955–77	M	2576	7	4.7	1.66	Shannon *et al.* (1984)
Rockwool/glass fibre	Canada: 2	1960–80	M	87	1	1.1	0.91	Finkelstein (1983)
Mineral wool	Denmark	1947–79	M	5543	9	4.3	2.09	Olsen and Jensen (1983)
Various	Europe	1976–81	M	25000	17	8.9	1.92	IARC (1983)
Fibrous glass	US: 1	1940–72	M	1448	16	20.2	0.79	Bayliss *et al.* (1976)
Rockwool	US: 2	1940–74	M	596	9	10.1	0.89	Robinson *et al.* (1982)
Mineral wool	US: 3	1945–77	M	1846	45	28.1	1.60	Enterline, Marsh and Esmen (1983)
Fibrous glass	US: 3	1945–77	M	14884	202	203.4	0.99	Enterline, Marsh and Esmen (1983)
Fibrous glass	US: 4	1968–77	M	6536	39	38.6	1.01	Morgan, Kaplan and Bratsberg (1981)
Totals					345	319.4	1.08	
95% CL							1.0–1.2	

*See text for description of method.

Europe

The annual report for IARC (1983b) described a study of 13 factories in 7 countries, involving follow-up of 25 000 men for an average of 5 years. National mortality rates were used to calculate expected deaths. Though there was a significant excess of lung cancer in those who had worked more than 30 years, there was no clear specificity for different types of fibre. No information was available on smoking of the men.

US: 1

Men who had worked in a major fibrous glass plant in the US for at least 5 years in 1940–49 were followed until 1972. All 1448 were traced and deaths were compared with expected, based on national rates. The men had been employed in fibrous glass production, packing, or maintenance work (Bayliss *et al.*, 1976).

US: 2

A mid-western US plant producing rockwool had been in operation since 1907, switching to blast furnace slag as raw material in the 1930s from limestone. A newer spinning process producing more uniform fibre size was introduced in the 1940s. Seven hundred and two white men employed for at least a year in the period 1940–48 were followed until 1974; 5% were lost to follow-up. Expected mortality was based on national rates (Ness *et al.*, 1979). Exactly the same criteria for entry to the study was used by Robinson *et al.* (1982), but they only include 596 workers who were again followed until 1974. Over 98% were traced. No explanation was given by Robinson, who does not even mention this duplication of publication.

US: 3

Fibrous glass and mineral wool workers employed prior to 1964 were identified at 17 plants in the US. The plants had opened in the period 1929–51, using a variety of raw materials and methods to produce glass fibre and mineral wool. Asbestos may have been used for some products in the mineral wool plants, but details of this were not available. All 16 730 men studied had had at least 1 year's exposure in the period 1945–63, except for those from 2 plants where this was 6 months; 98.0% were traced until 1977 (Enterline, Marsh and Esmen, 1983). Expected deaths were based on national mortality rates. There was no evidence of a dose–response in risk of cancer. Preliminary results were published by Enterline and Marsh (1980b).

US: 4

All males who had been employed at a plant for fibrous glass production in the US in 1968–77, who had worked for at least 10 years were followed to 1977; 98.1% were traced. Observed mortality was compared with expected based on national rates (Morgan, Kaplan and Bratsberg, 1981).

2.32.1 Conclusion

Milne (1976b) felt that the evidence pointed away from fibre glass being a substance with long-term hazards to workers. Hill (1977; 1978) reviewed available information and concluded that there was not evidence (at that time) of an increased risk to exposed workers. However, he pointed out the need for further epidemiological studies. A number of studies have been published since these comments; the results are in *Table 2.15* and show an increase in lung cancer of borderline significance.

2.33 Fibre (3): talc

There has been longstanding concern that exposure to talc dust might pose a health hazard. In a study of rubber workers using talc, Hogue and Mallette (1949) found no evidence that long exposure to the dust produced pathological changes in the lung. Subsequently, there was evidence of pneumoconiosis in exposed workers (*see* for example Klienfeld *et al.*, 1963). Twenty years later this was still an unresolved issue; Wegman *et al.* (1982) investigated a small group of workers exposed to asbestos/silica-free talc. They found loss of pulmonary function greater than could be accounted for by smoking. It was emphasized that longer follow-up was required to see if present dust levels are safe. However, there is difficulty in interpreting many of the earlier studies; Hildick-Smith (1976) emphasized that talc could be the label for very different dusts, with varying particle size and contaminated with many other minerals.

The following notes cover the main epidemiological studies of exposed workers, with key results being given in *Table 2.16*.

England and Wales

Preliminary results of follow-up of over 2000 workers at a factory in England making and packing cosmetic talc did not identify any health hazard. It was emphasized that further follow-up was required (Newhouse, Miller and Moore, 1976).

Italy

Rubino *et al.* (1976) studied miners and millers from
the Piedmont locality in Italy; the work involved
handling a pure type of talc compared with the
mixed exposure in New York workers. They
followed all workers employed for a minimum of 1
year and entering in the period 1921–50 until 1974;
about 90% were traced. Control subjects were
matched on age and drawn from the same social and
economic categories. In both miners and millers
they found a deficiency of lung cancer. Because of
the doubts about the comparison with an agricultural population, expected mortality for the period
1946–74 was recalculated using national rates
(Rubino *et al.*, 1979c). Again, the hazard from
pneumoconiosis was evident, but not a risk of lung
cancer in either miners or millers.

US: 1

The records of all (220) talc miners and millers in
northern New York State who had reached a total of
15 years exposure in the period 1940–65 were
obtained; the 91 deaths occurring amongst these
men were subjected to a proportional-mortality
analysis (Klienfeld *et al.*, 1967). All men dying from
lung cancer had worked before the introduction of
wet drilling (i.e. when dust exposure was high, with
talc mixed with other silicates such as serpentine and
tremolite). The follow-up was extended to 1969
(Klienfeld, Messite and Zaki, 1974). Two hundred
and sixty men had reached 15 years exposure and
108 deaths had occurred; again national rates were
used in a proportional-mortality analysis. The excess
of lung cancer remained. It is not clear why a

proportional analysis was used, rather than a
conventional person-years calculation.

US: 2

Annual X-rays of workers in dusty jobs began in
Vermont, New York in 1937. These records were
used to identify men who had worked for at least 1
year in the talc mining and milling industry in the
period 1940–69. Of 392 men, all but 4 (99%) were
followed until 1975. Observed mortality was contrasted with expected based on US rates, except for
respiratory causes for which state rates were used
(Selevan *et al.*, 1979a). The talc was free of asbestos
and significant quantities of free silica. Limited data
were presented on dust levels. Exactly the same
results are provided by Selevan *et al.* (1979b); no
cross-reference to this double publication is given.

US: 3

A talc mine and mill opened in Upper New York
State in 1947. All (398) white males employed in
1947–59 were identified; 96% were traced to
mid-1975. Observed mortality was compared with
expected based on national rates (Brown, Dement
and Wagoner, 1979). There was evidence of an
increase in risk of lung cancer with longer follow-up
from date of initial involvement.

US: 4

Stille and Tabershaw (1982) contrasted the causes of
death in 655 white male talc workers employed in
the period 1948–77 in New York State with
expected figures based on national mortality rates.

Table 2.16 Lung cancer in studies of talc workers*

Occupation	Country	Data–years	Sex	No. subj.	O	E	O/E	Author
Miners and millers	Italy	1946–74	M	1346	8	17.2	0.4	Rubino *et al.* (1979)
Millers	Italy	1946–74	M	438	4	6.1	0.7	Rubino *et al.* (1979)
Miners and millers	US: 1	1940–69	M	260	13	4.0	3.2	Klienfeld, Messite and Zaki (1974)
Miners	US: 2	1940–75	M	163	5†	1.1	4.5	Selevan *et al.* (1979a)
Millers	US: 2	1940–75	M	225	2†	2.0	1.0	Selevan *et al.* (1979a)
Miners and millers	US: 3	1947–75	M	382	9	3.3	2.7	Brown, Dement and Wagoner (1979)
Talc processing	US: 4	1948–72	M	655	10	6.4	1.6	Stille and Tabershaw (1982)
Talc mining and processing	USSR	1949–75	M	?	?	?	4.5‡	Katsnelson and Mokronosova (1979)
Talc mining and processing	USSR	1949–75	F	?	?	?	9.3‡	Katsnelson and Mokronosova (1979)
Total					51	40.1	1.27	
95% CL							0.9–1.7	

*See text for description of method.
†ICD 160–166.
‡RR, without basic data in publication.

There was an excess of lung cancer deaths which occurred predominantly in those who had had other jobs before working with talc.

US: 5

About 17 000 employees in 2 rubber companies in the US were identified from records as occupied or retired in 1964; 98% were traced to 1973. An excess of stomach cancer was observed (Blum *et al.*, 1979). A case-control study of 100 stomach cancer subjects and 4 matched controls used detailed occupational records. The jobs were classified into about 100 job titles; hygienists assessed the potential exposure to talc. In one company there was an increased risk of stomach cancer with high or medium exposure; it was not known if the talc had contained asbestos.

USSR

Katsnelson and Mokronosova (1979) used death records to identify workers from (*a*) 2 plants producing alumosilicate fire bricks, (*b*) a plant producing silica fire bricks, (*c*) a gold mine, and (*d*) a company mining, grinding, and processing talc. Deaths were identified from a variety of sources. Estimated populations at risk were obtained for the talc workers for the period 1940–75; data were also available on the local populations and their mortality. Death rates of those exposed to dusts were compared with age-standardized rates for the populations. The report only provides the RR based on these comparisons, and not the numbers of deaths.

2.33.1 Conclusions

Hildick-Smith (1976) reviewed animal and epidemiological data and concluded that exposure in modern mining of cosmetic grade talc did not appear to be a hazardous job. The *Lancet* (1977), although also concentrating on cosmetic talc, did not identify clear evidence of occupational hazards to miners or millers.

2.34 Fibre (4): other

The following notes indicate the recent epidemiological studies on some miscellaneous fibres.

Cane sugar farming

There is a high toll of lung cancer in southern Louisiana; Rothschild and Molvey (1982) studied 284 cases and controls matched on year of birth, sex, race, parish, and year of death. They identified an increased risk from sugar cane farming. After

adjustment for smoking this was 2.4 (95% CL = 1.7–3.6).

Beet sugar refining

Malker, Malker and Blot (1983) reported 4 male workers in a beet sugar refining plant developing mesothelioma. However, some asbestos exposure may have occurred from the machinery used.

Steinbeck *et al.* (1983) confirmed the excess of mesothelioma in sugar beet refinery workers in Sweden (O = 7, E = 0.62, O/E = 11.3, 95% CL = 4.5–23.2). However, they emphasize that this occurred in 'permanent' workers who were responsible for dismantling and servicing the equipment out-of-season, with known exposure to asbestos. Nearly half the workforce was only involved in processing and packing the product and no case of mesothelioma occurred in this group unexposed to asbestos.

Taconite mining

Follow-up of 5751 men who had worked for at least a year mining taconite in the period 1952–75 showed no increase in overall mortality from malignant disease, nor increase in those who had worked at least 15 years before the end of the period (Higgins *et al.*, 1983).

2.34.1 Conclusion

The above reports are inadequate to evaluate the possible cancer hazard from these fibres.

2.35 Fluorescent lighting

Though it has been suggested that outdoor work is associated with increased risk of melanoma (Klepp and Magnus, 1979), a number of studies have reported an excess risk for office workers, e.g. in the US (Williams, Stegens and Goldsmith, 1977), and Australia (Holman *et al.*, 1980). Using the occupation recorded for patients registered with melanoma and 19% of those with other skin cancers in England and Wales for 1970–75, Beral and Robinson (1981) noted that (*a*) office work was associated with a large excess of melanoma of the trunk and limbs, whilst (*b*) outdoor work was associated with an excess of melanoma of the head, face, and neck.

A case-control study of 274 women aged 18–54 with melanoma in Australia suggested that exposure to fluorescent light was higher in those who worked in offices (RR = 2.6) and elsewhere indoors (RR = 1.8). These findings could not be explained by differences in skin and hair colour, or sunlight exposure (Beral *et al.*, 1982). Carlton-Foss (1982) emphasized the preliminary nature of the results and the inverse relationship with proximity to lighting. Examination of the ultraviolet (UV) radiation from fluorescent tubes suggested that short-wavelength ultraviolet B around 290 nm was present, whereas that from sunlight is filtered out by the atmospheric ozone. In contrast, the amount of radiation from 300 nm wavelength and above from sunlight greatly exceeded the levels from artificial light (Maxwell and Elwood, 1983). Pasternak, Dubin and Moseson (1983) found an increased risk of melanoma with increased exposure to fluorescent light, whilst Rigel *et al.* (1983) did not. The latter authors pointed out that ultraviolet exposure from an average working year in fluorescent rooms was equivalent to about 40 minutes of sunshine exposure.

2.35.1 Conclusion

The above is an inadequate base to evaluate the association between exposure to fluorescent light and cancer in human beings.

2.36 Formaldehyde

Laboratory studies have suggested that formaldehyde at certain doses may be carcinogenic (*see* IARC, 1982c, for review). This has stimulated a number of epidemiological studies. The following notes refer to case reports briefly, and then deal with case-control studies. The main emphasis has been placed on prospective studies involving 3 groups potentially exposed: (*a*) morticians, (*b*) pathologists and anatomists, and (*c*) industrial workers. Available results are reviewed, and included in *Table 2.17*.

Two studies have concentrated upon examining workers for signs of ill health. One hundred and ninety-nine workers exposed for up to 42 years at a formaldehyde plant in Germany (Goldman *et al.*, 1982); 100 morticians in West Virginia carrying out about 1 embalming per week (Levine *et al.*, 1983b). Neither found evidence of cancer in these small groups that were carefully investigated.

2.36.1 Case reports

A report of nasal cancer in a man exposed to 'low' concentrations of formaldehyde for 25 years in a textile finishing plant is difficult to interpret. Helperin *et al.* (1983) point out that the man's employment had also involved exposure to other chemicals.

2.36.2 Case-control studies

A case-control study of 1967 patients with nasal cancer in Denmark, Finland, and Sweden diagnosed in 1978–80 and controls with colorectal cancer examined the association with occupation (Hernberg *et al.*, 1983a,b). Although the detail on potential exposure was limited, there was no evidence of an association with formaldehyde. Many case-control studies have been reported on nasal cancer; the above is the only one explicitly referring to formaldehyde, and even this study was in the analysis stage when it was decided to explore the possible exposure to formaldehyde.

2.36.3 Prospective studies

The results from the following studies are shown in *Table 2.17*.

2.36.3.1 Morticians and embalmers

Study of mortality in 1447 male undertakers licensed in 1928–57 in Ontario identified 331 deaths by 1977 (Levine *et al.*, 1983c). Expected deaths were based on US or province mortality rates. There was no evidence of increase in cancer of the buccal cavity, pharynx, or upper respiratory tract (O = 2, E = 3.7, O/E = 0.54, 95% CL = 0.1–1.9). There were non-significant increases in brain and RES tumours.

Licensure records for funeral directors and embalmers in California were used to identify 1050 men and 65 women who died in 1925–80. Proportional-mortality analysis, in comparison with state mortality, indicated a significant elevation in men of cancers of the colon, and brain, and of leukaemia (Walrath, 1983).

Records were available in New York to identify 1132 embalmers who had died in 1925–80. Proportional mortality, using national data to calculate expected figures, suggested a significant excess of cancer of the skin, kidney, and brain in those who had been licensed as embalmers, but not in those licensed as funeral directors (Walrath and Fraumeni, 1983a). Similar results, but based on only 1077 deaths, were provided by Walrath and Fraumeni (1983b).

2.36.3.2 Pathologists and anatomists

In the period 1943–76, there were 3 cases of nasal cancer in doctors registered in Denmark (Jensen, 1980). None had ever worked as pathologists or anatomists. Jensen and Anderson (1982) found no evidence of work involving possible formaldehyde exposure in 84 doctors developing lung cancer in Denmark in 1943–76. These 2 studies are using national cancer registration, and conceptually can be thought of as follow-up studies of all the medical profession, with case-control analysis of those developing the cancer of interest.

Membership lists were used to identify 2079 pathologists from 1955, and 12 944 medical laboratory technicians from 1963; they were traced until 1973 (Harrington and Shannon, 1975). Excess deaths from lymphoma occurred in the English pathologists (O = 6, E = 1.4, O/E = 4.29, 95% CL = 1.6–9.3), but not in Scottish pathologists nor in technicians in either country.

The records of the Royal College of Pathologists were used to follow-up 2307 male and 413 female pathologists in the UK in 1974–80 (Harrington and Oakes, 1984). There was no excess of RES neoplasms and no death from nasal cancer. A significant excess of brain tumours (O = 6, E = 2.0, O/E = 3.00, 95% CL = 1.1–6.5) and a reduced SMR for lung cancer were found.

In a follow-up study of 24 324 male doctors from 1951 until 1971, there was no evidence of relative excess mortality from cancer in those who had worked in laboratories (Doll and Peto, 1977). However, specific analyses by site are not presented for pathologists—due to the small number of deaths involved.

2.36.3.3 Industrial cohorts

Proportional mortality of 136 deaths of men who had worked for at least a month in formaldehyde-related areas in one of 5 chemical plants was reported by Marsh (1982). There was no abnormality in the pattern of mortality, in comparison with that expected on the basis of either US mortality or that of non-exposed workers in the plants. A more detailed analysis of causes of death is provided by Marsh (1983a).

Wong (1983) identified all 2026 white males employed at a formaldehyde-producing plant in the US at any time between the 1940s and 1977. Only 2.5% were lost to follow-up. Expected mortality was based on US rates. It was pointed out that potential exposure might have occurred to other hydrocarbons, benzene, asbestos, and a variety of pigments.

A cohort of 7680 men first employed before 1965 in 6 British chemical or plastic factories which made or used formaldehyde were traced to 1981. There was no death from nasal cancer (E = 1.07), nor any excess mortality for cancer of those sites reported as associated with formaldehyde exposure. One location had a modest excess of lung cancer, but this was only significant when using national rather than local rates for calculating the expected deaths (Acheson *et al.*, 1984b). Further analyses showed no relationship between lung cancer and cumulative estimates of exposure to formaldehyde (Acheson *et al.*, 1984c). There was no case of nasal cancer identified from national registration in this cohort (Acheson *et al.*, 1984d).

Table 2.17 Results for various malignancies reported in prospective studies of groups exposed to formaldehyde*

Occupation	Dig. syst.		Lung		Prostate		Bladder		Kidney		Leukaemia		Author
	O	E	O	E	O	E	O	E	O	E	O	E	
Morticians													
Canada			19	21.3	2	3.1			1	1.8	12	6.9	Levine *et al.* (1983c)
California	68	55.7	41	42.8			8	5.8	4	4.0	12	6.9	Walrath (1983)
New York	64	62.9	64	65.0	16	16.4	7	6.8	9	4.9	8	5.2	Walrath and Fraumeni (1983a)
Σ	132	118.6	124	129.1	18	19.5	15	12.6	14	10.7	20	12.1	
Pathologists													
England and Wales: 1	21	37.6	24	50.1			2	3.7			2	3.8	Harrington and Shannon (1975)
England and Wales: 2	9	16.8	9	22.7			2	2.0			2	1.2	Harrington and Oakes (1984)
England and Wales: 3			11	15.9									Doll and Peto (1977)
Σ	30	54.4	44	88.7			4	5.7			4	5.0	
Industry													
US: 1	8	6.3	6	7.1			2	0.6			1	1.2	Marsh (1983a)
US: 2	5	9.5	11	11.7	4	1.3	1	0.8	1	1.0	2	1.7	Wong (1983)
England and Wales			205	215.8									Acheson *et al.* (1984b)
Σ	13	15.8	222	234.6	4	1.3	3	1.4	1	1.0	3	2.9	
Grand total	175	188.8	390	452.4	22	20.8	22	19.7	15	11.7	27	20.0	
O/E	0.93		0.86		1.06		1.12		1.28		1.35		
95% CL	0.8–1.1		0.8–0.9		0.7–1.6		0.7–1.7		0.7–2.1		0.9–2.0		

*See text for description of method.

2.36.4 Hazard to the next generation

A postal questionnaire to all hospital staff in sterilizing rooms in Finland in 1980 and matching against hospital discharge records found no evidence that exposure to formaldehyde was associated with frequency of abortion (Hemminki *et al.*, 1982).

2.36.5 Conclusion

The toxicity review (Health and Safety Executive, 1981a) indicated that no evidence was available on a risk of cancer in humans, but studies were in progress. A review in the *Lancet* (1983b) suggested that it was 'very unlikely that occupational formaldehyde exposures prevalent today will be carrying risk of cancer'.

IARC (1982c) considered that though there was sufficient evidence that formaldehyde was carcinogenic to rats, there was insufficient epidemiological evidence to assess the hazard to man. The results published since 1978 are entered in *Table 2.17*; they do not show a significant increase in cancer risk.

2.37 Herbicides and pesticides

A variety of inter-related chemicals have been developed for use as herbicides and/or pesticides (as well as being used as intermediaries for many other industrial purposes). Much of the literature concentrates upon (*a*) phenoxy acids and (*b*) chlorophenols. Often the exposures are mixed, or the specific agent is not known. Due to the small number of workers involved and the interest in this subject, the following notes begin with case reports. There is then reference to use of mortality statistics and case-control studies of patients with various malignancies. Review is provided of the two main occupational groups potentially exposed: (*a*) manufacturing, and (*b*) use in agriculture and forestry.

The studies on farming (3.14) should also be considered, as the general occupational review overlaps with the present specific section.

2.37.1 Case reports

Jedlicka *et al.* (1958) reported development of acute paramyeloblastic leukaemia in 2 cousins aged 20. It was found that the 2 boys had worked for 8 months in an agricultural cooperative unloading sacks of an insecticide Gammexane (hexachlorocyclohexane).

Hardell (1977) reported that 7 patients with soft-tissue sarcoma treated at Umea, had had previous exposure to phenoxyacetic acids. Subsequently Hardell (1979) described the occupational histories of 17 consecutive patients treated at Umea

in 1978; 14 reported occupations consistent with exposure to chlorophenols or phenoxyacetic acids.

Johnson, Kugler and Brown (1981) provided case reports of father and son with soft-tissue sarcoma who both worked at a factory manufacturing chlorinated phenols.

Moses and Selikoff (1981) reported an American worker with a soft-tissue sarcoma. Though not directly involved in manufacture of trichlorophenol and trichlorophenoxy acetic acid (2,4,5-T), he had been exposed as a truck driver and maintenance man at the plant. They emphasized the need to include men potentially exposed, as well as the process workers.

2.37.2 Occupational mortality

Milham (1982c) examined the proportional mortality from soft-tissue sarcoma and various haematopoietic malignancies for 12 occupational groups likely to be exposed to phenoxy acid herbicides and chlorophenols in Washington State, for the period 1950–79. There was a slight increased risk of soft-tissue sarcoma (O = 49; E = 41; O/E = 1.20; 95% CL = 0.9–1.6).

2.37.3 Case-control studies

Soft-tissue sarcoma

Hardell and Sandstrom (1979) investigated 52 male patients (31 of whom were dead) diagnosed with soft-tissue sarcoma in Umea in 1970–77 and 208 matched controls. Exposure to phenoxyacetic acids or chlorophenols was reported significantly more frequently in the cases than the controls. There may have also been exposure to chlorinated dibenzodioxins and dibenzofurans. However, of the 12 cases reporting exposure, 7 had been included in the earlier case reports. The relative risks may have also been inflated by the method of excluding subjects with other exposures.

A comparable study was carried out in southern Sweden (Eriksson *et al.*, 1981). A detailed questionnaire was sent to patients registered with soft-tissue sarcoma in 1974–78, or next of kin for deceased patients. Controls, matched for locality, sex, and age, were selected from the population or death registers. Points of details in the occupational histories were clarified over the phone or in correspondence. A significant increase in risk occurred for those exposed to phenoxy acids (2,4,5-T or others) or to chlorophenols. There was no evidence of risk for those exposed only to other pesticides. Re-examination of the data for Hardell and Sandstrom (1979), Eriksson *et al.* (1981) and Hardell *et al.* (1981) (*see* next section on lymphoma) identified no evidence of observational bias. Investigation of patients with colon cancer showed no association with the use of herbicides, but a two-fold risk from exposure to asbestos (Hardell, 1981).

Smith *et al*. (1982) identified 102 patients with soft-tissue sarcoma treated in New Zealand in 1976–80 and 106 other male cancer patients matched for year of treatment and age. There was no evidence of increased risk in agricultural and forestry workers, though phenoxyherbicides had been used for many years in New Zealand.

Using data from national cancer registration, 1961 men with soft-tissue sarcoma diagnosed in England and Wales in 1968–76 were identified. Controls were men registered with other cancers and matched on age and region of residence. There was a significantly increased risk for farmers, farm managers, and market gardeners (RR = 1.7; 95% CL = 1.00–2.88). Other workers, potentially exposed to herbicides, had no increased risk: agricultural workers = 1.0; gardeners and groundsmen = 0.7; foresters and woodsmen = 1.0 (Balarajan and Acheson, 1984).

Using deaths in British Columbia in 1950–78, Gallagher and Threlfall (1984) examined the association of occupations potentially exposed to chlorophenols and certain sites of malignancy. There was no evidence of increased risk for soft-tissue sarcoma in any farming or other occupation.

Colorectal cancer

Ten out of 13 children with colorectal cancer treated at Memphis, Tennessee in 1974–76 came from rural areas with high pesticide use. However, levels of pesticide residues were not higher in blood samples from the patients than controls (Caldwell *et al*., 1981). A Swedish study (Hardell, 1981, described under Soft-tissue sarcoma) found no evidence of risk in colon cancer from herbicide exposure.

Liver

An increase in the proportion of cancer patients with primary liver lesions admitted to Hanoi hospitals was noted in 1962–68, in comparison with 1955–61. Though this was attributed to the spraying of herbicides with TCDD (Ton That *et al*., 1973), it was pointed out by IARC (1977b) that this could not be assessed from the available data.

Nasal cancer

A study of 44 patients with nasal cancer, 27 with nasopharyngeal cancer, and 571 controls from an earlier study of soft-tissue sarcoma in Umea, showed that prior exposure to chlorophenols was associated with a significant seven-fold excess of cancer at both sites. Exposure to phenoxyacetic acids was associated with a non-significant doubled risk of these cancers. Further analysis suggested that

this was an effect of the chemicals rather than occupation as woodworkers (Hardell, Johansson and Axelson, 1982).

One hundred and sixty patients with nasal cancer treated in North Carolina and Virginia in 1970–80 were matched to (*a*) hospital patients, (*b*) decedents if the index patients were dead (Brinton *et al*., 1984). There was a non-significant increase in risk for exposure to insecticides and pesticides: RR = 1.26, 95% CL = 0.7–2.2.

Gallagher and Threlfall (1984) found no evidence of risk for nasal or nasopharyngeal cancer from exposure to chlorophenols (*see* Soft-tissue sarcoma for details).

The Danish cancer registry was used to identify 839 patients with nasal cancer, and 2465 controls with other cancers in 1970–82. Linkage with pension fund records provided information on occupation back to 1960 (Olsen and Jensen, 1984). There was no evidence of increased risk from possible exposure to chlorophenols, but a significant risk from exposure to wood dust.

Brain

Gold *et al*. (1979), in a case-control study of 127 children under 20 with brain tumours treated in Baltimore in 1965–75, found no difference in parents' occupational exposure to chemicals, but a non-significant excess reported exposure to insecticides in the home. A study of 47 patients with glioma hospitalized in Milan in 1979–80 found an increased risk with agricultural work after 1960, when organic chemicals were introduced (Musicco *et al*., 1982).

Neuroblastoma

Amongst 14 patients treated for neuroblastoma in a paediatric hospital in 1974–76, there were 5 in whom antenatal or childhood exposure to chlordane formulations had occurred (Infante, Epstein and Newton, 1978). In addition, these authors reported 3 patients with aplastic anaemia and 3 with leukaemia who had been exposed to chlordane; these patients had been identified at several hospitals. Review of the literature identified 25 other reports of blood dyscrasias associated with chlordane alone or in combination with other drugs. It was pointed out that such data were inadequate to quantify the health risks from such exposure (from either lawn care or termite extermination in homes).

Lymphoma

Hardell *et al*. (1981) identified every patient treated in Umea for malignant lymphoma in 1974–78; this included the 17 patients reported by Hardell (1979). Controls were matched from the population register

84 Agents which cause occupationally induced cancers

for living patients and from the death register for deceased patients. A detailed self-completion questionnaire was completed by subjects and relatives, which was then coded blind; particular emphasis was paid to chemical exposure. Of 169 patients, 60 had Hodgkin's disease and the remainder non-Hodgkin's lymphoma. Raised risk was found to each of the chemicals which formed the focus of the enquiry: phenoxy acids 4.8; high-grade exposure to chlorophenols 8.4; low-grade exposure 2.9; organic solvents 2.4. There was an indication that exposure to trichloroethylene, perchloroethylene, styrene, benzene, and other solvents may all be implicated; the numbers involved were insufficient to calculate risk ratios for specific solvents.

In a further note, Olsson and Brandt (1981) emphasized that cutaneous manifestations of non-Hodgkin's lymphoma were particularly associated with herbicide exposure.

Lymphoma

Examination of mortality from non-Hodgkin's lymphoma in Wisconsin in 1968–76 (Cantor, 1982) showed an increased risk of reticulum cell sarcoma in young decedents in counties with a high proportion of acres treated with insecticides: RR = 6.6, 95% CL = 2.8–15.6.

In their study of workers exposed to chlorophenols, Gallagher and Threlfall (1984—see Soft tissue subsection) found a significant risk of non-Hodgkin's lymphoma in male sawmill and pulp workers.

Leukaemia

Though Blair and Thomas (1979) found an increased risk for leukaemia in farmers in Nebraska in 1954–74, this was not related to level of insecticide use in the different counties.

A case-control study of 1675 deaths of white males aged 30 or more from leukaemia in Iowa in 1964–78 showed an increase in counties with the largest number of acres treated by herbicides (Burmeister, Van Lier and Isacson, 1982).

Aplastic anaemia

A case-control study of 60 males aged 15–65 dying from aplastic anaemia in 1968–77 showed an increased risk for prior work with potential exposure to pesticides (Wang and Grufferman, 1981).

2.37.4 Manufacture

Out of a group of 78 workers exposed to tetrachlorodibenzo-*p*-dioxin (TCDD) for 5–6 years, follow-up was available on 55; 4 had died from cancer, 2 from

primary lung cancer (Jirasek *et al.*, 1974). The IARC (1977b) pointed out that an estimate of expected deaths for lung cancer, based on national rates for 1965, was 0.12.

Amongst 1403 males employed in the manufacture of pesticides, chlordane and heptachlor, in the US in 1946–76 there was no significant excess deaths from malignancy (Wang and MacMahon, 1979a). Ditralgia *et al.* (1981) followed up workers employed for at least 6 months prior to 1964 at 4 plants manufacturing pesticides in the US to the end of 1975. Two of the plants were those studied by Wang and MacMahon. The chemicals handled differed in the plants, though all involved organochlorine. No excess of cancer that was significant was found in the 2 plants not involved in the other study.

Follow-up of 55 workers exposed during the production of 2,4,5-T from trichlorophenol in Czechoslovakia from 1970 to 1980 identified 52 with chloracne, but only 2 deaths from cancer (E not given) and no soft-tissue sarcoma were identified (Pazderova-Vejlupkova *et al.*, 1981).

Ott, Holder and Olson (1980) followed up 204 persons exposed to 2,4,5-T in its manufacture from 1950 to 1971. There was no evidence of adverse mortality effects, though this was based on small numbers; cancers showed O = 1, E = 3.6, O/E = 0.28, 95% CL = 0.004–1.5.

A small group of workers processing trichlorophenol developed chloracne in 1964; 61 (who were thought to have been exposed to TCDD) were followed until 1978. There were 3 deaths from cancer with 1.6 expected (Cook *et al.*, 1980). Subsequently (Cook, 1981), it was reported that there had been 2 deaths from soft-tissue sarcoma in this group. The second was only identified after review of the material. Honchar and Halperin (1981) pointed out that there were 4 small groups of workers being followed in the US, and that only by pooling the results could the possible hazard be assessed. One of the studies was unpublished and there were 3 soft-tissue sarcomas amongst 105 deaths. (This becomes 4 with the additional death reported by Cook, 1981.)

Monitoring the health of 158 workers employed in a plant manufacturing pentachlorophenol (in which homologues of dioxin were present as contaminants up to 300 ppm) identified 2 patients with non-Hodgkin's lymphoma of the skin in 1978–81. The expected figure was about 0.28 (Bishop and Jones, 1981).

2.37.5 Manufacturing: accidents
1949: US

An accident occurred in 1949, exposing a small group of workers to tetrachlorodibenzodioxin; Zack and Suskind (1980) followed 121 who developed chloracne until 1978. There were no excess deaths from malignant disease in this small group of workers (O = 9; E = 9), but one patient developed a soft-tissue sarcoma.

1953: Germany

Follow-up of 73 workers potentially exposed in 1953 following an accident in a German trichlorophenol plant identified 42 with chloracne. By 1978, there were 6 deaths from cancer (E = 4), but no soft-tissue sarcoma had been identified (Thiess and Frentzel-Beyme, 1978).

1963: Netherlands

Follow-up of 141 men potentially exposed to dioxin in an explosion in 1963 showed no evidence of excess or atypical cancer mortality 20 years later (Dalderup and Zellenrath, 1983).

1968: England

During the manufacture of 2,4,5-trichlorophenols (2,4,5,-TCP) an accident occurred in the plant, with release of dioxin. Seventy-nine workers developed chloracne; 41 of the 46 workers still employed in 1978 were investigated together with others possibly not exposed to dioxin (May, 1982). No cancer was identified in the study population. Blank, Cooke and Potter (1983) found no evidence of chromosome changes in 93 of the individuals exposed in 1968, compared with samples from non-exposed employees studied in 1977–78.

2.37.6 Users of herbicides/pesticides

Finland

A cohort of 1926 men exposed to 2,4- and 2,4,5-T in 1955–71 when working as sprayers in Finland were followed until 1980. In comparison with national rates, there was no increase in mortality from all neoplasms and no death from soft-tissue sarcoma or lymphoma (Riihimaki, Asp and Hernberg, 1982). Caution is needed as there were only 45 deaths in all.

Germany

A study of 316 subjects exposed to long-term agricultural use of pesticides in East Germany followed through the period 1950–74 identified 30 tumours, of which 11 were lung cancer. The latter was reported to be twenty-fold higher than age-specific estimates from the population (Barthel, 1976). There had been very mixed exposure, including 2,4-dichlorophenoxyacetic acid (2,4-O), dinitro-*o*-cresol (DNOC), DDT, chloromethylphenoxyacetic acid (MCPA), hexachlorocyclohexane (HCH), parathion, as well as copper and organic fungicides. Some of the workers had been exposed to arsenic in 1950–56. No conventional person-years at risk was provided.

Sweden: 1

As a result of publicity in newspapers, a study was mounted in Sweden on the mortality of 735 railroad workers who had been using herbicides and were followed for an average of 8.0 years. There were problems in interpreting the results, due to the relatively small number of individuals involved and the mixed exposure to a variety of different herbicides, or the lack of any quantified information about ambient air concentrations. Expected figures were based on national rates. It was suggested that those who had been exposed to amitrole showed an excess of lung cancer (O = 2, E = 0.33, O/E = 6.1, 95% CL = 0.7–21.9). There was no evidence of increased mortality in workers exposed to phenoxy acids including 2,4,5-T (Axelson and Sundell, 1974). Extension of follow-up of 348 of these sprayers to 1978 showed no significant differences for cancers, though results were still based on very small numbers. There was a suggestion that an excess of cases was more marked in those with exposure in the earlier period of use of these chemicals (Axelson *et al.*, 1980).

Sweden: 2

Hogstedt and Westerland (1980) followed up 1396 lumberjacks and 148 foremen who had been potentially exposed to herbicides in Sweden in 1954–78. In comparison with 2649 non-exposed subjects there was no clear evidence of increase in cancer; only 8 neoplasms were identified in the men and no reference was made to specific tumours involved.

Sweden: 3

Records of the Swedish Forestry Workers' union identified 1030 male deaths occurring in 1968–77. Proportional-mortality analysis compared deaths with national mortality showed fewer deaths from cancer; in comparison with other cause mortality in a form of case-control study, Edling and Granstam (1980) suggest there was excess deaths from kidney cancer and lymphatic/haemopoietic malignancy.

US: 1

Wang and MacMahon (1979b) followed over 16 000 pesticide applicators who had worked at least 3 months between 1966 and 1976. Deaths were traced through Social Security administration and an excess was found for: lung: O = 24.3, E = 21.2, O/E =

1.15, 95% CL = 0.8–1.7; skin: O = 3.5, E = 2.0, O/E = 1.73, 95% CL = 0.6–4.7; bladder: O = 3.5, E = 1.3, O/E = 2.77, 95% CL = 1.0–7.6. (The O are not whole numbers, due to the distribution of 42 deaths according to the known causes for 269 deaths.)

US: 2

Follow-up of 3827 white workers licensed in Florida to apply pesticides showed an excess of deaths from leukaemia (O = 4, E = 3.0, O/E = 1.3, 95% CL = 0.4–3.4); brain (O = 5, E = 2.5, O/E = 2.0, 95% CL = 0.6–4.7) and lung cancer (O = 34, E = 25.1, O/E = 1.3, 95% CL = 0.9–1.9). The increase in risk of lung cancer was associated with length of exposure; the SMR was 100, 175, and 186 in three lengths of exposure (Blair *et al.*, 1983a).

2.37.7 Hazard to the next generation

A correlation was found between use of 2,4,5-T in Australia and the incidence of neural tube defect in New South Wales (Field and Kerr, 1979). Monitoring the incidence of cleft lip and palate in the county part of Western Australia showed an increase in 1978, with a lower proportion of subjects having either a familial or medical factor in their history, and a higher proportion conceiving in the spring and summer than in earlier years. It was suggested that this might be associated with exposure to herbicides, though there does not seem to be any hard evidence to support this view (Brogan, Brogan and Dadd, 1980).

2.37.8 Conclusions

Due to the paucity of epidemiological studies on individual substances it is necessary to use those that have involved multiple exposures. There are also problems as the agriultural workers that have been studied have a rapid turnover in staff, changing patterns of chemical use, exposure to other quite different agents, and lack any environmental measures of exposure. In contrast, the industrial workers are a more stable workforce and may have less extent of mixed exposures, but the environmental levels in manufacture may be less than when mixing and using the substances in farms and forests.

The quality of the history of exposure in the case-control studies may not be of the standard that is desirable, and some of the studies have examined a mixture of pathological types of tumour—especially for soft-tissue sarcoma and RES tumours.

The *Lancet* (1979a), in discussing the possible hazard from 2,4,5-T, pointed out that 'journalists and public are easily misled by campaigning toxicologists who seek to persuade their audience that all is well and no chemical compound could possibly harm the public, or that the products of industry are poisoning us all'.

In a review of hazards from pesticides (WHO, 1982), it was noted that 2 cases of leukaemia had been reported in individuals exposed to lindane— but the reported studies did not permit evaluation of this (due to the numbers of persons exposed occupationally). No general conclusion on cancer risk from pesticides was provided in this report.

Coggon and Acheson (1982) reviewed the epidemiological evidence on phenoxyherbicides and cancer in man. They acknowledged the positive Swedish and US studies on soft-tissue sarcomas and the unsupported Swedish evidence on risk of Hodgkin's disease and non-Hodgkin's lymphoma. They concluded that further studies were required to confirm or refute the associations.

A toxicity review on pentachlorophenol (Health and Safety Executive, 1982b) indicated that a causal relationship could not be established with lymphoma, but that further studies were in progress. The Advisory Committee on Pesticides (1983) concluded that formulations of 2,4,5-T herbicides and other phenoxy acid herbicides and related wood preservatives do not pose a safety hazard, whether used in agriculture, forestry, the home and garden, or elsewhere.

Acheson, Pannett and Pippard (1984) pointed out that nasal cancer had been reported in men who had left the furniture, and boot and shoe industry before the introduction of chlorophenols in either industry.

A working group (IARC, 1977b) concluded that the limited data then available were insufficient to evaluate the carcinogenicity to man of 2,4-D, 2,4,5-T, or the chlorinated dibenzodioxins. In a further review (IARC, 1983a), it was concluded that there was inadequate evidence to evaluate the carcinogenic effect of organic pesticides. There was thought to be limited evidence of carcinogenicity from phenoxy acids and chlorophenols, but the specific compounds involved could not be unequivocally identified.

Gloag (1981c) emphasized that a large number of active ingredients in pesticides had been shown to be mutagenic or carcinogenic in the laboratory.

2.38 Hydrazine

Follow-up of 427 men exposed to hydrazine at a plant in the east Midlands for an average of 19.6 years showed no evidence of excess cancers. Wald *et al.* (1984) pointed out that the results for a small number of men could only rule out a gross hazard. This was a more extensive follow-up of the group previously studied by Roe (1978).

2.38.1 Conclusion

IARC (1974a) had no epidemiological data on which to base an evaluation of carcinogenicity to man. The above study does not appreciably alter the situation.

2.39 Irradiation

There are four occupational groups where evidence has accumulated of a hazard: (*a*) staff involved in medical care and laboratory research, (*b*) luminous dial painters, (*c*) miners exposed to radon, and (*d*) the nuclear power industry. Each of these is discussed in further detail below.

Other jobs have been suggested as hazardous, such as use of artificial radionuclides in activation analysis, oil well drilling, testing the viability of metal welds, tracer chemistry, or astronauts exposed to cosmic rays (Archer, 1977). No epidemiological data have demonstrated the risks in such workers. Very few countries provide comprehensive summaries or estimates of doses due to industrial uses. It was pointed out in a report from the United Nations Scientific Committee on the Effects of Atomic Radiation (UNSCEAR) that industrial radiography gives rise to some of the highest average individual doses and a large proportion of individual overexposures (UNSCEAR, 1977).

2.39.1 Health professionals

The pioneer radiologists and radiographers, working without clear guidance on safe levels of radiation, developed skin changes (telangiectasia, pigmentation, atrophy) that were followed by multiple skin cancers often leading to tragic deaths (Ingram and Comaish, 1967). However, such complications do not occur below a total life time exposure of 1000 rad—well above the levels that should occur with present day safety measures. There has also been a suggestion that the 'early' radiologists had nine-fold increased risk of mortality from leukaemia (March, 1950). This was based on a comparison of the cause of death for radiologists and all other medical practitioners in the period 1929–48.

Warren (1956) studied the age at death of physicians in the US and observed that radiologists died on average 5.2 years earlier than other physicians. No information on death rates by cause was provided, but the average age at death was lower for non-malignant as well as malignant causes.

Lewis (1963) used the death certificates of 425 radiologists aged 35–74 dying in the US in 1948–61. He suggested that there was a significant excess of deaths from leukaemia (none of which were chronic lymphatic leukaemia), multiple myeloma, and aplastic anaemia. The latest reports (Matanoski *et al.*, 1975a,b) have looked at the mortality in US radiologists up to 1969 and compared their experience with that of their contemporaries who were physicians, ophthalmologists and otolaryngologists. Amongst those joining their respective colleges in 1920–29 and 1930–39, the radiologists had the highest mortality from cancer and from all other causes; the later cohort joining in 1940–49 still had the highest mortality from cancer but the lowest mortality from all other causes. A very high mortality from leukaemia and excess deaths from lymphoma and multiple myeloma were observed in the first two cohorts but not in the later one. The *British Medical Journal* (1975) in reviewing this and earlier publications suggested that further follow-up is required of the more recent cohort in order to quantify the final mortality from malignant disease and other causes, and that the statistical techniques for calculation of overall mortality could be improved. They conclude that 'until this has been done, there seems to be no reason to change our 1958 belief that the case has not been proved'.

Using professional society registers, Court Brown and Doll (1958) identified 1377 male British radiologists who had worked in the period 1897–1957 and whose vital status was known. There was evidence of excess mortality from cancer of the skin (O = 7, E = 0.8), pancreas (O = 7, E = 3.2), and leukaemia (O = 3, E = 1.4). The expected values were based on mortality in social class 1. There was no evidence of the excess in those who had only worked after 1920. This study was extended until 1976. The observed mortality was compared with (*a*) all men in England and Wales, (*b*) men in social class 1, and (*c*) male medical practitioners. Radiologists entering the profession before 1921 had a 75% higher death rate from cancer than other doctors. The excesses were significant for pancreas (O = 6, E = 1.9, O/E = 3.2, 95% CL = 1.1–6.9); lung (O = 8, E = 3.7, O/E = 2.2, 95% CL = 0.9–4.3); skin (O = 6, E = 0.8, O/E = 7.5, 95% CL = 2.7–16.3); leukaemia (O = 4, E = 0.7, O/E = 5.7, 95% CL = 1.5–14.6). There was no excess of specific sites of cancers for those entering after 1920 (Smith and Doll, 1981).

Miller and Jablon (1970) followed 6560 US army radiological technologists and other laboratory technologists for the period 1946–73. There was virtually no difference in cancer mortality in the two groups. Extension of this study (Jablon and Miller, 1978) to 1974 showed no overall increase in cancer deaths in the radiological technologists, nor any significant increase for a specific site of malignancy.

2.39.2 Laboratory staff

In the period 1972–77, 19 out of about 5000 employees in a high energy physics laboratory developed malignant melanoma. This was significantly more than expected, but no reasons for the excess were identified (Austin *et al.*, 1981). A case-control study of 31 employees with melanoma diagnosed in 1969–81 subsequently indicated some job-related risks, but no association with exposure to irradiation was reported (Reynolds, Austin and Thomas, 1982).

However, there was no evidence of increased incidence among 11 308 workers of the Los Alamos National Laboratory from 1969 to 1978 (Acquavella *et al.*, 1982).

2.39.3 Luminous dial painters (luminizers)

Martland. Conlon and Knef (1925) described the occurrence of 'chronic leukopenic anaemia of pernicious type' in a luminous dial painter, which could lead to death from anaemia or terminal infection.

Martland (1929) reviewed the hazards to those painting luminous watch dials in the US. The majority of his article deals with the severe acute effects of 'occupational poisoning' from radioactivity in the paint. In a small group of 15 patients dying from the acute effects, there were two with osteogenic sarcoma; he suggested this was too high to be mere coincidence. He referred to the mode of death being like benzene poisoning or leukaemia, but did not discuss whether any of the subjects may have had leukaemia.

Hasterlik, Finkel and Miller (1964) reported the occurrence of 15 osteosarcoma, 11 tumours of the cranial structures, and 3 leukaemias in about 400 dial painters who had worked before 1925. Two of the leukaemias were myeloid and it was suggested that the expected, based on national figures, was about 1. There had been no further subject identified with leukaemia in the subsequent 25 years.

Aub *et al.* (1952) described 30 patients with internally deposited radioactive material; 14 had been dial painters, 3 chemists, and 2 physicists. Three of the dial painters developed nasal sinus cancer, but no expected figure was provided. It was also reported by Rowland (1975) that exposure to radium from painting dials has resulted in cancers of the upper respiratory tract in addition to the more usual osteosarcoma.

Follow-up of 94 female dial painters from 1925 to 1976 identified 43 who had died. There were 5 osteosarcomas, 2 sarcomas, 7 mastoid or nasal sinus cancers, and 1 leukaemia in this group, but no expected values were provided (Brues and Kirsh, 1977).

Polednak, Stehney and Rowland (1978) used company records to identify 634 women who had worked in the US radium dial painting industry in 1915–29; they were followed until 1971. There were significant excesses of death from: cancer of the colon (O = 10, E = 5, O/E = 2.0, 95% CL = 1.0–3.7), bone cancer (O = 22, E = 0.3, O/E = 73.3, 95% CL = 45.9–110.0), cancer of other and unspecified sites (O = 18, E = 2.6, O/E = 6.9, 95% CL = 4.1–10.9). Compared with those employed in 1915–24, women first employed in 1925–29 had low cause-specific mortality ratios. A more detailed analysis of the risk of bone cancer (Polednak, 1978) showed a consistently higher incidence with higher dose, but no apparent effect of age at irradiation. Rowland, Stehney and Lucas (1978) derived a dose–response relationship between bone sarcoma and body burden of ^{226}Ra and ^{228}Ra for these workers.

Adams and Brues (1980) followed 1180 white women working as radium dial painters in the US before 1930, who were known to be alive in 1935 (the majority of whom had their body radium content measured). US national rates were used to calculate expected deaths and Connecticut incidence rates expected cancers. There was a significant excess incidence and mortality amongst women who had a radium intake of at least 50 curies (Ci).

Baverstock, Papworth and Vennart (1981) reported follow-up of 1110 women who worked as luminizers in the period 1936–61 in the UK. Estimates of dose were available, based on calendar period and duration of work though the authors emphasized the lack of specific information about an individual's dose.

There was an excess of breast cancer in the higher dose group of women that was not significant ($P = 0.077$ on a one-sided test). However, there was a significant excess of breast cancer in those under 30 when commencing work. The risk was compatible with 20–500 deaths from breast cancer per 10^4 women exposed to 1 gray (Gy). There was no excess of other cancers and a deficiency of deaths from all causes that decreased with increasing duration of follow-up.

A study of 1418 dial painters exposed before 1930, 1244 exposed in 1930–49, and 279 exposed after 1950 in the US identified 10 patients with leukaemia when 9.24 were expected (Spiers *et al.*, 1983).

Pochin (1983), in considering luminizers, suggested that the dose relationship for bone cancer was:

Dose	Risk
2 Gy	= No risk (though based on few observations and not accepted by all workers in this field)
2–100 Gy	= Proportional to (dose)^2—though linear risk is possible, as results are based on small numbers
100 Gy	= Risk decreases (cell kill)

2.39.4 Miners

Towards the end of the nineteenth century a strikingly high proportion of deaths from respiratory neoplasms were reported amongst miners in the Schneeberg and Joachimsthal area of Europe (Harting and Hesse, 1879). Previously this had been known as 'mountain disease' for several centuries. Lorenz (1944) provided a full review. Various causes were advanced for this; in the 1920s the radioactivity in the mines was suggested as the hazard. Lorenz suggested that radon inhalation could not be considered the sole cause and that chronic respiratory disease from dust exposure, arsenic, other radioactive substances, and genetic susceptibility might all play a part. He did not present appropriate epidemiological data to substantiate these points. More recent studies have quantified the risk for those mining uranium, iron-ore, fluorspar, tin and possibly gold.

2.39.4.1 Uranium mining

Wagoner *et al.* (1964) presented data on the mortality of US uranium miners from the Colorado region; those who had worked for 5 or more years underground had a ten-fold increased risk of lung cancer. Subsequent work (Wagoner *et al.*, 1965) showed that there was a relationship between risk of lung cancer and estimated airborne radiation; the age-standardized incidence ranged from 3.10 per 10 000 miners per year at the lowest level of exposure to 116.12 at the highest cumulative exposure category. Examination of the histology of the malignancies showed an atypical distribution, with undifferentiated carcinomas being most common in the high exposure subjects (small cell undifferentiated carcinoma predominating). Further follow-up (Archer, Gillam and Wagoner, 1976) of over 4000 workers confirmed the excess respiratory cancer rate; a proportion of the workers were Indians and it was demonstrated that they had a high respiratory cancer rate despite their low level of smoking. This finding has now been confirmed by Samet *et al.* (1984).

Lundin *et al.* (1969) followed underground uranium miners in the peiod 1950–67. There were 62 deaths from respiratory neoplasms with only 10 expected, and increasing excess for increasing exposure. There was some evidence of increased risk for those miners who smoked compared with non-smokers. A subsequent study in Colorado miners (Lundin, Wagoner and Archer, 1971) indicated that the highest exposure group of men had small cell undifferentiated lung cancers more frequently than the US population (i.e. in three-quarters of their tumours compared with a more usual proportion of one-quarter).

Examination of the histology for tumours from 121 American uranium miners and 138 age/smoking matched non-miners suggested that there was an increased risk of small cell undifferentiated tumours in exposed subjects. The latent interval was shorter for subjects with this histological type (Saccomanno *et al.*, 1971).

Study of Indians admitted to hospital in south-western US showed that 16 out of 17 with lung cancer were uranium miners, with a mean cumulative radon exposure of 1139.5 working level months. Sixty-five per cent of the lesions were small cell undifferentiated cancers, and 14 out of 16 miners were non-smokers (Gottlieb and Husen, 1981).

Workmen's Compensation Board records in Ontario were used to identify deaths from lung cancer in uranium miners (it was not clear how complete these records were). Data were available on the exposure of the general workforce (expressed as working-level months) for 135 lung cancer deaths. The results showed an increase in risk of lung cancer with increase in exposure. There was limited evidence that different levels of exposure altered the risk of histological type of tumour (Chovil, 1981). It was suggested that there was a greater risk of oat cell small/undifferentiated histology.

Uranium miners in Czechoslovakia who worked initially in 1948–52 were followed to 1975; their exposure to radiation was quantified and related to lung cancer incidence. There was a linear increase in risk with increase in cumulative exposure, but a complex effect of duration and intensity of exposure. Particularly with small cell undifferentiated lung cancer, there appeared to be a greater sensitivity to the sterilizing effect of radiation, and thus a decrease in incidence with increase in exposure rate (Kunz *et al.*, 1979).

In 1974, periodic sputum cytology examination was offered to residents of Uranium City, Saskatchewan; 80% of the uranium workers and 50% of the general population participated. Miners who smoked had a significantly higher incidence of abnormal cytology than 'control' smokers. The frequency of abnormality in the miners was related to the duration of both smoking and uranium mining (Band *et al.*, 1980).

Analysis on data of lung cancer mortality and smoking in Colorado uranium miners suggested there was a multiplicative effect between cumulative radon exposure (in working level months) and cumulative cigarette smoking (in packs). Thus the differences in risk between miners and non-miners was substantially higher for smokers than non-smokers (Whittemore and McMillan, 1983).

Three thousand six hundred and sixty-nine men who had worked in 1942–60 in a uranium mine in Canada were traced to 1975. Of 73 who had worked underground for more than 5 years 10 had developed lung cancer (RR = 36.3), compared with either the rate for those working less than 5 years or the 'unexposed' surface workers (Grace, Larson and Hanson, 1980). However, the age distribution of these 3 groups was quite different and no age adjustment was carried out. No data were available on smoking.

2.39.4.2 Iron-ore miners

Faulds and Stewart (1956) reviewed the records for 240 male postmortems for Cumberland for 1932–53. One hundred and eighty had been haematite miners and 17 (9.4%) had had cancer of the lung; this compared with 20% of the remaining autopsies. The number of autopsies in haematite miners had increased in 1948–53 and also the proportion with lung cancer. In a subsequent study, proportional-mortality analysis of those dying in the Cumberland area indicated a nearly two-fold increased proportion of deaths from lung cancer in those who had worked in the haematite mines, when compared with local or national mortality (Boyd *et al.*, 1970). A review (*Lancet*, 1970) discussed the possible relationship with either radon contamination or other dust in the mines and concluded that the study could give no definite explanation of the increased risk, though this was clearly demonstrated.

Metal miners in the US followed from 1937 to 1959 had an excess of deaths from respiratory tract cancer (O = 47, E = 16.1, O/E = 2.9, 95% CL = 2.1–3.9). No non-occupational explanatory variable could be identified (Wagoner *et al.*, 1963).

An increased risk of lung cancer has also been reported in iron-ore miners in France (Roussel *et al.*, 1964), but again the factor responsible has not been identified. When discussing the five-fold excess of lung cancer in iron-ore miners in Lorraine, it was emphasized that the level of radiation in the miners was not raised at all (Anthoine *et al.*, 1979).

In the locality of an iron-ore mine in Sweden there had been 52 deaths from lung cancer among underground miners in 1957–80; estimates of the exposed population were obtained from census reports. It was calculated that there were about 30–40 excess cases of lung cancer per 10^6 person-years and working level month (Edling and Axelson, 1983).

A case-control study of 604 deceased males with lung cancer, an equal number dead of other conditions and 467 living controls was conducted in northern Sweden (Damber and Larsson, 1982). History of occupation and smoking were obtained. There was a lower level of smoking in the lung cancer subjects who had worked underground in iron-ore mines. This was considered evidence of a multiplicative effect. In particular there was a higher proportion of small cell undifferentiated tumours in the miners, suggesting that the environmental factors especially increased the risk of this tumour.

Using the death register in Grangesberg, Sweden, Edling (1982) identified iron-ore miners dying in 1957–77 from lung cancer and other causes, and matched controls. Those miners who smoked appeared to have a shorter latent period from first working as a miner to death from lung cancer than the non-smoking miners.

2.39.4.3 Other types of miners

Fluorspar miners in Newfoundland were found to have an increased risk of lung cancer; this was about 30-fold the expected for those working for a 10-year period in 1952–61 underground (Villiers and Windish, 1964). Levels of radon and daughter products were well in excess of the suggested maximum permissible air concentrations.

Axelson and Sundell (1978) identified 29 males dying from lung cancer in Hammar, Sweden in 1956–76; 6 controls dying from other cancers were selected from the local death register. Twenty-one of the 29 cases had worked in the local zinc/lead mines, but only 19 out of 174 controls (RR = 16.4). Though based on small numbers, there was some evidence of higher risk in non-smokers; it was suggested that an increased mucus layer in smokers might protect against inhaled particles and radiation. This was an extension of earlier reports by Axelson *et al.* (1971) and Axelson and Rehn (1971).

A study of 1974 gold miners in Western Australia followed in 1961–75 (Armstrong *et al.*, 1979) documented a relatively high mortality from lung cancer: O = 59, E = 40.8, O/E = 1.45, 95% CL = 1.1–1.9. This was inconclusively related to underground miners experience and might possibly be related to excess smoking reported in these miners. The level of radon was much lower than in some of the other studies where this was thought to be a factor; the level of arsenic in the rock was also low, with no evidence of arsenism in the miners. No results were presented for stomach cancer.

A historical prospective study of Cornish tin miners identified a two-fold excess of cancer of the lung in underground miners. This was thought to be associated with exposure to radon and its daughter products (Fox, Goldblatt and Kinlen, 1981).

Mixed metal miners working with copper, gold, iron, lead, tin, and zinc in Canada who developed silicosis in 1969–77 were followed and 11 deaths from lung cancer identified. There was a higher proportion of these deaths in miners with early silicosis, than in those with advanced silicosis. Enzenwa (1982) suggested that there was an increased risk of lung cancer from the work environment.

In a case-control study in northern Sweden, lung cancer cases exposed to underground (non-uranium) mining had a lower average tobacco consumption than other lung cancer cases. It was suggested that there was a synergistic effect of smoking and underground mining (Larsson and Damber, 1982). This view is also supported by Radford and Renard (1984).

Other studies of the cancer risks in miners appear in 3.22.

Pochin (1983) suggested that the lung cancer hazard from high linear energy transfer (LET) particle irradiation was:

Uranium mines	300–750 per 10^4 per Gy
Metal mines	230 per 10^4 per Gy
Fluorspar mines	150 per 10^4 per Gy

2.39.5 Nuclear power

Though a number of different locations have been studied, interest has focused on two quite different locations in America, (a) a large nuclear plant—Hanford, and (b) a naval shipyard servicing nuclear submarines—Portsmouth. The reports on these two locations are discussed below, followed by a subsection on other more general aspects.

Bonnell and Harte (1978) utilized data on the occurrence of cancer in the general population and risk factors published by ICRP to assess the increment from irradiation. They suggested that even an individual worker exposed for a long time at the dose limit (50×10^3 sievert (Sv)/year) would only have a small increment in cancer risk, whilst the population risk was also very small.

2.39.5.1 Hanford Nuclear Plant, US

Mancuso, Stewart and Kneale (1977) analysed 3520 deaths amongst workers at a large nuclear plant in the US (Hanford Works). Identification particulars were available for all workers, details of annual radiation exposure for monitored workers, and cause of death for those dying in 1944–72. They suggested that there was an increase in cancer deaths in those with low level exposure, especially from myeloma.

This work was subject to major criticism. For example, Anderson (1978) drew attention to the unconventional analyses that had been used, which had resulted in undue stress being placed on a radiation effect because of a few abnormally high exposure figures. Reissland (1978) reviewed a range of comments that had been made on the Hanford study: the low level of exposure being similar to background radiation; the highly skewed distribution of doses; the correlation of length of service with lifetime dose; the men dying of leukaemia had below average exposure; there was no information on exposure to other hazards; not all deaths were identified (92%); the International Classification of

Diseases of the observed and expected deaths was different; there were problems of proportional-mortality analyses; no adjustment for age and calendar year of death was made; the calculated doubling dose leads to a negative value for the natural incidence; the data on internal irradiation were valueless. Riessland concluded that there were unexplained excesses of cancer of the pancreas and multiple myeloma.

Darby and Reissland (1981) re-analysed the Hanford material (a) by relating risk of deaths to levels of radiation doses, and (b) comparing the observed mortality with that expected from US national mortality rates. They concluded that there was no evidence that ICRP estimates were too low, but confirmed that there was evidence of increased deaths from multiple myeloma in the higher dose categories.

An independent study of the Hanford data (Gofman, 1979) suggested that the confidence limits of the doubling dose of radiation were so wide, that it could not be concluded that the results were incompatible with other (higher) estimates. It was suggested that the myeloma risk may be partly a reflection of the multiple probes of the data (50 categories of cancer were explored) rather than confirmation of a specific tissue sensitivity.

Analyses were carried out for the US (Controller General, 1981), which indicated that there had not been a significant increase in cancer deaths.

Tolley *et al.* (1983) extended the study of Hanford workers to include those employed after 1964 for a minimum of 2 years, and to include deaths up to the end of 1978. The relationship of risk to myeloma to irradiation dose remained significant, that for pancreas was non-significant, and that for stomach nearly significant.

Two important method issues have stemmed from further analysis of data from Hanford. Though most production work is done by annual workers, 40% of the most dangerous jobs are performed by professional or technical staff. These trained staff have mortality risks which correlate with work irradiation; the manual smokers, who have higher mortality, show an inverse relation with dose. It is suggested that the latter was an artefact of recruiting more skilled workers for more dangerous work (Kneale, Mancuso and Stewart, 1984a). A further paper discussed some of the problems of allowing for (a) job-related mortality risks, (b) lack of information on how specific jobs are related to education and income (Kneale, Mancuso and Stewart, 1984b).

2.39.5.2 Portsmouth Naval Dockyard, US

Najarian and Colton (1978) scanned all death certificates for the years 1959–77 in the mortality register for Maine, Massachusetts, and New Hampshire, searching for those indicating prior employment at the Portsmouth Naval Shipyard. Next of kin were contacted for about one-third of such individuals and asked if the deceased had worked with radiation or worn a radiation badge. (The men were thought to have had a lifetime exposure of about 10 rem.) On the basis of this information an analysis suggested that there was a significantly increased proportion of deaths from cancer, especially leukaemia. However, the method of identifying shipyard workers, the very low proportion of contacts with next of kin, and the method of assessing exposure to radiation cast doubt on the findings.

Rinsky *et al.* (1981) collected further data for 7615 radiation workers at the same naval shipyard, together with mortality for other non-irradiated workers. Deaths due to leukaemia, all lymphatic and haematopoietic neoplasms, and all neoplasms was slightly lower in the total cohort than expected. There was no leukaemia excess when the radiation workers were compared with the non-radiation workers at the same shipyard. They suggest their result may be due to more complete ascertainment and more accurate classification of radiation exposure than in the earlier study by Najarian and Colton (1978).

2.39.5.3 Other aspects of nuclear power

When national mortality data have been used to calculate expected figures for mortality in men who have been employed by the UK Atomic Energy Authority there is no indication that the leukaemia mortality is raised and the overall mortality appears to be 'low' (Duncan and Howell, 1970). There have been reported cases, including those where legal action has been taken, where workers after even a short period of industrial exposure have developed leukaemia. However, there appears to be no clear indication that there is a raised risk to such workers.

Dolphin (1976) presented data on mortality from haematopoietic and lymphatic system malignancy amongst workers at Windscale (British Nuclear Fuels Ltd) from 1950 to 1974. There was no significant difference in leukaemia observed and expected deaths for the radiation workers (O = 4, E = 2.83, O/E = 1.43, 95% CL = 0.4–3.7). A further study of all employees in the period 1948–75 traced about 14 000 employees, with a loss of about 2%. There was no excess of all cancers; for bone, thyroid, plus leukaemia: O = 7, E = 9.2, O/E = 0.76, 95% CL = 0.3–1.6; for multiple myeloma O = 4, E = 2.7, O/E = 1.48, 95% CL = 0.4–3.8 (Clough, 1983).

In an attempt to put the hazards from nuclear power stations in perspective, Rothschild (1978) discussed risk accountancy for various sources of power. He concluded that energy was produced for uranium or natural gas at lower risk than when using coal, oil, wind or the sun. He also suggested that risk of 8 forms of 'disaster' from nuclear power stations was very remote.

Enstrom (1983) calculated infant mortality rates and age-adjusted rates for various cancers for the population located round a major nuclear power plant, which began operation in 1968, for the period 1960–78. There was no evidence of change in leukaemia, lung cancer, or all cancers compared with California and US rates.

A symposium was held by the New York Academy of Medicine on the health aspects of nuclear power plant incidents. No hard epidemiological data were presented on carcinogenesis following examples of such incidents (Shils and Bramnick, 1983).

2.39.6 Other 'occupational' exposure

Since 1951, sandlike residue from uranium mills had been used as construction fill material in Colorado. (This contains radioactive material giving off low level radiation.) Examination of trends of cancer mortality in 1950–67 in the localities showed no evidence of an irradiation effect (Mason, Fraumeni and McKay, 1972).

Mention was made in an earlier paragraph of those workers testing metal welds for faults; this has been suggested as a potential hazard but no documented data are available on the mortality of such workers in comparison with a control or contrast group. A recent report (UNSCEAR, 1977) states that 'Very few countries provide comprehensive summaries or estimates of doses due to industrial uses ..... but industrial radiography gives rise to some of the highest average individual doses and to a large percentage of over-exposures'.

Polednak, Stehney and Lucas (1983) studied the mortality of 3039 men employed in production of thorium in 1940–70 in the US. In the total group there was an increase in deaths from all neoplasms (O = 99, E = 81.75, O/E = 1.21, 95% CL = 0.99–1.48). Though no specific site showed a significant increase in the total group, those who had worked for at least a year in jobs with highest exposure had a significant excess of pancreatic cancer (O = 5, E = 1.21, O/E = 4.13, 95% CL = 1.34–9.63). This was thought to be due to excess smoking in part.

2.39.7 Laboratory studies

In a study of English nuclear-dockyard workers, Evans *et al.* (1979) showed a significant increase in chromosome damage with increasing exposure, though most workers had less than the accepted maximum level of 5 rem/year. However, Savage (1979) pointed out that the result did not equal a specified hazard to health; until information was available on effects in other tissues (such as the testis) no evaluation could be made.

Examination of chromosome aberrations in lymphocytes from 47 thorium workers and controls shows 'a non-significant increased frequency of two-break aberrations in the exposed workers' (Hoegerman and Cummins, 1983).

2.39.8 Conclusions

There is no dispute over the carcinogenic properties of ionizing irradiation, whatever the source. The argument has focused on the shape of the dose–response curve and whether the present permissible level of exposure is soundly based. The queries have arisen from suggested findings of risk in those receiving low-level exposure in two US studies (the Hanford and Portsmouth Naval Dockyard reports discussed above). However, a report to the US Congress (Controller General, 1981) emphasized the great difficulty of quantifying the effect of low-level LET radiation. It had been estimated that if 10 000 people each received an extra rad there would be one extra cancer death—when about 1670 cancers from other causes would occur. To obtain a firm estimate of such a small level of risk, a study on 100 million subjects would be required.

2.40 Isopropyl alcohol

Four studies of workers from isopropyl alcohol plants are briefly described.

Study of 71 men who had worked for at least 5 years manufacturing isopropyl alcohol using the 'strong acid' process identified 4 with paranasal sinus cancer (Weil, Smyth and Nale, 1952). It was suggested this was at least 3 times the expected (IARC, 1977b).

Eckhardt (1974) mentioned an earlier finding that workers in an isopropyl alcohol plant had developed 2 nasal cancers and 2 laryngeal cancers. He referred to this as a 'non-significant' finding, but gave no expected figure. The data were not published when initially collected. IARC (1977b) suggested that the combined incidence from the 2 sites was about 21 times that in the general population.

Employees working for at least 1 month on an isopropyl and ethyl alcohol plant at Baton Rouge, US were followed in the period 1950–76; this was extended to include all who had worked for any length on the plant in 1950–78 (Lynch *et al.*, 1979). Follow-up was complete for 89.6% of 744 employees. A proportional-mortality analysis used US national incidence and mortality data to calculate

expected figures. There was an excess of upper respiratory cancer; the results for larynx used a conventional person-years at risk analysis. For all workers: O = 7, E = 2.20, O/E = 3.18, 95% CL = 1.3–6.6. Examination of the detailed results suggested that the hazard was associated with work on the strong acid ethanol unit, rather than the weak acid isopropyl alcohol unit.

All men who worked on an isopropyl alcohol plant at Shell Stanlow, in England 1950–75 were traced. Expected deaths were based on national rates (Alderson and Rattan, 1980). There was a questionable excess of nasal cancer, based on very small numbers (O = 1, E = 0.02, O/E = 50.0, 95% CL = 0.6–278.2).

2.40.1 Conclusions

IARC (1977b) accepted that there was a risk of cancer of the paranasal sinuses and possibly larynx in those working on isopropyl plants using the strong acid process. Lynch *et al.* (1979) have argued that it is the alkyl sulphates produced in the strong acid process that are the specific carcinogens.

2.41 Lead

Though there had been some evidence of an association between lead intake and risk of certain malignancies, Dingwall-Fordyce and Lane (1963) pointed out that the emphasis in occupational studies had been upon the toxic effects, rather than risk of malignancy. This note indicates 2 case reports, and then briefly reviews 7 prospective studies carried out on workers in 3 countries.

2.41.1 Case reports

A cerebral tumour was reported in a lead worker by Portal (1961). A renal cancer in a man, who had worked for 22 years as a furnace tender and had been exposed to lead, bore a similarity to the histology of renal tumours induced in animals with prolonged lead exposure (Baker *et al.*, 1980).

2.41.2 Prospective studies

Australia

McMichael and Johnson (1982) followed 241 male smelter workers in south Australia who had been diagnosed as suffering from lead poisoning in 1928–59, until 1977. Out of 140 deaths only 9 were from cancer with a PMR of 0.59.

England and Wales: 1

Deaths were identified in men working in an accumulator factory in England in 1946–61 and in pensioners following at least 25 years service in a group of companies employing men with lead exposure in the period 1926–60 (Dingwall-Fordyce and Lane, 1963). Using national rates, expected figures were calculated which showed no excess of deaths from cancers. In the highest band of exposure: O = 27, E = 31.0, O/E = 0.87, 95% CL = 0.6–1.3.

England and Wales: 2

A survey of sickness in 955 lead workers in the 1965–72 period reported no evidence of increased rates of malignant disease (Shannon, Williams and King, 1976).

England and Wales: 3

Pension records for 4 lead acid battery factories in England and Wales were used to study mortality of 754 pensioners in 1925–76. Comparison was made with expected based on national rates. In addition, a proportional-mortality analysis was carried out on deaths occurring in employees in the largest of the factories (Malcolm and Barnett, 1982). There was no overall excess of deaths from malignant disease: male pensioners: O = 157, E = 159.5, O/E = 0.98, 95% CL = 0.8–1.1; female pensioners: O = 7, E = 10.9, O/E = 0.64, 95% CL = 0.3–1.3; male employees: O = 136, E = 118.3, O/E = 1.15, 95% CL = 1.0–1.4; female employees: O = 18, E = 14.1, O/E = 1.28, 95% CL = 0.8–2.0. The only more specific data presented were for male employees, who had an excess of gastrointestinal cancer in those with the greatest lead exposure: O = 21, E = 12.6, O/E = 1.67, 95% CL = 1.0–2.5.

England and Wales: 4

Follow-up of 57 chromate pigment workers who suffered from clinical lead poisoning mostly in 1930–45 until 1981 showed a slight excess of deaths from lung cancer: O = 4, E = 2.77, O/E = 1.45, 95% CL = 0.4–3.7. This could have been a reflection of the chromate exposure or smoking (Davies, 1984b).

US: 1

Men who had worked in (*a*) 6 lead production plants (1 primary smelter, 2 refineries, 3 recycling plants) and (*b*) 10 battery plants in the US were traced to examine their mortality (Cooper and Gaffey, 1975). Using national rates to calculate expected figures there was an excess of respiratory cancers; group (*a*)

O = 22, E = 15.8, O/E = 1.48, 95% CL = 0.9–2.1; group (*b*) O = 61, E = 49.5, O/E = 1.32, 95% CL = 0.9–1.6. This result is significant if the 2 groups of workers are pooled. It was suggested that there was no evidence of increased risk of alimentary tract, genito-urinary cancer, or leukaemia.

More detailed discussion of the findings on cancer mortality in these workers was provided by Cooper (1976). Kang, Infante and Carra (1980) suggested that the first paper had used an inappropriate test of the SMRs. Re-analysis indicated that the SMR was significantly raised for lead smelter workers for respiratory cancer, and for battery workers for digestive organ cancers.

The study was extended, by follow-up of the 5400 men alive at 31/12/70 until the end of 1975. Again there was an excess of lung cancer in this 5-year period, though not statistically significant.

US: 2

The health of a small group of 139 men exposed to tetraethyl lead for at least 20 years was compared with that of workers not so exposed but matched on age and length of employment. There was no appreciable difference in the incidence of skin cancer in the 2 groups (7/139 in the exposed and 4/139 in the controls); no other cancers were identified in the paper (Robinson, 1976).

2.41.3 Hazard to the next generation

A case-control study of 149 children reported to the Connecticut cancer registry in 1935–73 with Wilms' tumour showed an association with paternal occupations related to lead (Kantor *et al.*, 1979). These included drivers, motor vehicle mechanics, service station attendants, welders, solderers, metallurgists, and scrap-metal workers. There is confusion between these job titles and other exposures, such as to hydrocarbons. However, another study (Fabia and Thuy, 1974) of 71 tumours reported in children whose fathers worked in hydrocarbon-related jobs did not include any with Wilms' tumour, although 25 (6.5%) of the total cases had this diagnosis. Nor was there any association between hydrocarbon-related occupations found with Wilms' tumour by Zack *et al.* (1980).

2.41.4 Conclusions

IARC (1980) found the available epidemiological evidence inadequate but concluded that lead acetate and phosphate were carcinogenic in rats and these compounds should be regarded as presenting a risk to humans.

The more recent studies have still not clarified the hazard to workers. However, control of environment of workers potentially exposed to lead may be an important contribution to future negative findings.

2.42 Metals

Whenever possible, these reviews have allocated references to specific sections. With metals these cover: aluminium (3.2), arsenic (2.7), beryllium (2.11), cadmium (2.13), chromates (2.19), copper refining (2.7.3), electroplating (3.13), lead (2.41), nickel (2.44), and zinc (2.60). The section on mining includes material on metal miners (3.22.4). However, a number of studies have been less specific and these are collected here.

This section begins with studies of occupational mortality; a number of prospective studies relate to various groups of metal workers. Case-control studies have been of two types: (*a*) selecting occupations and searching for raised risks of any site of malignancy, i.e. 'fishing studies', and (*b*) examining a range of aetiological factors, including occupation, for a specific site of malignancy. Both these categories of study are briefly described.

2.42.1 Occupational mortality

Analysis of death certificates for lung cancer in England and Wales in 1920–29 by reported occupation showed an increased risk in those working as 'metal grinders' (Kennaway and Kennaway, 1936).

Statistics for England and Wales for 1970–72 (Registrar General, 1978) indicate raised SMRs for various categories of metal worker for: stomach, rectal, pancreas, larynx, lung, and bladder cancer.

Blair and Fraumeni (1978), in their examination of prostate cancer mortality by counties in the US, observed elevated rates of mortality in those counties with metal industries.

Using data from the Third National Cancer Survey in the US, Flanders and Rothman (1982) found increased risk ratios for larynx cancer in grinding wheel operators.

2.42.2 Prospective studies

Canada

Data on all deaths in British Columbia in 1950–78 indicated 10 036 were male metal workers. The total material was used to calculate PMRs (Gallagher and Threlfall, 1984). Significantly raised deaths occurred for: rectal cancer in metal mill men; lung cancer in metal millers, boiler makers, sheet metal workers, welders, plumbers, and machinists; RES neoplasms in metal millers, welders, and machinists.

Sweden: 1

Englund (1980) used employees' certificates to identify plumbers in 1965, who were followed to 1974 in the Swedish mortality files. Expected events were calculated from national rates. There was a significant excess of deaths from cancer of the stomach: O = 35, E = 25.1, O/E = 1.39, 95% CL = 1.0–1.9; larynx: O = 8, E = 3.2, O/E = 2.45, 95% CL = 1.1–4.9; lung: O = 38, E = 23.7, O/E = 1.61, 95% CL = 1.1–2.2. Use of the linked cancer environment files also suggested an excess of liver, nasal sinus, larynx, and lung cancers in 1960–73.

Sweden: 2

Follow-up of 86 men who had worked as steel polishers for at least 5 years in Sweden showed an excess of deaths from gastric cancer: O = 4, E = 0.44, O/E = 9.09, 95% CL = 2.4–23.3. This was thought to indicate a possible cancer hazard amongst such workers (Jarvholm, Thiringer and Axelson, 1982).

US: 1

Radford (1976) presented proportional-mortality analyses for deaths occurring in steel mill workers in 1973–74, including pensioners. The local metropolitan area mortality was used to calculate expected values. There was a significant excess of lung cancer (O = 44, E = 29.6, O/E = 1.49, 95% CL = 1.1–2.0).

US: 2

Mortality in 8679 members of a metal trades union employed in shipyards, metal fabrication shops, small boat yards, and field construction in the Seattle area, US, was studied in 1950–76. Expected figures were based on national rates. There was no significant increase in any site of cancer, but further examination of respiratory cancers showed an increased risk in those workers with longer latent interval and increased duration of work (RR by latent interval were: 3−years = 0.59; 10−years = 0.98; 20−years = 1.26; 30−years = 1.69; 40+years = 1.42). Beaumont and Weiss (1980) do not give actual values for O and E for these results.

US: 3

Union records were used to identify 1292 deaths in 1951–69 in males who had worked in the metal polishing and plating industries in the US. There was a non-significant excess of liver cancer (O = 5, E = 1.8, O/E = 2.78, 95% CL = 0.9–6.5) and oesophageal cancer (O = 10, E = 5.4, O/E = 1.85, 95% CL = 0.9–3.4). However, the numbers were small and there will have been multiple exposures to metals and chemicals, including trichloroethylene in degreasing (Blair, 1980).

US: 4

Union records identified 3369 deaths in white male plumbers and pipefitters in the US in 1971; a proportional-mortality analysis used national rates to calculate expected values (Kaminski, Giessert and Dacey, 1980). Plumbers had significantly raised mortality from cancer of the oesophagus, respiratory system, and lymphatic system.

US: 5

A cohort of males employed for at least 1 year in 1946–75 in 9 US zinc and copper refineries was traced (Logue, Konitz and Hattnick, 1982). In such electrolytic refineries, the men may have been exposed to low levels of arsenic, acid mists, and various metals such as antimony. However, some of the workers may have previously been employed at smelters with very different work environments. Vital status was determined for 88% and 355/423 death certificates were located. Expected deaths were calculated from national rates. There was no clear increase in risk of malignancy for any site.

2.42.3 Case-control studies

Multiple site exploratory studies

Detailed occupational histories were obtained for all patients admitted to Roswell Park hospital in 1956–65; these were subsequently used to calculate relative risks for various occupations. Houten *et al.* (1977) used the material to check for raised risks in men exposed to metals. The following RR were significantly raised: stomach—mill wrights (5.5), metal moulders (1.9), primary metal workers (2.6); prostate—blacksmiths (6.7), mechanics and repairmen (2.1); bladder—fabricated metal workers (2.1), furnacemen, smeltermen and pourers (2.4); leukaemia—machinists (2.9). Though these were based on records for 14 000 patients, many of the specific results only involve a few individuals. Slightly different results are also given in some of the other papers published on this material.

Pancreas

Occupation was reviewed for all patients diagnosed with pancreatic cancer in 1935—74 in Olmsted county, US (Maruchi *et al.*, 1979). Of the 70 male patients, 8.6% had worked with metal (including sheetmetal workers, welders, plumbers, tinners), but only 1.6% of the male population in the 1970 census.

Nasal

A collaborative study investigated patients with nasal cancer in Denmark, Finland, and Sweden diagnosed in 1978–80 and controls with colorectal cancer, matched for age and sex (Hernberg *et al.*, 1983a). There was a significantly increased risk for metal exposure from welding and electroplating.

Larynx

Burch *et al.* (1981) in a case-control study investigated 204 patients with laryngeal cancer diagnosed in Ontario in 1977–79. Controls were individually matched neighbourhood controls, interviewed at home by a trained interviewer. There were increased risks for metal processors, pipefitters, and plumbers.

Data from the Third National Cancer Survey in the US indicated an increased risk for larynx cancer in automobile mechanics and sheet metal workers (Flanders and Rothman, 1982).

All patients under 75 with laryngeal cancer diagnosed in Denmark in 1980–82 at 5 cancer therapy units were compared with population controls, matched for age, sex, and residence (Olsen, Sabroe and Lajers, 1984). Workers exposed to welding fumes had a slightly increased risk of this cancer after adjustment for alcohol and smoking (RR = 1.30, 95% CL = 0.9–2.0). This was significant for the subglottic region (RR = 6.3, 95% CL = 1.8–21.6).

Lung

One thousand and fifty-nine male welders followed in 1943–73 in 3 plants in Oak Ridge, Tennessee had an increased risk of lung cancer: RR = 1.50, 95% CL = 0.87–2.40. There were higher lung cancer risks in subgroups, but none were significant (Polednak, 1981).

Lymphosarcoma

In a follow-up of the US cancer mortality maps, Goldsmith and Guidotti (1977) examined the occupation for 484 deaths from lymphosarcoma in California in 1971–72. There was an increased risk of these neoplasms in 'engineers': O = 28, E = 18.8, O/E = 1.50, 95% CL = 1.0–2.1; and 'craftsmen': O = 131, E = 96.0, O/E = 1.36, 95% CL = 1.1–1.6.

Multiple myeloma

The occupations of 149 patients diagnosed with multiple myeloma in Hamburg in 1935–65 suggested an increased risk for those with exposure to heavy metals (Dorken and Vollmer, 1968). No expected figure was provided and many subjects had had several different jobs with quite different exposures.

2.42.4 Laboratory studies

There was no difference in the chromosome abnormalities found in 23 welders of stainless steel and 22 control subjects, though smokers in both groups had significantly raised sister chromatid exchanges compared with non-smokers (Husgafvel-Pursiainen, Kalliomaki and Sorsa, 1982).

2.42.5 Hazard to the next generation

Using hospital discharge data and census information, Hemminki *et al.* (1983b) showed that women who had worked in a textile factory in Finland had an increased spontaneous abortion rate. This appeared to be further affected by husbands' working in a metallurgical factory.

2.42.6 Conclusions

In a review of the hazard from metals, Hernberg (1977) stated that apart from arsenic, beryllium, cadmium, iron, and nickel there was no evidence of a carcinogenic effect from any other metal. It is not clear from the above notes whether this no longer holds. The results are not consistent between different studies, and the environmental factors varied considerably apart from a somewhat ill-defined exposure to metals.

2.43 Mustard gas

Case and Lea (1955) followed over 1000 British soldiers exposed to mustard gas in the First World War, whilst Beebe (1960) studied an equivalent group of US veterans. Both reported a significant excess of lung cancer over expected. Norman (1975) extended the follow-up of the US veterans to 1965, but found a non-significant excess of lung cancer. There have subsequently been studies of workers manufacturing the gas.

2.43.1 Prospective studies

Japan

Wada *et al.* (1968) identified former workers of a mustard gas factory by: local enquiry, questioning individuals about their coworkers, questioning in-patients about employment, a house-to-house survey of the neighbourhood, announcements on the television. This located 2620 former employees, of whom 495 had manufactured mustard gas in 1929–45; 361 had died by 1967. There were 37 deaths from respiratory cancer, with only 0.9 expected from national rates. This included 8 deaths from laryngeal cancer and 3 from cancer of the

pharynx, but no expected figure was given for these sites; there was a possible excess of nasal cancer.

England

Tracing was successful for 428 (84%) of 510 men and women employed in mustard gas manufacture in 1939–45 in England (Manning *et al.*, 1981). Expected deaths were based on national rates. There were 2 deaths from larynx cancer and 1 from the trachea, with 0.40 expected for the 2 sites combined: O/E = 7.5, 95% CL = 1.5–21.9. There was also an excess of lung cancer (O = 21, E = 13.4, O/E = 1.6, 95% CL = 1.0–2.4).

2.43.2 Conclusions

IARC (1982d) concluded there was sufficient evidence of carcinogenicity to humans, which appeared to be particularly in those with chronic rather than sporadic occupational exposure. The above reports suggest that the upper respiratory tract is affected as well as the lung.

2.44 Nickel

This section provides the background on the initial observations of nasal cancer hazard in nickel refinery workers. There follow brief notes from case reports and case-control studies; a number of prospective studies have been reported from different countries and these are reviewed.

2.44.1 Background

The production of nickel began in a refinery in South Wales in 1902. Bridge (1933) reported that, over the previous 11 years, 9 cases of carcinoma of the nose in workers at this plant had been brought to the notice of the Chief Inspector of Factories. Pathological specimens had been studied and an oral surgeon examined a group of men; no further cases came to light with this first probe of the problem and no clue was identified as to the cause. The work's surgeon examined the sickness statistics for the past 20 years and looked at death records for the preceding 27 years (Bridge, 1934). Subsequent reports noted a steady increment in the number of nasal cancers in these workers, and also lung cancers. It was pointed out that no similar cases had been recorded in Germany, though there was a hint that this might be due to the absence of adequate checks on the existence of a problem. It was suggested that arsenic might be responsible for the cancers (Amor, 1939).

Further studies of the South Wales workers are under the Prospective studies subsection (2.44.3)— England and Wales: 1.

2.44.2 Case reports and case-control studies

Nasal cancer

Andrews (1983) described 9 patients with nasal cancer in former employees of a nickel sintering plant in Canada. No estimate of the person-years in the exposed workforce was provided.

A collaborative study investigated patients with nasal cancer in Denmark, Finland, and Sweden diagnosed in 1978–80 and controls with rectal cancer, matched for age and sex (Hernberg *et al.*, 1983a). There was a non-significant increased risk for exposure to nickel: RR = 2.4, 95% CL = 0.9–6.6.

Larynx

A case-control study of 204 newly diagnosed patients with laryngeal cancer diagnosed in 1977–79 in Ontario used individually matched neighbourhood controls. All were interviewed at home by trained interviewers (Burch *et al.*, 1981). There was an increased risk for prior exposure to nickel (RR = 1.4), but this disappeared when controlled for smoking.

A case-control study of laryngeal patients in Denmark in 1980–82 showed a raised risk for those exposed to nickel: RR = 1.7, 95% CL = 1.2–2.5 (Olsen and Sabroe, 1984).

2.44.3 Prospective studies

Canada

Workers employed in a Canadian nickel refinery in 1930–57 were classified by job into 8 exposure groups. Amongst 2000 workers there were 7 deaths from nasal cancer, with high risk in work on the furnace and sinter plant; there was no clear evidence that exposure solely to the calcining furnace contributed to sinus cancer (Mastromatteo, 1967).

England and Wales: 1

In follow-up of the original observations, discussed above under background, a series of papers have been published. Hill (1939) used estimates of the number of workmen, including pensioners from the company's book for 1931 and 1937, to estimate expected deaths in the workforce and compare these with observed deaths by cause. These were nasal cancer: O = 11, E<1, O/E = 12, 95% CL = 6.1–21.9; lung cancer: O = 16, E = 1; O/E = 16.0, 95% CL = 9.1–26.0. It appeared that this excess was restricted to process workers in the refinery.

Morgan (1958) provided a detailed description of the process. No deaths had been recorded amongst workers who had been engaged after 1924, when increased precautions had been instituted against dust.

Further studies were reported by Doll (1958), Doll, Morgan and Speizer (1970), and Doll, Mathews and Morgan (1977). This latter extension indicated that the risk had persisted until about 1930, which accorded better with environmental changes in the plant. The hazard appeared to be associated with dust from the calcination of the impure nickel copper sulphate, rather than exposure to nickel carbonyl or arsenic (which had occurred particularly at an early phase of operation from contamination in one source of sulphuric acid).

England and Wales: 2

Burges (1980) followed up 850 nickel platers from a plant in England in the period 1945–78. Expected figures were based on national rates. Only limited data were provided in a brief conference report: stomach cancer O = 8, E = 4.0, O/E = 2.0, 95% CL = 0.9–3.9; lung cancer O = 10, E = 8.2, O/E = 1.22, 95% CL = 0.6–2.2.

England and Wales: 3

Follow-up of 1925 men who had worked for at least 5 years in a plant manufacturing nickel alloys from metallic nickel in Hereford in 1953–78 was reported by Cox *et al.* (1981). Only 22 men (1.1%) were untraced. Expected values were based on national rates corrected for the local urban mortality. There was no evidence of increased deaths from respiratory or other cancers.

Japan

Tsuchiya (1965) obtained the number of deaths and numbers of employees by questionnaire from 200 large organizations in Japan in 1957–59. There was an excess of lung cancer in comparison with national-based expected figures, for those exposed to chrome and nickel. These two exposures were not analysed separately.

Norway

Pedersen, Hogetveit and Andersen (1973) followed 1916 men who had worked at a nickel refinery in Norway for at least 3 years in 1953–60 until 1971. Expected deaths were based on national rates. There was an excess of nasal, laryngeal, and lung cancer. The cohort was increased to those employed in 1953–65; 2247 men were followed up to 1979. Collection of smoking histories suggested there was an additive effect of nickel exposure and smoking (Magnus, Andersen and Hogetveit, 1982).

US

Men at a nickel refinery in the US who had worked between 1922 and 1947 were followed until 1977. Two developed a sinonasal cancer, whilst 2 others in the company also developed such tumours—one had worked on a nickel conversion plant, and the other on maintenance of the plant (Enterline and Marsh, 1982b).

2.44.4 Conclusions

In a clear review of the literature, Mastromatteo (1967) emphasized that respiratory cancer had only been in excess for workers exposed to furnace dusts and fumes containing nickel; there was no evidence that the metal or its compounds used in subsequent activities had been associated with any hazard.

IARC (1976a) stated that epidemiological studies conclusively demonstrated that there was an excess risk of cancer of the nasal cavity and lung cancer in workers in nickel refineries. This was also the view expressed in a detailed review by Sunderman (1976). There is an indication from the above material that laryngeal cancer may also be increased.

2.45 Nitrate fertilizers

Cohorts of men working at the time of the 1961 and 1971 censuses in fertilizer manufacture in England and Wales (thus potentially exposed to nitrate-containing dust) were followed until 1978. The 1961 cohort showed no excess of cancer mortality, whilst that of 1971 had excess deaths from lung and digestive tract cancer. This was surprising, as industrial conditions had improved between 1961 and 1971 (Fraser, Chilvers and Goldblatt, 1982).

2.45.1 Conclusion

The disparate findings are an inadequate base to consider that there is a genuine risk of these cancers in the industry.

2.46 Paint

A few studies have explored the cancers developing in those exposed in (*a*) manufacturing, and (*b*) using paints.

2.46.1 Manufacture

Morgan, Kaplan and Gaffey (1981) followed over 16 000 workers who had been employed for at least 1 year in paint and varnish manufacture. Increased mortality was noted for large bowel, rectal, liver, and skin cancer. Of the 12 skin cancers, there was a significant excess of melanoma: O = 10, E = 4.76, O/E = 2.10, 95% CL = 1.0–3.9.

2.46.2 Painters

Occupational mortality for England and Wales in 1970–72 (Registrar General, 1978) showed a raised SMR for painters and decorators for myeloid leukaemia.

Prospective studies

Chiazze, Ference and Wolf (1980) obtained the cause of death for men who had worked as spray painters in 10 car assembly plants in the US and died in 1970–76. PMRs showed no excess risk of lung cancer, and a case-control study was also negative with adjustment for length of exposure.

Englund (1980) used union records to identify painters in 1966 in Sweden, who were followed until 1974. Expected deaths were calculated from national rates. There was a significant excess of cancer of the oesophagus: O = 24, E = 12.3, O/E = 1.95, 95% CL = 1.2–2.9; lung cancer: O = 124, E = 97.6, O/E = 1.27, 95% CL = 1.1–1.5. There were non-significant excesses for biliary tract and larynx cancers.

These findings for intrahepatic biliary tract and oesophagus cancers were supported by an analysis from the National Cancer Environment files linking census information in 1960 with cancer registrations up to 1973.

Case-control study

The occupational history of patients attending Roswell Park hospital in 1956–65 facilitated examination of relative risk for various cancers. Houten *et al.* (1977) found an increased risk of kidney cancer in painters.

In the review of bladder cancer (*see* 4.23.1), 5 studies reported risks >1.0, and 4 risks <1.0. None of the differences were significantly different from 1.0.

2.46.3 Hazard to the next generation

Children registered with cancer in Finland in 1959–75 were identified and about 70% of the pregnancy records traced of the whole group and controls. This provided 2659 pairs of parental occupations for analysis (Hemminki *et al.*, 1981). There was increased risk for children whose fathers had worked as painters: RR = 2.75, 95% CL = 1.0–6.2.

2.46.4 Conclusion

The above studies do not show a consistent pattern of results, the positive associations are of only borderline significance, and the subjects will have been exposed to a variety of agents. They are insufficient to consider that manufacture or use of paint increases the risk of cancer.

2.47 Peat

A case-control study of 152 males with head and neck cancers treated in Ireland involved 7 with paranasal sinus cancer. Of these 7, 3 had been involved in peat production, a highly significant excess compared with the other cancers or the controls (Herity, 1984).

2.47.1 Conclusion

Though this is an isolated report for this specific (but restricted) occupation, it parallels the other studies showing excess risk of nasal cancer on exposure to vegetable dust (*see* 3.20, 3.38).

2.48 Plastics

The majority of studies on this area of work have been more specific, dealing with known or suspect exposures to vinyl chloride (VC), polyvinyl chloride (PVC), or closely related compounds (*see* 2.58). Two more general studies are briefly described in this section.

Using occupation recorded at death certification in 1970–72 in England and Wales, a proportional-mortality analysis was performed for male plastic workers. About 60% of these workers would have been wholly or partially engaged in work with PVC. With a total of 707 deaths there was a significant excess of stomach cancer: O = 24, E = 16.4, O/E = 1.5, 95% CL = 0.9–2.2 (Baxter and Fox, 1976).

A historical cohort study of 2490 males employed in plastics production in Massachusetts in 1949–66, followed over 99% until 1976. Expected deaths were based on US mortality rates. This showed a significantly raised mortality for genito-urinary cancers (RR = 1.54). There was no clear association with a particular plant for these cancers. However, with 21 different categories of occupational environment, these detailed analyses were based on small numbers of events. There was a suggestion that the development of rectal cancer in cellulose production workers and prostate cancer in polystyrene processing should be under surveillance (Marsh, 1983b).

2.48.1 Hazard to the next generation

Holmberg (1977) reported CNS defects in 2 children of mothers exposed to chemicals in the reinforced plastics industry. It was indicated that further studies were in progress, but Holmberg (1979) presented the same results.

2.48.2 Conclusion

There is no consistency between the findings of these 2 prospective studies, and no adequate evidence of a cancer hazard.

2.49 Polychlorinated biphenyls (PCBs)

Three prospective studies and one cross-sectional survey of workers exposed to PCBs are briefly reviewed.

2.49.1 Prospective studies

Bahn *et al.* (1976) reported preliminary findings of malignancies occurring in a plant in the US which had handled PCBs. Out of 92 workers, 3 developed melanomas; 31 men were heavily exposed and, in these, 2 melanomas had occurred, and 3 other cancers. The authors suggested that this was unlikely to have occurred by chance (though, as their P value was not from a specific test of an hypothesis, it is difficult to interpret). In a subsequent letter, Bahn *et al.* (1977) acknowledged that multiple exposures had been involved of other chemicals, and that further investigations were in progress.

Male and female employees working for at least 3 months in 2 plants (one in Massachusetts, the other in New York State) where PCBs were used in the manufacture of capacitors, were followed in the period 1940–76. Of 2567, the vital status was found for 98%. Expected deaths were calculated from US mortality rates (Brown and Jones, 1981). There was no death from melanoma, nor significantly raised risk for any other site of malignancy. There was also no clear relationship to length of exposure for any cancer. There were only 39 deaths from all neoplasms; thus results for specific sites were based on very low numbers.

Bertazzi *et al.* (1982) followed, until 1978, 1310 male and female workers employed for at least 6 months in 1946–70 in a plant north of Milan that manufactured electrical capacitors and used PCBs. Three cases of chloracne had occurred in 1954. There was an excess of RES neoplasms: O = 4, E = 0.91, O/E = 4.40, 95% CL = 1.2–11.2.

2.49.2 Cross-sectional survey

Eighty workers exposed to PCBs in manufacture or testing of electrical capacitors underwent clinical and laboratory investigation (Maroni *et al.*, 1981). Their average exposure had been 12 years at a plant in Italy. Four had chloracne, and 2 had fast growing haemangiomas; one of the latter workers also had chronic myelocytic leukaemia.

2.49.3 Conclusions

IARC (1978b) considered the epidemiological evidence suggestive of a relationship with malignant melanomas. Jensen (1982) proposed that PCBs might be the factor associated with office risk of melanomas, as the concentration was higher in offices than out of doors. However, this was advanced on very slender grounds.

The most recent studies fail to provide consistent evidence of risk of malignancy at a particular site.

2.50 Polynuclear aromatic hydrocarbons

The following note indicates the long-standing evidence of the hazard from various sources of polynuclear aromatic hydrocarbons (PAH), and then reviews more recent studies. A rather arbitrary division of sources of exposure has been drawn up, with the subsections arranged in alphabetical order. Many studies have involved the petroleum industry; however, as there can be other petrochemicals of very different natures involved, these studies are all dealt with in another chapter (*see* 3.23), rather than with PAH.

2.50.1 Background

Pott (1775) identified scrotal cancer as a tumour occurring predominantly in chimney sweeps, ascribing this to contact with soot. Bell (1876) described scrotal cancer in a man in the Scottish shale oil industry, whilst Wilson (1910) observed that 28 patients out of 35 with scrotal cancer in Manchester were or had been employed as mule spinners in the cotton industry. In an extension of this work, Southam and Wilson (1922) reviewed all admissions for cancer of the scrotum to the Manchester Royal Infirmary for the period 1902–22. Of 141 patients the occupations were: mule spinner 69, tar/paraffin workers 22, sweep 1, various (with no specific hazard identified) 38, not stated 11. They emphasized that cotton spinning had not hitherto been

considered an industry of importance. They described how a mule spinner worked so as to saturate the left side of his trousers with oil, particularly at waist height.

A Home Office (1926) report declared prolonged exposure to mineral oil as the prime cause of scrotal cancer. Scott (1922) described the incidence of epithelioma in the Scottish shale oil industry. It appeared that such cancers were more common in the paraffin workers than in other jobs involving distillation of shale oil and refining of products.

Kennaway and Kennaway (1946) examined the mortality of 17 occupations 'of the higher professional classes' in England and Wales for 1911–40. Only one death from scrotal cancer was found, when 22 were expected (and this individual's main job would place him in social class 4). This is indirect evidence of the powerful influence of some environmental factors affecting the manual, but not 'office' workers. In contrast, they found no evidence of a social class trend in cancer of the penis.

Henry (1946) found no increased risk in metal workers, but Cruickshank and Squire (1950) quantified the hazard from mineral oil used in the engineering industry, and also indicated the hazard from tar and pitch exposure. Cruickshank and Gourevitch (1952) also noted an increase in scrotal cancer in metal workers.

Lione and Denholm (1959) described 10 cases of cancer of the scrotum in wax pressmen. The age of onset was from 47 to 62 years; exposure varied from 14 to 32 years. No information was given about the population at risk and it is impossible to estimate the risk in these workers.

2.50.2 Atmospheric pollution

Stocks (1952) discussed the epidemiology of cancer of the lung in England and Wales. He presented a map of the London County Council, showing an appreciable difference in age-standardized mortality in males in 1946–49 in the metropolitan boroughs. There was an excess of lung cancer mortality in the East End of London and Stocks remarked 'it can hardly be supposed that the people of north-east London smoke 50% more tobacco than those in south-west London, though they might tend to smoke different brands'. He also presented data on the county boroughs in the country and at the end advanced the hypothesis that the results were not incompatible if it be supposed that the effects of tobacco and atmospheric pollution are additive. One of the main constituents of atmospheric pollution is PAH. This and comparable work (Stocks, 1960) indicates the indirect effect of industry on risk of lung cancer. The literature on the association of atmospheric pollution is extensive (*see* Royal College of Physicians, 1970).

2.50.2.1 Conclusion

Though there is evidence of increased risk of lung cancer in localities with marked air pollution, an appreciable component of atmospheric pollution has been soot from coal burned in domestic grates—the data are only tangential evidence of a possible 'neighbourhood' effect of pollution from past industrial practice.

2.50.3 Carbon black

Using data from 4 carbon black producers in the US, men were identified who had been employed in 1935–74; the analyses were based on nearly 35 000 person-years by 1974, but 2% of these in persons 65 and over. Expected deaths were calculated from state mortality rates (Robertson and Ingalls, 1980). There was a decreased risk for digestive cancer (O = 6, E = 9.6, 95% CL = 0.46–2.72) and respiratory cancers (O = 13, E = 14.7, 95% CL = 0.58–1.88). This brought up-to-date the results published by Ingalls (1950) and Ingalls and Risquez-Iribarren (1961). Exposure to carbon black also occurs to rubber workers (*see* 3.30), and printing workers (*see* 2.50.12).

2.50.3.1 Conclusion

IARC (1984) emphasized that only a small proportion of the person-years was accumulated at age 65 and over. This restricts the power to detect cancers with an appreciable latent interval. It was concluded that the data were inadequate to evaluate the carcinogenicity to humans of carbon black.

2.50.4 Chimney sweeps

Union records identified 2071 men who had been chimney sweeps for at least 10 years in Sweden; 2048 were traced in the period 1961–79. Expected mortality was calculated from the national rates. There was a significant excess lung cancer: O = 16, E = 2.3, 95% CL = 1.3–3.8 and of oesophageal cancer: O = 6, E = 0.9, O/E = 6.6, 95% CL = 2.4–14.5 (Hogstedt *et al.*, 1982).

In a report on mortality in chimney sweeps in Denmark, Hansen (1983) referred to only one specific site of cancer—lung, in which there was a significant excess of deaths (O = 5, E = 1.6, O/E = 3.12, 95% CL = 1.0–7.3).

2.50.4.1 Conclusion

Since the percipient report of Pott (1775), there has never been any doubt about the risk of skin cancer in chimney sweeps. The above reports are compatible with increased hazard from lung cancer; without

information on dose and smoking habits the results are difficult to interpret.

2.50.5 Coke plants

Coke plants are of two different designs: (*a*) for the production of metallurgical coke to be used in blast furnaces, with the secondary purposes of recovery of chemical byproducts, and (*b*) vertical or horizontal retorts for the production of gas for household or industrial use. Though the methods of coal carbonization differ, the workers may be exposed to common volatiles and chemical byproducts. This section therefore covers both types of plant.

Henry, Kennaway and Kennaway (1931) noted an excess of skin and bladder cancer in gas workers. Kuroda and Kawahata (1936) reported an excess of oesophageal, liver and gallbladder, and lung cancer deaths in coke oven workers; insufficient data were provided to assess the degree of risk. Kennaway and Kennaway (1947), using death certificates for lung cancer in England and Wales from 1921 to 1938, showed an excess risk in coal gas workers.

2.50.5.1 Prospective studies

The following notes describe prospective studies carried out on workers in coke plants in England and Wales and the US. Case-control and other laboratory studies are then briefly mentioned. *Table 2.18* shows the risk of various cancers from prospective studies of coke workers.

England and Wales: 1

A large London gas company had records of all men who became pensioners. Doll (1952) identified those taking a pension and being over 60 years of age in the period 1939–48; there were 80 deaths in this group of men. About two-thirds of the men who died had been employed in the works (e.g. on gas production and handling residues). The age 60 was used to exclude the majority of those retiring on health grounds. Expected deaths were calculated from mortality rates for Greater London. Apart from an excess of lung cancer, there was no other finding of note; employees on production of gas and waste treatment seemed particularly at risk of lung cancer.

England and Wales: 2

The cause of death was ascertained for all employees at coking plants in the UK dying in 1949–54 (Reid and Buck, 1956). Job histories were obtained and compared with those for a sample of all employees. A special census of 1952 provided an estimate of the age and job of present employees;

rates for a large (unspecified) industrial organization were used to calculate expected figures. There was an excess of lung cancer in men who had worked in the ovens. Proportional mortality of deaths in pensioners who had worked on coke ovens provided no evidence of an excess of lung cancer.

England and Wales: 3

Men employed in 4 regional gas boards in England for at least 5 years were followed from 1/9/53 for 8 years (Doll *et al.*, 1965). There were 11 499 men who had worked (*a*) on coal carbonizing, (*b*) with intermittent or other exposure to the gas-producing plant, and (*c*) on byproduct processing, maintenance, meter reading, and gas fitting; 99.6% were traced. A substantial excess of lung cancer occurred in comparison with nationally based figures; this varied from board to board (when comparisons were made with expected based on the mortality rates in the different regions). When the ratio of O/E deaths was compared across the 3 categories of exposure there was a significant trend for lung cancer ($P<0.01$) and a near significant trend for bladder cancer ($P = 0.06$).

More extensive data were reported by Doll *et al.* (1972) based on 12 years mortality in the original group and follow-up of 4687 men working in 4 other boards followed for 7–8 years. It was clear that the risk of lung cancer was greatest in the men at the top of the ovens, but the data could not distinguish difference in risk between the types of retort. There was no evidence of a hazard in men working on byproducts from the coke plants, nor was there evidence of an excess of leukaemia in the total workforce (O = 9, E = 11.3, O/E = 0.80, 95% CL = 0.4–1.5).

England and Wales: 4

Davies (1977) identified 610 men employed in 2 coke plants of the steel industry in South Wales in 1954 who were traced until 1965. It was not possible to distinguish the particular job carried out by the men. Expected deaths were obtained from national rates for 1960–63. There was no clear evidence of an increase in death from malignancy in this small group of workers.

England and Wales: 5

Nearly 7000 coke workers in plants in (*a*) British Steel, and (*b*) a branch of the Coal Board were followed over the period 1967–79 in Great Britain. Expected values were obtained from national rates and a case-control study was carried out within the study population. An excess of lung cancer was found: O = 167; E = 142.3; O/E = 1.17, 95% CL = 1.0–1.4; there was no difference between oven and non-oven workers (Hurley *et al.*, 1983).

Japan

A cohort of 504 workers employed at a gas generator plant and 25 760 workers at the location not employed on the plant were followed from 1953 to 1965. There were 6 deaths from lung cancer with only 0.135 expected in those exposed in the gas generator. The risk increased with increased duration of work (Kawai, Armamoto and Harada, 1967).

US

In a series of papers Lloyd and his colleagues examined the mortality of American steel workers. The general method and results are described in 3.16 about foundry workers.

Table 2.18 Risk of various cancers in coke workers*

Occupation	Country	Lung		Skin		Bladder		Author
		O	E	O	E	O	E	
Gas worker	England and Wales: 1	25	10.4	4	2.4	9†	5.8	Doll (1952)
Coke plant	England and Wales: 2	21	23.0			4	5.0	Reid and Buck (1956)
Gas workers	England and Wales: 3	189	140.0	3	0.5	16	10.9	Doll *et al.* (1972)
Coke ovens	England and Wales: 4	8	9.8			3†	1.2	Davies (1977)
Coke plants	England and Wales: 5	167	142.3					Hurley *et al.* (1983)
Gas generator	Japan	6	0.1					Kawai, Armamoto and Harada (1967)
Coke plants	US: 1	37‡	21.8					Lloyd (1971)
Coke ovens	US: 2	69	41.5	1	1.5	9†	4.1	Redmond *et al.* (1972)
Total		522	388.9	8	4.4	41	27.0	
O/E			1.34		1.82		1.52	
95% CL			1.2–1.5		0.8–3.6		1.1–2.1	

*See text for description of method.
†Urinary organs.
‡Respiratory system.

Lloyd *et al.* (1970) noted an increased risk of lung cancer in men working in the coking plants. A more detailed study (Lloyd, 1971) examined the lung cancer risk in 2552 men working on these plants in 1953 and followed until 1961; he also included 998 men who had been on the coke oven plant prior to 1953, but were then working elsewhere in the steel plant. Results were presented for white and non-white and compared with expected mortality for the whole population of 58 828 steel workers. Because the risk was concentrated in the coke oven operators, the study population was extended to include a sample of 3305 men working at 10 steel coke ovens elsewhere in Canada or the US for a minimum of 30 days from 1951 (Redmond, Strobino and Cypress, 1976). The mortality follow-up was extended for all men until 1966; about 1.2% were lost to follow-up. Again the expected deaths were calculated from the mortality of all the steel workers. The excess risk of lung cancer was concentrated in men working in the tops of the coke ovens; it was 10-fold in those employed there full time for more than 5 years. There was confounding of colour and place of work within the coke ovens, that resulted in an earlier reported lower risk in white workers on the plants. An increased risk of pancreatic cancer was also reported.

Mazumdar *et al.* (1975) combined the mortality data from the preceding study with analyses of work environment, based on an extensive survey of 10 installations in Pennsylvania in 1965. From 319 samples, it was possible to categorize the exposure to coal-tar-pitch volatiles. Over the period 1951–66, the age-adjusted mortality from lung cancer showed the following relationship:

	Cumulative exposure (mg/m³)			
	199	200–499	500–699	700+
Non-white	4.0	12.9	24.9	54.6
White	15.4	10.5	13.5	—

The risk was 2–3 times higher for top oven men.

2.50.5.2 Laboratory studies

Examination of lymphocytic cultures for sister chromatid exchange frequencies showed a significantly greater proportion per cell examined for 12 coke oven workers compared with 12 controls (Miner *et al.*, 1983).

Repeated sputum cytology and lung function tests were carried out on 3799 male coke-oven workers for a 3-year period. Those with persistent metaplasia evident had reduced lung function. It was suggested that sputum cytology could thus identify those at risk of both chronic obstructive lung disease and lung cancer (Madison, Afifi and Mittman, 1984).

2.50.5.3 Case-control studies

In the review of 16 case-control studies on bladder cancer (*see* 4.23.1), only 2 mentioned gas production and these had RR of OC and 2.0, but neither were significantly raised. No occupation indicating coke work was provided in the other 14 studie.

A study of 74 patients with renal pelvis cancer showed an increased risk for men who had been exposed to coal or natural gas: RR = 2.9, 95% CL = 1.0–8.2 (McLaughlin *et al.*, 1983).

2.50.5.4 Conclusion

The 8 reports included in *Table 2.18* provide clear evidence of increased risk of lung cancer in coke workers. Other data indicate particular parts of the plant in which the risk may be especially high. Five of the studies combined provide a significantly raised risk of bladder cancer, though this has not been strongly supported by case-control studies.

2.50.6 Diesel fumes

Deaths in 235 110 Ohio railway workers in 1953–58 were compared with the expected, based on national age, sex, and calendar specific rates. The deaths from lung cancer were subdivided by exposure to fumes:

	O	E	O/E	95%CL
Regularly exposed				
to fumes	49	56.0	0.87	0.6–1.2
Occasionally exposed	67	93.5	0.72	0.6–0.9
Non-exposed	38	42.5	0.89	0.6–1.2

The workforce included males and females, though no lung cancer deaths occurred in the females (Kaplan, 1959). No reason was given for the deficiency of lung cancer.

Follow-up of 43 826 male pensioners from the Canadian National Railway from 1965 to 1977 showed an elevated risk from lung cancer (O = 993, E = 881.0, O/E = 1.06, 95% CL = 1.1–1.2). When this was split into not/possibly/probably exposed to diesel fumes, the RR values were 1.0/1.20/1.35 (Howe *et al.*, 1983).

A study of London Transport maintenance workers is discussed in 2.50.11. A proportion of the men were those working at night tuning running diesel engines; they would have been exposed to fumes.

2.50.6.1 Conclusion

The above studies provide no evidence of an increased risk of lung cancer in those exposed to diesel fumes.

2.50.7 Mineral oil

2.50.7.1 Scrotal cancer

The background section referred to the identification of the hazard of scrotal cancer in mule spinners working in the cotton industry and then the recognition that other workers were also at risk.

Fife (1962) reported the development of scrotal cancer in 2 machine tool setters working in the same machine shop. Waterhouse (1971) compared the death rate for scrotal cancer in the Birmingham region with that for the whole of England and Wales; there was an ascending trend in the Birmingham region, with the reverse for the country. This was compatible with the growth of the number of skilled metal workers in the Birmingham locality, and the decline of mule spinning elsewhere.

Full occupational histories were obtained for 88 of 103 men with scrotal cancer in the Manchester region in 1962–68. Fifty-one had worked as mule spinners, 11 had been exposed to cutting oils, 6 to tar products, and 14 to oils and other agents. Only 5 subjects failed to identify any aetiological agent (Lee, Alderson and Downes, 1972). Comparable data were obtained for 109 out of 253 men with scrotal cancer registered in the Birmingham region in 1950–72. Ninety-four had been exposed to oils, predominantly in tool setting and machine operating. About half of these had been exposed to neat oil and most of the remainder both neat and soluble oils (Brown, Waldron and Waterhouse, 1975).

Kipling and Waldron (1976) showed that in the period 1936–72, the proportion of scrotal cancers thought to be due to oil exposure had steadily risen whilst those associated with pitch and tar had fallen.

Kipling (1971) described the relatively high incidence of scrotal cancer in the Savoy Alps, and commented on appreciable international variation in incidence or mortality of scrotal cancer. One small Swedish factory was noted to have 8 men with oil-induced scrotal cancer (Avellan *et al.*, 1967), although collection of occupational histories for subjects from the Swedish National Cancer Register failed to identify oil exposure in two-thirds of a small sample (Wahlberg, 1974).

A case-control study of 45 men with scrotal cancer diagnosed in Connecticut in 1935–75 showed a marked risk for potential exposure to cutting oils (RR = 10.5; 95% CL = 4.0–36.9). The risk persisted to the period after 1966 and 'accounted' for over half of the cancers (Roush *et al.*, 1982).

The history of scrotal cancer has been reviewed by Waldron (1983). He drew attention to the shift in hazard from cotton workers to engineering workers exposed to cutting oils, and noted that the number of notifications and deaths in England and Wales had fallen to a low level.

Analysis of data on 95 men with scrotal cancer from the Connecticut cancer registry for 1935–79

did not indicate any decline in risk of this tumour. Review of the published data confirmed a change in the occupations contributing to risk from mule spinning, oil and wax refining, and exposure to tar and soot, to increasing risk from metal working (Roush, Schymura and Flannery, 1984).

2.50.7.2 Other sites of malignancy

Kinnear *et al.* (1955) examined 3023 persons employed for an average of 16 years in the jute industry in Dundee at 7 firms. In 219 (7.2%) there were premalignant skin changes, oil acne in 465 (15.4%), and both changes in 8 (0.3%). This survey had been prompted from clinical observation of skin changes in elderly jute workers and skin cancers seen at the outpatients in jute workers in 1952–53.

Mastromatteo (1955) reported 6 cases of skin cancer in one Canadian plant particularly drawn from automatic machine operators. On follow-up of patients with scrotal cancer registered in the Birmingham region, Waterhouse (1971; 1972) showed they developed a significant excess of second primary skin cancers (*see also* Lung cancer in next subsection on Oil mists).

Using occupational histories for patients admitted to Roswell Park in 1956–65, Decoufle *et al.* (1977) reported that those potentially exposed to cutting and mineral oils had increased risk for: buccal cavity and pharynx (RR = 2.58 in print workers); prostate (RR = 2.09 in mechanics and repairmen); leukaemia (RR = 2.85 in machinists).

Ninety-eight workers exposed to an antirust oil in 1954–57 at a Swedish plant were followed until 1976; all were traced. Expected cancers were based on national rates. Of the 78 women, 12 had developed cancers by 1973 (E = 3.9). However, the study was mounted because 3 of these cancers were reported amongst the staff in the packing department (Jarvholm and Lavenius, 1981).

The case-control studies on aetiology of bladder cancer (*see* 4.23.1) indicate a number of results in workers potentially exposed to mineral oils. Four of 5 reports of machinists showed significantly raised risks; of 7 reports of exposure to cutting oils, gasoline, grease, or oil, 5 showed a raised risk, but only 2 were significant.

2.50.7.3 Conclusions

IARC (1984) concluded that there was sufficient evidence that mineral oils (containing various additives and impurities), which had been used in occupations such as mule spinning, metal machining, and jute processing, were carcinogenic to humans. The results presented above confirm the continuing hazard of skin cancer.

Table 2.19 Lung cancer in men exposed to oil mists at work*

Occupation	Country	Data–years	No. subj.	O	E	O/E	Author
Machine operators	US	1942–61	343	10	11.0†	0.91	Ely *et al.* (1970)
Various	England and Wales	1930–67	228	32	11.6	2.75	Waterhouse (1971)
Machine operators	US	1938–67	2485	38	33.9	1.12	Decoufle (1978)
Metal industry	Sweden	1958–76	788	3	5.4	0.56	Jarvholm *et al.* (1981)
Total				83	61.9	1.34	
95% CL						1.1–1.7	

*See text for description of method.
†Not corrected for age or calendar period.

2.50.8 Oil mists

A particular aspect of exposure to lubricating and other oils is the risk of exposing the worker to fine droplets from oil mist thrown off from lubricants on various high-speed pieces of machinery. This subsection describes a number of studies of workers exposed to this possible hazard. The section on printing workers (*see* 2.50.12) is also relevant, as it has been suggested that the lung cancer excess in such workers is a reflection of oil mist exposure.

The main emphasis of the published studies has been on lung cancer. These are reviewed first, in chronological order. The main results are given in *Table 2.19.* This is followed by notes relating to other sites of cancer.

2.50.8.1 Lung cancer

Kennaway and Kennaway (1947) found a deficit of lung cancer deaths in 'cotton spinners and doublers' in England and Wales in 1921–28, despite the suggestion that these workers were exposed to oil mists.

Huguenin, Fauvet and Mazabraud (1950) reported 2 cases of oil pneumonia in association with lung cancer, whilst amongst 144 cases of pulmonary carcinoma occupations involving regular exposure to oil sprays and vapours were 'frequently represented'. (These data are hard to interpret without specific observed and expected figures.)

Jones (1961) reported on the health of 19 workers exposed to oil mists in a steel rolling mill in South Wales for 9–18 years. None had developed lung cancer—but this should not be considered a negative finding, because of the very small number of men involved and the very low probability of detecting cancers in those fit for work.

Ely *et al.* (1970) identified 343 deaths in men exposed to oil mists and 3122 deaths in other workers in Kodak plants in Rochester, US in 1942–61. There were 10 deaths from respiratory cancer in the exposed (2.9% of all deaths) and 99 (3.2%) in the non-exposed. No allowance was made

for age or calendar period of deaths; no information was given for smoking.

Waterhouse (1971) followed 187 men who had developed scrotal cancer in the Birmingham area in 1950–67. There were 22 who developed lung cancer, with only 8.3 expected. Waterhouse (1972) extended these findings to all men developing scrotal cancer in the period 1935–49. There were an additional 41 subjects of whom 10 had second primaries, with 3.34 expected. The excess seemed to involve skin, lung, and upper gastrointestinal tract.

Two thousand four hundred and eighty-five white men exposed to cutting oil mists for at least 5 years from various metal machining processes at one plant in the US were followed in the period 1938–67 (Decoufle, 1978); 98% were traced to the end of 1967, but it was not explained why this was not continued to a later date. Expected deaths were based on national rates. The plant had used soluble, insoluble, and synthetic cutting fluids at different times. Jobs were divided into those in metal machining with heavy exposure, and others with moderate or minimal exposure. (A preliminary analysis, based on 5189 workers who had been employed for one year at least was presented by Decoufle, 1976.) There was a slight increase in deaths from lung cancer.

Cancer developing in 788 men exposed to oil mist for at least 5 years in the metal industry in Sweden in 1958–76 was compared with expected numbers based on national rates. Only 22 (3%) were lost to follow-up. There were 3 who developed lung cancer, with 5.4 expected. In contrast, there were 4 with scrotal cancer, but none expected (Jarvholm *et al.*, 1981).

2.50.8.2 Other cancers

Henry, Kennaway and Kennaway (1931) found a two-fold excess of deaths from bladder cancer in 'cotton spinners and doublers' in England and Wales in 1921–28. It had been suggested that these workers were exposed to oil mists.

Coggon, Pannett and Acheson (1984) used occupation recorded at death registration in England and Wales in 1975–79 to examine the risk of bladder cancer via a job-exposure matrix. This identified effects with exposure to cutting oils (RR = 1.5, 95% CL = 0.8–2.8).

Proportional-mortality analysis was used to compare 232 deaths from cancer in the optical manufacturing industry and control workers in a Massachusetts town (predominantly textile workers) in 1956–75. Cardiovascular deaths were used as the reference disease. There was an excess of cancers particularly of the lower gastrointestinal tract; risks were 3.2 and 2.6 for medium and long-term workers. This was the only site for which results were presented. Wang, Wegman and Smith (1983) suggested that the result may reflect exposure to abrasives or cutting oil mists.

A case-control study of patients with nasal cancer in the United States showed an increased risk for those exposed to cutting oils (Roush *et al.*, 1980): RR = 2.8, 95% CL = 1.4–5.7. However these results were dependent on exclusion of some jobs with possible exposure to oil mist.

2.50.8.3 Conclusions

Hendricks *et al.* (1962) reviewed the available data at that time and suggested that the cancer risk from oil mists was 'unknown'. There have been a number of published studies since then. The pooled results are shown in *Table 2.19* and indicate a statistically increased risk of lung cancer. However, in the absence of hard data on smoking, and more detail of the work environment, it is not conclusive that the oil mist exposure is the causal factor.

The evidence of risk of other cancers is less convincing.

2.50.9 Hazard to the next generation

Fabia and Thuy (1974) examined the occupation reported for fathers at the time of birth of children who subsequently died of malignant disease in Quebec province in 1965–70. The occupations were compared with those reported for a control group of birth registrations. These authors identified an excess of fathers in hydrocarbon-related occupations, compared with controls (RR = 2.1). These occupations included motor vehicle mechanic, machinist, miner, and painter; the leukaemia excess was found particularly in the motor vehicle mechanic and machinist groups. Using a slight variation in technique, Hakulinen, Salonen and Teppo (1976) failed to find any excess of fathers reporting hydrocarbon-related occupations in children registered with malignant disease in Finland.

Children born in 1947–59 and 1963–67 in Massachusetts who died of cancer by the age of 15 were identified, and controls selected from the birth registers. To check the earlier findings, Kwa and Fine (1980) particularly searched for an associated parental occupation: (*a*) motor vehicle mechanic and service station attendant; (*b*) machinist, miner, and lumberman; (*c*) painters, dyers, and cleaners. No excess risk for these occupations was identified.

Zack *et al.* (1980) compared the occupational histories of parents of 296 children with cancer, with those of the children's uncles and aunts, the parents of neighbourhood children, and the parents of children without cancer attending the same hospital. There was no evidence of a relationship between cancer and parental occupation involving hydrocarbon exposure.

2.50.9.1 Conclusion

IARC (1984) emphasized that the above 4 studies had covered a range of different potential exposures and that their results were inconsistent.

2.50.10 Pitch and tar

Kennaway (1925) drew attention to the high risk of scrotal and facial skin cancer in men exposed to pitch and tar. An examination of occupation for all lung cancer deaths in England and Wales in 1921–32 showed an increased risk in those exposed to coal tar (Kennaway and Kennaway, 1936).

Men applying hot pitch or asphalt to roofs and buildings were identified by union records in the US and 5939 working in 1960 followed to 1971. Expected deaths were obtained by using national mortality rates. There were significant excess deaths for buccal cavity and pharynx (RR = 1.68), colorectal cancer (1.35), lung (1.40), prostate (1.47), and leukaemia (1.68). There were also non-significant excesses of stomach and bladder cancer (Hammond *et al.*, 1976).

2.50.10.1 Conclusion

Though there is no doubt of the carcinogenic potential from exposure to pitch and tar, the workforce potentially exposed is likely to be difficult to identify and follow-up. There has been only the one US study of such workers in the recent past providing estimates of the risk for various malignancies.

2.50.11 Other

Putoni *et al.* (1979) showed an increase in lung and bladder cancer in shipyard workers in Genoa. This was possibly associated with high levels of PAH in the work environment (Valerio *et al.*, 1982).

Rushton, Alderson and Nagarajah (1983) examined the mortality patterns of 8490 maintenance workers employed by London Transport in 1967–75. There was no clear evidence of any increase in a specific malignancy; after adjusting the expected deaths for Greater London rates, there was a deficiency of lung cancer (O = 102, E = 117, O/E = 0.87, 95% CL = 0.7–1.1).

A study of aluminium workers by Theriault *et al.* (1984) (*see also* 3.2) suggested that the bladder cancer risk was associated with tar and PAH exposure levels in one specific process.

Examination of the SMR for cervix cancer in married women by husbands' social class and potential exposure to soot, tar and mineral oil showed no consistent evidence of increased ratios for higher exposure within social class (Zakelj, Fraser and Inskip, 1984).

2.50.11.1 Conclusion

These miscellaneous reports cover a range of possible exposures and fail to provide evidence of a consistent set of results. However, because of the undoubted carcinogenicity for animals and humans of PAH in general, the results from the aluminium and shipyard workers are consistent with other evidence.

2.50.12 Printing workers

Ask-Upmark (1955) pointed out that in a group of 125 patients with lung cancer diagnosed in Stockholm, 8 (6.4%) were printing workers, all of whom had been exposed to printing ink. In the general population only 1.14% were printing workers, about one-third of whom would be exposed to printing ink. There have subsequently been a number of studies of printing workers, which have indicated an increased risk of lung cancer. Because of the possible increase in risk in other sites of malignancy in these workers and the lack of clear proof that it is the oil mist that is the important factor, the studies are reviewed here rather than in the section on oil mist (*see* 2.50.8).

2.50.12.1 Prospective studies

Eight studies of groups of printing workers are briefly described; the results being presented in *Table 2.20*. A number of case-control studies have included analyses of the risk of various cancers for printing workers; these studies are mentioned with their key results.

England and Wales: 1

Eleven London newspaper printing companies and 5 from Manchester identified 3485 deaths occurring to workers and pensioners in 1952–66. Proportional-mortality analysis was performed, using mortality rates for the region of residence to calculate the expected figures (Greater London and the Manchester conurbation). The only cancer presented was lung; for all workers there was an excess. In Manchester, but not in London, the excess appeared to be concentrated in the machine room (Moss, Scott and Atherley, 1972).

England and Wales: 2

In order to investigate an anecdotal report of excess bladder tumours, Greenberg (1972) obtained death certificates for 670 men in 1954–66, who had worked in a London newspaper printing firm (one of the ones also studied by Moss, Scott and Atherley). Greater London mortality rates were used to calculate expected deaths, using proportional analysis. There was no evidence of an excess risk of bladder cancer, but a significant excess of stomach and lung cancer.

Italy

Follow-up of 700 newspaper printing workers in Italy in 1956–75, in comparison with expected based on national rates, showed a significant excess of lung cancer in 'packers and forwarders'. It was not clear whether this was due to some specific environmental factor, or a chance finding in the subset of workers (Bertazzi and Zocchetti, 1980).

US: 1

Goldstein, Bendit and Tyroler (1970) traced the deaths in about 460 pressmen exposed to oil mists and about 700 unexposed compositors in New York in 1947–62. There were 3 deaths from lung cancer in the pressmen and 6 in the compositors in this period. No information on smoking was collected, though pressmen could not smoke whilst working on a press run. The age distribution of the workers is also not provided; unless there were extreme differences in the proportion of the elderly between the two groups of workers, the lung cancer mortality seems very similar.

The above study was extended by Pasternak and Ehrlich (1972), who followed 778 printing pressmen and 1207 compositors in New York in the period 1958–69. They compared the deaths in the two groups, but used an unconventional analysis which makes it impossible to judge the risk of specific causes of death in the pressmen.

Table 2.20 Risk of various cancers in follow-up of printing workers*

Country	Buc.cav.phar		Stomach		Colorectal		Liver		Pancreas		Larynx		Lung		Prostate		Bladder		Leukaemia	
	O	E	O	E	O	E	O	E	O	E	O	E	O	E	O	E	O	E	O	E
England and Wales: 1													85	60.3						
England and Wales: 2			29	20.5									93	70.0					4	3.3
Italy											3	1.5	13	8.8						
US: 2	22	13.6	26	26.5	74	60.7	28	27.0	20	19.8	9	6.9	138	129.6					20	18.7
US: 3	11	13.9	23	21.2	50	42.4	13	8.9	5	3.9	3	7.5	84	95.0	38	30.5	17	12.1	16	11.6
US: 4	2	2.2	3	4.3			1	0.9					22	14.8	4	5.4	2	2.4	7	2.8
US: 5	17	6.8	13	20.8	34	39.0			12	12.5	5	4.1	72	54.8	25	16.3	14	9.4	10	6.9
Total	52	36.5	94	93.3	158	142.1	42	36.8	37	36.2	20	20.0	507	433.3	67	52.2	33	23.9	57	43.3
O/E	1.42		1.01		1.11		1.14		1.02		1.00		1.17		1.28		1.38		1.32	
95% CL	1.1–1.9		0.8–1.2		0.9–1.3		0.8–1.5		0.7–1.4		n.a.		1.1–1.3		1.0–1.6		0.9–1.9		1.0–1.7	

*See text for description of method.

US: 2

A proportional-mortality analysis was carried out on 2604 deaths recorded in 1966–68 in printing pressmen from union records in the US. The men could be separated into newspaper and commercial pressmen, and paper handlers (Lloyd, Decoufle and Salvin, 1977). Expected figures were based on US white males in 1967. Though there was no significant excess of lung cancer, there was for buccal cavity and pharyngeal cancer.

US: 3

A proportional-mortality analysis of 347 deaths of male employees in a printing plant in Washington in the period 1948–77 showed a significant excess of colon cancer, Hodgkin's disease, and multiple myeloma. Expected figures were based on the mortality rates for the District of Columbia (Greene *et al.*, 1979).

US: 4

Follow-up of 1361 newspaper web pressmen working for at least 1 year in 1949–65 in Los Angeles until 1978 showed a significant excess of leukaemia and kidney cancer compared with national statistics (Paganini-Hill *et al.*, 1980).

US: 5

Using union records, 1769 men employed in 1950 (or formerly employed) as pressmen in New York were identified. Many had been employed prior to 1930. Follow-up was completed for 98.6%. Expected mortality was based on rates for New York City white males. Analysis of the overall pattern of deaths suggested that the respiratory cancer excess could not be accounted for by a 20% excess in smoking (Nicholson *et al.*, 1981).

2.50.12.2 Case-control studies

The following general studies have been included as they provided brief mention of risk in printing workers.

Buccal cavity and pharynx

The Roswell Park study of occupations for patients admitted in 1956–65 led to analysis of risks for various occupations exposed to mineral oils (Decoufle *et al.*, 1977). Print workers had a significantly increased risk of cancer of the buccal cavity and pharynx (RR = 2.58), which remained after adjustment for smoking.

Nasal cancer

A general survey of patients registered with nasal cancer in England and Wales in 1963–67 obtained information on occupation from hospitals, patients, or next-of-kin (Acheson, Cowdell and Rang, 1981). A non-significantly raised risk was found for printers.

Lung cancer

Deaths from lung cancer in Los Angeles in 1968–70 and registrations in 1972–73 were analysed by reported occupation (Menck and Henderson, 1976). There was a significantly increased risk for 'pressmen' (O = 20; E = 7.2, O/E = 2.76; 95% CL = 1.7–4.3).

Skin, other than melanoma

Whitaker, Lee and Downes (1979) obtained detailed occupational histories from 598 patients with skin cancer in north-west England, with more restricted information from 148 patients. Comparing the histories with the distribution of workers by occupation reported in the 1931 and 1951 censuses, they found an increased risk from paper and printing work. There did not appear to be any effect from eye colour, previous residence in the tropics, or smoking.

Bladder

Six case-control studies of bladder cancer (*see* 4.23.1) have reported risks for printing workers; only 2 had a significantly raised risk, whilst 2 had a risk well below 1.0.

2.50.12.3 Conclusions

Table 2.20 indicates that the lung cancer excess has been consistently found in different studies; there is also a significant excess of buccal cavity but not laryngeal cancer. IARC (1984) does not comment specifically whether the risk of lung cancer in printing workers is due to oil mists, or other environmental factors.

Some of the other raised risks are based on small numbers, but the pattern of results does not just appear to reflect differences in smoking habits.

2.51 Silica exposure

A number of different occupational groups are exposed to silica, particularly as dust which may be inhaled or swallowed in phlegm. Sections have dealt with the individual occupations: foundry workers (3.16), miners (3.22), quarrymen (3.28).

Table 2.21 Risk of lung cancer in workers exposed to silica in various occupations*

Occupation	Country	Data years	Sex	No. subj.	O	E	O/E	Author
Foundry workers	See Table 3.2		M		805	525.5	1.5	Various
Granite workers	US	1952–78	M		62	52.6†	1.2	Davis *et al.* (1983)
Miners	See Table 3.4		M		1627	1344.5	1.2	Various
Pottery workers	US	1955–77	M		178	146.6†	1.2	Thomas (1982)
Pottery workers	US	1955–77	F		15	16.0	0.9	Thomas (1982)
Quarry‡	England and Wales	1970–72	M		56	40.3	1.4	Registrar General (1978)
Sandblasters	Italy	1960–75	M	190	16	4.2	3.8	Putoni *et al.* (1979)
Silicosis register	Sweden	1931–69	M	3610	49	17.5	2.8	Westerholm (1980)
Silicosis register	Canada	1940–75	M	1190	45	22.7	2.0	Finkelstein, Kusiack and Suranyi (1982)
Fettlers/metal dressers	England and Wales	1970–72	M		70	54.3	1.3	Registrar General (1978)
Total					2923	2224.2	1.3	
95% CL							1.2–1.4	

*See text for description of method.
†PMR.
‡Surface workers in non-coal mines and quarries.

2.51.1 Lung cancer

Goldsmith, Guidotti and Johnson (1982) reviewed a number of studies on workers exposed to silica and demonstrated wide agreement from different occupations in various countries of an increased risk of lung cancer. The results from a number of these studies are presented in *Table 2.21*. Some of the reports are based on occupational-mortality statistics, whilst others have already been reviewed in the discrete sections on the relevant industry. Two studies relate to workers known to have silicosis.

Westerholm (1980) examined the mortality of 3610 males known to the Swedish silicosis register in 1931–69. Expected deaths were calculated for lung cancer using national mortality rates. Although this was a major analysis, data were only presented for this site, other cancers, and all causes of mortality.

Using compensation records, Finkelstein, Kusiak and Suranyi (1982) identified 1910 miners registered with silicosis in Ontario in 1940–75, who were followed until 1978. Expected deaths were based on province mortality rates. There was a two-fold excess of lung cancer deaths in those awarded compensation in 1940–59, but no increase in those diagnosed after this period.

All deaths occurring in Vermont granite workers in 1952–78 were identified and the observed distribution compared with expected proportions based on US mortality (Davis *et al.*, 1983). Industrial information was available and work histories, thus enabling estimates to be made of dust exposure. For lung cancer, O = 62, E = 52.6, O/E = 1.2, 95% CL = 0.9–1.5. There was no indication of increased risk with increased dust exposure.

2.51.2 Stomach cancer

In an analysis of occupational histories of all patients admitted to Roswell Park Institute in 1948–51, Kraus, Levin and Gerhardt (1957) found an association of stomach cancer with exposure to inorganic dusts with free silica, in a case-control study of inpatients at Rothwell Park Hospital, US. For those exposed for more than 10 years, RR = 2.56, 95% CL = 1.2–5.7.

Kurppa, Koskela and Guobergsson (1982) found an excess of gastrointestinal cancer on follow-up of over 1000 males who had worked for at least 3 months in the granite industry and been exposed to quartz particles. There was a significant excess of these tumours (O = 15, E = 7.4, O/E = 2.03, 95% CL = 1.1–3.3).

2.51.3 Pottery workers

Union records were used to identify deaths of 2924 male and 946 female pottery workers dying in the US in 1955–77. Expected figures were based on national data, and PMRs were calculated. There was a significant excess of lung cancer, which was restricted to males making ceramic plumbing fixtures (Thomas, 1982).

2.51.4 Conclusions

Maillard (1980) pointed out the difficulty of assessing the lung cancer hazard in those exposed to silica. In Switzerland, the miners also worked in an atmosphere with radon contamination and low level benzpyrene.

The above reports and the data in *Table 2.21* show a clear excess of lung cancer in those exposed to silica. However, it is by no means clear whether this is a marker of exposure to a range of other relevant but unspecified carcinogens. The data on gastro-intestinal cancer is insufficient to consider an evaluation.

2.52 Solvents

Other sections have dealt with potential exposure to specific solvents: benzene (2.8); petrochemical industry (3.23); rubber industry (3.30). The following is based on a more general report of environmental pollution.

Capurro and Eldridge (1978) reported an excess of RES tumours in a small group of individuals living near a chemical recycling plant in the US. There had been evidence of solvent exposure in the atmosphere since 1961, which was reduced in 1971; this included ketones, alcohol, aromatic hydrocarbons, and other compounds. In the period 1968–74 there was an excess of deaths from non-Hodgkin's lymphoma, compared with expected based on local mortality rates: O = 3, E = 0.04, O/E = 75.0, 95% CL = 15.1–29.1.

2.52.1 Hazard to the next generation

A case-control study of 120 mothers of children with CNS defects registered in Finland in 1976–78 showed an increased risk from exposure to organic solvents in the first trimester: RR = 6.5, 95% CL = 1.8–23.6 (Holmberg, 1979).

A questionnaire of pregnancy outcome was completed by 782 women employed in laboratories in Gothenberg university in 1968–79. There was a non-significant increase in miscarriage rate in those exposed to solvents: RR = 1.31, 95% CL = 0.9–1.9. There was no evidence of a solvent effect on perinatal mortality or congenital malformations (Axelsson, Lutz and Rylander, 1984). The validity of the data was assessed by Axelsson and Rylander (1984). For 12% of the reported miscarriages, confirmation was not obtained from hospital records, and in these unverified ones there was a high reported exposure to solvents.

2.52.2 Conclusions

The US geographical study is difficult to evaluate in the absence of other studies of such exposed populations. The studies on pregnancy outcome

require repeating with more specific definition of exposure.

2.53 Styrene

2.53.1 Prospective studies of manufacturing plants

A study of 563 workers employed for at least 5 years in a styrene polymerization plant in Pennsylvania (Lilis and Nicholson, 1976) identified 3 deaths from leukaemia and lymphoma. However, no expected figures were provided and there had also been exposure to benzene. It is not clear whether the following report also relates to the same plant. Union records identified all who had worked for at least 5 years by 1960 at a large styrene monomer and polymerization plant in the US. All 560 males were followed from 1960 or the tenth anniversary of first exposure until 1975. Expected deaths were based on national mortality rates. Though there were obvious increases in cancer deaths, this was based on small numbers (Nicholson, Selikoff and Seidman, 1978). Reference is made in the text to possible increase in leukaemia and other RES neoplasms, for those working at least 6 months in the plant; however, expected numbers were not provided and further follow-up was stated to be in progress.

Frentzel-Beyme, Thiess and Weilland (1978) studied 1960 men employed on a German plant manufacturing styrene and polystyrene for at least 1 month in 1931–75; 93% of the German workers were traced, but only 29% of foreign workers. A proportional-mortality analysis, using national mortality, showed no increase in malignant deaths for the total group (O = 11, E = 13.6, O/E = 0.81, 95% CL = 0.4–1.4). Though subgroups of the workforce were analysed, these were based on very small numbers of deaths. The absence of any evidence of risk in German workers employed for more than 5 years does not provide a conclusive negative.

Ott *et al.* (1980) used company records and hygiene measurements in a study of the mortality of nearly 3000 workers employed for at least 1 year on styrene production in a Michigan plant from 1937 to 1970, followed up to 1975. Only 88 individuals were lost to follow-up, but the persons-years at risk or average follow-up was not quoted. US mortality and incidence rates were used as well as company statistics to calculate expected figures. There were 6 deaths from leukaemia; the expected value was 3.4 using US rates for all men, and 2.9 for those in production and non-technical research, but only 1.6 when using company rates. (The later differences were statistically significant.) An increase in lymphatic leukaemia in those exposed to polymer extrusion, solvents, and colourants was observed, but had no relation to duration or intensity of exposure. The study was complicated by multiple exposure and small numbers.

Werner (1980, unpublished observations) examined the patterns of mortality of 622 workers from 1945 to 1974 who had at least 1 year's history of work in a UK styrene plant. There were 3 deaths from lymphoma with an expected of 0.64, based on England and Wales mortality statistics with a regional correction (RR = 4.7, 95% CL = 0.9–13.7). However, there was only short exposure for 2 of the 3 deaths, with probable mixed exposure to other chemicals.

2.53.2 Rubber workers

A number of studies of rubber workers have commented on possible hazards to those exposed to styrene, but interpretation is difficult due to mixed exposure (*see* 3.30). For example, in the study of over 8000 white male workers (Andjelkovic *et al.*, 1977), a subgroup were exposed on the synthetic rubber plant to styrene–butadiene. There was an excess of lung cancer in 1964–73 (O = 3, E = 0.73, O/E = 4.09, 95% CL = 0.8–12.0). This is the Akron Company B in the rubber section (3.30.1).

Case reports of various RES neoplasms in workers from styrene–butadiene rubber plants were provided by Spirtas (1977) and Block (1977).

Spirtas (1977) reported a case-control study of workers developing RES neoplasms at the Akron rubber plant (the data years were not given). There were 60 cases, with 180 matched controls. Review of job histories showed an increased risk for those on styrene–butadiene production: RR = 2.4, 95% CL = 0.6–9.2.

In order to explore the possible associations of work with styrene–butadiene, Taulbee *et al.* (1977) carried out 3 studies at the Akron rubber plants: (*a*) using the 1964 cohort, the mortality of men spending the longest portion of their working time on synthetic latex production was compared with that of all workers; there was no RES death in the synthetic group of workers; (*b*) a case-control study of leukaemia deaths in those who had spent time in various sections of the plants; there was no clearly increased risk for potential exposure to styrene; (*c*) a case-control study of RES other than leukaemia in the same departments showed some association with work in the synthetic latex production area, though the added risk was small if it did exist. The details of this report are very limited.

Meinhardt, Young and Hartle (1978) reported 9 patients with leukaemia who had worked at 2 plants producing styrene–butadiene rubber in Texas in 1967–78. No information was given of the total workforce or the expected incidence. Some information was given on the environmental exposures of workers on the plants.

2.53.3 Laboratory studies

Blood samples were taken from 16 men aged 21–51, who had worked as styrene laminators in 2 plants in Finland for 1–15 years. There was an excess of abnormal chromosomes (especially breaks) compared with controls. There was no evidence of increased frequency of sister chromatid exchanges compared with the controls (Meretoja *et al.*, 1978).

Fleig and Theiss (1978b) reported an excess of chromosomal aberrations in a small group of workers involved in manual finishing processes on styrene products, which involved a higher exposure to styrene than those men working on the initial manufacturing stages. The workers were also exposed to solvents (especially methylene chloride and acetone), and to epoxide resin and their hardeners.

2.53.4 Conclusions

Zielhuis (1979) and the Health and Safety Executive (1981b) reviewed the health hazards from styrene; neither found evidence from epidemiological studies of carcinogenicity to man. IARC (1979a) pointed out that various studies of workers potentially exposed to styrene–butadiene polymer were based on small numbers of subjects, with mixed exposures. It was concluded that these results could not be evaluated.

2.54 Tetrachloroethane

Norman, Robinette and Fraumeni (1981) followed 1099 white US males who had been exposed to tetrachloroethane whilst impregnating clothing in the Second World War. Overall cancer mortality was increased: RR = 1.26 (based on 1319 non-exposed workers). The risks of genital cancer, leukaemia, and lymphoma were moderately but not significantly raised.

2.54.1 Conclusion

IARC (1979b) concluded that there was limited evidence of carcinogenicity to animals, but insufficient evidence to evaluate the hazard to man. The above study does not alter this conclusion.

2.55 Tetrachloroethylene

Exposure to tetrachloroethylene has usually occurred with mixed exposure to other solvents.

Union records identified 330 deaths occurring amongst laundry and dry-cleaning workers in the Kansas area in 1957–77 (Blair, Decoufle and

Grauman, 1979). Compared with national statistics, there was an excess of deaths from malignancies: O = 87, E = 67.9, O/E = 1.29, 95% CL = 1.0–1.6. Significant excesses were noted for lung: O = 17, E = 10, O/E = 1.7, 95% CL = 1.0–2.7 and cervix cancer: O = 10, E = 4.8, O/E = 2.08, 95% CL = 1.0–3.8. The workers would have been exposed to mixed solvents; although tetrachloroethylene was likely to have been the predominant fluid used, exposure probably occurred to carbon tetrachloride and benzene.

Other studies included in the section on trichloroethylene (*see* 2.56) also involved some exposure to tetrachloroethylene.

2.55.1 Conclusion

IARC (1982d) considered the epidemiological data inadequate, whilst there was limited evidence of carcinogenicity from animal experiments.

2.56 Trichloroethylene

A few limited studies have been reported on the mortality of workers exposed to trichloroethylene. Also one case-control study included questions about exposure to this chemical.

2.56.1 Prospective studies

Biological monitoring of Swedish workers identified 518 exposed to trichloroethylene in various work places in 1955–70, who were followed to 1975. There were 11 deaths from malignant disease with 14.5 expected from national rates (Axelson *et al.*, 1978b).

Union records identified 330 deaths occurring amongst laundry and dry-cleaning workers in the Kansas area in 1957–77 (Blair, Decoufle and Grauman, 1979). Compared with national statistics, there was an excess of deaths from malignancies (O = 87, E = 67.9, O/E = 1.28). Significant excesses were noted for lung: O = 17, E = 10, O/E = 1.7, 95% CL = 1.0–2.7 and cervix: O = 10, E = 4.8, O/E = 2.08, 95% CL = 1.0–3.8. The workers would have been exposed to mixed solvents.

Men working for at least 1 year in dry cleaning in Prague in 1950–75 were identified and 57 (86%) traced until 1975. There was no evidence of atypical mortality in this very small group (Malek, Kremarova and Rodova, 1979).

Follow-up of over 2000 workers exposed to trichloroethylene in Finland in 1963–75 indicated an SMR of 77 for malignant disease in comparison with national rates. Though there was no evidence of increased risk of cancer, the follow-up period of this young cohort was very short (Tola *et al.*, 1980b).

Other studies on metal workers, including metal polishers may have involved use of trichloroethylene for degreasing—*see* 2.42.2

2.56.2 Case-control study

Occupational histories from pensioners records for 59 patients treated in 1972–74 with liver cancer showed none were employed in dry cleaning or degreasing (Novotna, David and Malek, 1979). However, the job histories were limited and this study cannot be used to rule out a risk.

2.56.3 Conclusions

IARC (1979b) only had available the study of Axelson *et al.* (1978b); it was considered, due to the small size of the group and the short time since onset of exposure, that no assessment could be made.

The Health and Safety Executive (1982c) concluded that all the studies then reported had serious limitations and that there was no evidence of a cancer hazard in man.

2.57 Ultraviolet light (UV)

It is generally accepted that exposure to UV is associated with increased risk of melanoma and other skin cancers. There are 2 occupations where increased exposure to UV occurs, which are reviewed in the next chapter—farming (*see* 3.14), and fishermen (3.15). The section on fluorescent lighting should also be consulted (2.35).

There is increased exposure to UV of other occupational groups (e.g. aircraft crews), but no adequate data have yet been reported on the risk of cancer in such persons.

2.57.1 Conclusion

The material presented elsewhere is thought to reflect an increased risk of skin cancer from exposure to natural UV. No definitive studies are available of the hazard from artificial UV.

2.58 Vinyl chloride and polyvinyl chloride

The following notes cover the background to concern of the carcinogenicity of vinyl chloride, stemming from case reports of angiosarcoma in workers in a number of countries. This was amplified by the establishment of angiosarcoma registers in a number of countries. Limited results stem from geographical studies, whilst the main contribution comes from a number of prospective studies. Studies are reviewed of workers potentially exposed to vinyl chloride monomer (VCM), and polyvinyl chloride (PVC) in fabrication plants.

2.58.1 Case reports of angiosarcoma

Creech and Johnson (1974) described how 3 men who had worked for one chemical company in the US had died from angiosarcoma of the liver, having been treated by different physicians. It then transpired that all 3 had been working on the same PVC plant. This immediately resulted in further enquiries and early publication of these findings. Falk *et al.*(1974) reported on hepatic disease amongst workers in a vinyl chloride polymer plant which had begun operation in 1942. About 250–300 workers had been employed at any one time, together with 850 working elsewhere on the site. The turnover or population at risk was not provided, nor any estimate of expected cancers. However, in this relatively small group of workers they had identified 7 with hepatic angiosarcoma.

These initial reports were soon followed by others from a number of countries: England (Lee and Harry, 1974); Lange *et al.* (1975) reported that 2 autoclave cleaners from Germany had died of liver angiosarcoma; 3 workers were reported from Sweden (Byren and Holmberg, 1975); further reports came from the US (Thomas *et al.*, 1975), Wales (Smith, Crossley and Williams, 1976), and France (Roche *et al.*, 1978); Delorme and Theriault (1978) reported 10 subjects with angiosarcoma who were all vinyl chloride workers in Quebec.

Ghandur-Mnaymneh and Gonzalez (1981) provide a case report of a man with low level VC exposure who developed hepatic angiomas and an angiosarcoma of the penis. They concluded that the role of VC in this case could not be determined.

By 22/1/75, 38 angiosarcomas of the liver in vinyl chloride or polyvinyl chloride workers were known, reported from 10 different countries (Lloyd, 1975). By October 1977, there were 64 polymerization workers known to the US reported from 12 countries (Spirtas and Kaminski, 1978). A review (*British Medical Journal,* 1981) noted that less than 200 deaths from this rare liver tumour had been reported worldwide; the majority were of unknown aetiology, with arsenic and thorotrast accounting for more than vinyl chloride.

Thomas *et al.* (1975) discussed the histological findings of liver disease in VC workers. They had identified 15 subjects with angiosarcoma and also reported 5 with hepatic fibrosis but with no cancer. They discussed whether exposure to VC resulted in fibrosis and subsequently cancer. All the cancer subjects had fibrosis but their data did not indicate the proportion with fibrosis that will progress to cancer.

2.58.2 Registers of angiosarcoma patients

Brady *et al.* (1977) obtained information from all patients developing angiosarcoma of the liver in New York in 1958–75 and controls from the cancer register matched on age, sex, race, and county of residence. The known associations with arsenic, thorium and vinyl chloride were found, but no direct exposure was found for 19 (73%) of the 26 patients. However, 5 of the cases lived within 1 mile of VC fabrication or polymerization plants but none of the controls.

Baxter and Fox (1975) examined the 34 certified deaths from angiosarcoma in England and Wales in 1963–73; there was evidence that some deaths from the malignancy were not identified by death certificates. Subsequently Baxter *et al.* (1977) investigated 41 deaths certified from angiosarcoma in Great Britain in 1963–73; in addition to these deaths, there were 9 published cases and 1 reported to them directly. Histology was obtained for 36 of these and reviewed by a panel of pathologists. Only in 14 was the angiosarcoma of the liver confidently confirmed; there was a query for 7; 12 were definitely excluded; in 3 the material was of such poor quality the lesions were unclassifiable. In a review of the occupational histories only 1 subject was confidently associated with VC exposure. These data were updated to 1977 (Baxter *et al.*, 1980) with identification of 8 further patients treated by thorotrast and 2 workers exposed to VC. There was also a suggestion of risk in the electrical and plastics fabrication industries.

2.58.3 Environmental studies

Mason (1975) identified counties in the US where there was a concentration of plastics and related industries (using VC). An excess of multiple myeloma was associated with location of synthetic rubber and fibre production.

Infante (1976) examined the cancer mortality in residents over 45 in the vicinity of the VC polymerization plants in Ohio in 1970–73. There was an unexplained excess of CNS neoplasms in males (O = 27, E = 14.3; O/E = 1.89, 95% CL = 1.2–2.7).

Saric *et al.* (1976) investigated the incidence of liver and lung cancer in persons living in a city in Yugoslavia with a PVC plant in the period 1968–71. There was no liver cancer in workers from the plant or in residents in the vicinity of the plant. The lung cancer incidence near the PVC plant was similar to that elsewhere in the city.

The proximity of 5 patients with angiosarcoma to VC plants in New York was mentioned in the previous subsection (Brady *et al.*, 1977).

2.58.4 Prospective studies

The following notes cover the key points on the method for the various studies, which are listed by country and chronological order. The main results are given in *Table 2.22*.

Canada

All men who had worked at a chemical plant in Quebec in 1948–72 for at least 5 years were identified from company and union records. Those who had worked at least 5 years on VCM or PVC production, and those whose maximum duration was 5 months on these plants were followed to 1977. The trace was 99%. Expected deaths were based on the province mortality; comparisons were also made between the exposed and unexposed groups (Theriault and Allard, 1981).

Great Britain: 1

Fox and Collier (1977) examined the mortality of over 7000 men working between 1940 and 1974 on VC polymerization in the 4 companies involved in Great Britain. Over 99% of the men were traced; expected deaths were based on national rates. Relatively few men had long-term exposure to VC. Additional analyses of the risk of lung cancer by length of exposure were given by Fox and Collier (1976b). There was no evidence for a dose–response relationship in risk of lung cancer.

Great Britain: 2

Duck, Carter and Coombes (1975) presented the mortality amongst 2100 males who had worked on a polymerization plant at anytime in the period 1948–74. Deaths in those under 75 were compared with expected based on national mortality rates. It should be noted that the handling of the analyses for years of exposure by these authors was incorrect (Berry and Rossiter, 1976; Fox, 1976; Wagoner, Infante and Saracci, 1976). It is likely that the men in the study were also included in the previous report by Fox and Collier.

Norway

Company records identified 454 men who had been first employed before 1970 for at least 1 year in a plant producing VCM and PVC in south-east Norway. The men were followed until 1979, identifying the incidence of cancer and deaths from all causes; expected figures were based on national rates (Heldaas, Langard and Anderson, 1984).

Sweden: 1

Company records identified 771 individuals who had worked from the 1940s until 1974 at a factory producing VCM and PVC in Sweden. Excluding 21 foreign workers, all were traced and cancer registrations and deaths identified. Expected figures were based on national rates (Byren *et al.*, 1976).

Table 2.22 Risk of various cancers in workers exposed to vinyl chloride*

Country	Liver (155)		Lung (162–3)		Brain (191)		RES (200–207)		Author
	O	E	O	E	O	E	O	E	
Canada	8	0.7†	2	5.8	0	0.6	1	1.7	Theriault and Allard (1981)
GB: 1	1	0.7	46	51.2	2	3.7	9	9.0	Fox and Collier (1977)
GB: 2			16	15.5					Duck, Carter and Coombs (1975)
Norway			5	2.8					Heldaas, Langard and Anderson (1984)
Sweden: 1	4‡	1.0	3	1.8	2	0.3			Byren *et al.* (1976)
US: 1			25	23.9			9	9.8	Tabershaw and Gaffey (1974)
US: 2	0	—	4§	5.2					Ott, Langner and Holder (1975)
US: 3	8	0.7	13	7.9	5	1.2	5	1.5	Monson, Peters and Johnson (1974)
US: 4	3	0.0							Nicholson *et al.* (1975)
US: 5	7	0.6	12	7.7	3	0.9	4	2.5	Waxweiler *et al.* (1976)
US: 6	6	4.2	193	165.6	16	13.8	61	55.7	Chiazze, Nichols and Wong (1977)
US: 7			4	1.5					Buffler *et al.* (1979)
Total	37	7.9	323	288.9	28	20.5	89	80.2	
O/E	4.68		1.12		1.37		1.11		
95% CL	3.3–6.5		1.0–1.2		0.9–2.0		0.9–1.4		

*See text for description of method.
†Estimated from other studies.
‡Liver and pancreas.
§Excluding arsenic-exposed subjects.

Sweden: 2

Follow-up of 1771 workers employed at the 4 PVC producing plants in Sweden involved those who had worked for at least 3 months in 1945–74 until 1976. Expected figures were based on national rates; the only cancer results were for alimentary tract (Molina *et al.*, 1981).

US: 1

Tabershaw and Gaffey (1974) obtained records for males who had worked for at least 1 year in 33 plants in the US with potential exposure to VC. This included 43% working prior to 1960; 85% were traced to 1972. Expected mortality was based on the US rates. Only limited information was available on extent of exposure.

US: 2

Production workers employed in 1942–60 on VC plants in Michigan were followed to 1973 (Ott, Langner and Holder, 1975). Of 594 only 1 was not traced; 72 individuals also had exposure to arsenicals. Expected mortality was based on US rates. An unspecified number of the men were included in the study by Tabershaw and Gaffey, but more details were provided on length and intensity of exposure. There were relatively few men with long periods of low-level exposure.

US: 3

Company records identified 161 deaths occurring in active or retired employees from 2 VC production and polymerization plants in Kentucky in 1947–73. Deaths in those leaving before retirement were not identified. A proportional-mortality analysis was performed, using national data to generate expected figures (Monson, Peters and Johnson, 1974). Details of the degree of exposure to VCM were not available.

US: 4

Company records were used to identify 257 men employed at a New York State VC production plant, who had worked for at least 5 years in 1946–63. The men were followed to April 1974, only 2 being untraced; the analysis was restricted to deaths occurring at least 10 years after first employment. Expected deaths were based on state mortality rates (Nicholson *et al.*, 1975).

US: 5

Waxweiler *et al.* (1976) studied selected facilities which had been engaged in polymerization of VC for at least 15 years and had a sizable workforce.

Four plants were included in the survey which employed a total of 825 men in 1974; 1294 men had at least 5 years exposure, which began at least 10 years before the start of the survey; only 7 were not traced. This study was extended to all male workers on the total plant sites; 4806 had been employed at some time from 1942 and were followed to 1973. Sixty-three per cent had first been employed prior to 1954; only 1.5% were lost to follow-up. Expected deaths were based on national rates. The histology was reviewed for all lung cancers and there appeared to be an excess of adenocarcinoma and large cell undifferentiated neoplasms. Detailed job histories permitted an examination of the risk from exposure to various chemicals. PVC dust was the only substance with a significant risk of lung cancer (Waxweiler *et al.*, 1981).

US: 6

Company records were used to identify 4341 deaths in men who had worked in 17 PVC fabrication plants in the US in 1964–73. A proportionate analysis was performed, using national data to produce expected figures (Chiazze, Nichols and Wong, 1977).

US: 7

Company records identified 464 men who had worked at least 2 months on a VC monomer production plant in Texas in 1948–77; 100% were traced, and observed mortality was compared with expected based on state mortality rates. Though there were no deaths from liver tumours, there was a significant excess of lung cancer; there was no clear dose–response, but this may be a reflection of small numbers of deaths (Buffler *et al.*, 1979).

2.58.5 Hazard to the next generation

Infante (1976) reported that mothers living in the vicinity of 3 PVC production plants in Ohio in 1970–73 had an increased proportion of babies with congenital abnormalities (especially of the CNS), for which no explanation was found.

Men employed in VCM polymerization, PVC fabrication, and rubber manufacture at plants in Ohio in 1974 were interviewed and detailed histories of previous pregnancy outcome of their wives obtained (Infante *et al.*, 1976). The response rate varied from 62 to 77% in the different groups. There appeared to be a significant excess of fetal loss in the wives of men after exposure to VCM. Paddle (1976) emphasized that the results were based on small numbers and would be influenced by adjustment for maternal age.

2.58.6 Conclusions

The initial observation of angiosarcoma of the liver was chiefly from workers in the polymerization of VCM with high atmospheric levels of exposure to vinyl chloride (possibly up to 10 000 ppm in the worst conditions in autoclaves). Heath, Falk and Creech (1975) estimated that the 13 US workers developing this tumour had a 400-fold increased risk of this rare tumour.

IARC (1979a) concluded that VC was a human carcinogen affecting liver, lung, brain, and the haemolymphopoietic systems. There was no evidence of a level of exposure below which no increased risk would occur. The evidence of possible hazard to workers exposed to PVC was insufficient for evaluation.

The *British Medical Journal* (1974) had pointed out that PVC may contain 200–400 ppm of VC and processed plastic contains 0.5–20 ppm VC. There is no hard evidence of a hazard from the secondary processing of the products.

2.59 Vinylidene chloride

Two small studies have reported on the development of cancer in workers exposed to vinylidene chloride.

Company records identified 138 men who had worked in production or processing of vinylidene chloride at a Dow US chemical plant in 1945–73. The men were followed until 1974; expected deaths were calculated from national rates for the period 1945–73 (Ott *et al.*, 1976). There was only 1 death from respiratory cancer with 0.3 expected.

In a preliminary report mortality was available on 629 workers from a German vinylidene chloride production and polymerization plant (Thiess, Frentzel-Beyme and Penning, 1979). There were 7 deaths from malignant tumours, which was not greater than expected; in those aged 35–39 there was an increase of lung cancer: O = 2, E = 0.08, O/E = 25.0, 95% CL = 2.8–90.3. The results were based on small numbers and there was no such excess at other ages.

2.59.1 Conclusion

IARC (1979b) considered that the human data did not permit adequate evaluation and further results from laboratory studies were awaited.

2.60 Zinc refineries

A cohort of 4802 males employed for at least 1 year in 1946–75 in one of 9 US zinc and copper refineries were traced. Vital status was obtained for 88% and 353/423 death certificates were obtained. Using national rates, expected deaths were calculated (Logue, Koontz and Hattwick, 1982). There was no evidence of a significant increase in any specific site of malignancy.

2.60.1 Conclusion

The trace rate, including that of actual death certificates was below the level usually considered acceptable. For this reason, and because the findings have not been replicated in other reports, these negative results require confirmation.

Recommended reading

COLE, P. and MERLETTI, F. (1983) In *The Epidemiology of Cancer*. Ed. G.J. Bourke. pp. 260–291. London: Croom Helm

DECOUFLE, P. (1982) In *Cancer Epidemiology and Prevention*. Eds D. Schottenfeld and J.F. Fraumeni, pp. 318–334. Philadelphia: Saunders

INTERNATIONAL AGENCY FOR RESEARCH ON CANCER (1972–1985) *IARC Monographs on the Evaluation of the Carcinogenic Risks of Chemicals to Humans*. Lyon: IARC. (Volumes 1–33 have already been published)

MILLER, G.L. (1975). *Indexes to Selected Literature on Occupational and Environmental Carcinogenic Hazards*. Philadelphia: Franklin Institute Research Laboratories

SIMONATO, L. and SORACCI, R. (1983). In *ILO Encyclopedia on Occupational Safety and Health*, 3rd edn. Ed. L. Parmeggiani. pp. 369–375. Geneva: ILO

3

Occupations associated with increased risk of cancer

This chapter complements the material in the previous one on specific agents causing cancer in various occupations. Reviews are provided of the processes, occupations, or industries for which epidemiological studies have indicated an increased incidence or mortality from cancer. Sometimes the analyses of risk in relation to the work processes involved may suggest the agent involved (e.g. the risk of nasal cancer increasing with higher levels of exposure to dust in leather workers). However, an arbitrary judgement has been made to include such topics in this rather than the preceding chapter, as the specific agent has not been agreed. The occupations are presented in alphabetical order; should a particular occupation not be readily located, the index should be consulted.

The points in the introduction to Chapter 2 apply equally to the present chapter on: the ordering of the material within the sections, the key items presented for any study that is reviewed, the need to refer to Chapter 1 in order to judge the weight to be placed on different studies, and the provision of a conclusion for each occupation discussed.

3.1 Alcohol industry

Due to the access to free or reduced-price beer/ wine/spirits, there is potential excess 'exposure' to alcohol in those working in the production, distribution, or sales side of the industry. Though this is a rather different concept to environmental exposure than in other groups of workers, this section is included as it is work related. Brief comments are provided about the indications of cancer hazard to such workers.

Newsholme (1903) described how the Registrar General's statistics for England and Wales for 1880–1890 stimulated him to consider that occupations associated with intemperance had higher mortality from cancer. Analysis of 18 280 death certificates for larynx and lung cancer in males in England and Wales in 1921–32 showed an excess of laryngeal cancer in those working in the supply of alcohol (Kennaway and Kennaway, 1936). Support for this has come from case-control studies. Herity *et al.* (1981), in a study of 200 Dublin patients with head and neck cancer have confirmed the importance of combined smoking and drinking. There was a significant excess of occupations involving exposure to alcohol in the cases (i.e. brewery workers, publicans, barmen, and hotel workers).

Dean *et al.* (1979) examined the patterns of mortality between 1954 and 1973 for over 4000 workers and pensioners who had been employed in an Irish brewery. There was a significantly increased risk of death from rectal cancer, but no increased risk for cancer of the oesophagus, pharynx, or liver. A similar study was carried out in Denmark by Jensen (1979), involving all individuals who had worked for at least 6 months in a brewery from 1939 to 1963; over 15 000 individuals were traced to the end of 1976. Morbidity was increased for pharynx, oesophagus, liver and larynx cancer. The risk of these tumours was highest amongst those workers who had had a ration of free beer for 30 years or more of employment. There was a modest increase in lung cancer that was comparable to that found in other individuals of equivalent low socio-economic class. No increased risk was found for cancer of the colon or rectum.

3.1.1 Conclusion

Brief comments about the evidence that consumption of alcohol increases the risk of cancer are provided in the next chapter (*see* 4.1, 4.3, 4.5, 4.6, 4.8).

The above results are compatible with the other work on the cancer risk from alcohol consumption; they suggest that occupations which are associated with ready access to increased alcohol consumption expose workers to head and neck and possibly liver cancer.

3.2 Aluminium industry

The findings from 4 prospective studies of aluminium industry workers are presented. There has recently been a case-control study of bladder cancer occurring to men in the industry.

3.2.1 Prospective studies

Gibbs and Horowitz (1979) followed 5406 workers employed at one aluminium smelter in 1950, and 485 workers employed at another until 1973. There appeared to be an increased risk of lung cancer for workers exposed to higher tar levels or those who had worked for long duration; for exposure of 20 years: O = 23, E = 9.5, O/E = 2.41, 95% CL = 1.5–3.6, with values for all lengths of exposure of O = 68, E = 50.2, O/E = 1.35, 95% CL = 1.0–1.7. (The tar was derived from the burning of the anode in the cell of the smelter.)

An historical prospective study of 2103 workers employed for a year in 1946–72 in an aluminium reduction plant in north-western US followed the subjects until 1976 (Milham, 1979). Expected deaths were based on national rates. There was a significant excess of lympho/reticulosarcoma (O = 6; E = 0.9; O/E = 6.43; 95% CL = 2.4–14.5), and a non-significant increase in lung cancer (O = 16; E = 12.4; O/E = 1.29; 95% CL = 0.7–2.1).

Anderson *et al.* (1982) followed 7410 male employees of the Norwegian primary aluminium industry in 1953–79. There were 428 cancers with 412.2 expected, with a significant excess of lung cancer (O = 57; E = 35.9; O/E = 1.60; 95% CL = 1.2–2.1). This was particularly in (*a*) those working for a short time in the industry, and (*b*) those with long duration of work in the older plants.

The mortality of 21 829 men working for at least 5 years in 14 aluminium reduction plants in the US in 1946–77 was compared with the expected based on national rates (Rockette and Arena, 1983). There was no site showing a significant excess in the exposed workers, with observed lung cancer being slightly below expected (O = 272, E = 289.2, O/E = 0.94, 95% CL = 0.8–1.1).

Chan-Yeung *et al.* (1983) studied the prevalence of respiratory disease in aluminium smelter workers in British Columbia. There was no information on cancer risk in the men examined.

3.2.2 Case-control study: bladder

Theriault *et al.* (1984) mounted a case-control study of men with bladder cancer who had worked in 5 aluminium plants in Quebec in 1970–79 and controls in the same industry matched for age and date of employment. There was a significant risk for those working in a particular part of the plant—the Soderborg reactor rooms (RR = 2.70; 95% CL = 1.64–4.43); this risk increased with duration of work and estimated level of tar and benz(a)pyrene exposure, and was not explained by differences in smoking.

3.2.3 Conclusion

Pooling the results for the 4 prospective studies gives a borderline significant excess of lung cancer (O = 413, E = 387.7, O/E = 1.07, 95% CL = 1.0–1.2). This result is particularly affected by the deficiency found in the largest of the 4 studies. Though there is no clear evidence of an increase of cancer in these workers, there is sufficient evidence to indicate the need for further carefully conducted studies.

3.3 Bakers

There are 2 studies which include reference to nasal cancer in bakers. Engzell, Englund and Westerholm (1978) report exposure to flour in 1 of 127 males and 3 of 85 females with nasal cancer registered in Sweden in 1961–70. No expected figures were provided.

A general survey of nasal cancer patients in England and Wales in 1963–67 obtained information on occupation from hospital records, patients, and next of kin (Acheson, Cowdell and Rang, 1981). An increased risk was recorded for bakers and pastrycooks, but not flour millers, in comparison with expected based on the census. The specific figures were not quoted.

3.3.1 Conclusion

The above is insufficient as a basis from which to evaluate the hazard of cancer in exposed workers.

3.4 Beekeeping

McDonald, Li and Mehta (1979) used 3 journals of the beekeeping industry for 1949–78 to identify deaths in beekeepers. Using proportional-mortality analysis, there were significantly fewer deaths from lung cancer than expected (O = 14; E = 24; O/E = 0.58; 95% CL = 0.3–1.0), but no other significant differences.

3.4.1 Conclusion

The above study is compatible with the hypothesis that repeat immunostimulations from bee stings reduce the risk of the common cancers in man. However, further studies would be required to confirm this, particularly using more specific information of frequency of bee stings and exposure to other known carcinogens.

3.5 Butchers

Fox, Lynge and Malker (1982) used routine mortality and incidence statistics to highlight excess risk of lung cancer in butchers in England and Wales, Denmark, and Sweden. This had shown in data for England and Wales in 1930–32 (Wynne Griffith, 1982), and also was then reflected in that for Scotland in 1969–73 (Registrar General, Scotland, 1981). Further data for Denmark (Lynge, Andersen and Kristensen, 1983) showed an excess in butchers from lung cancer in 1975–80 (SMR for skilled or self-employed butchers of 152). The SMR for unskilled workers in slaughter houses was about the average for economically active men in the period 1970–80.

In response to these communications, which were all based on routine data, results were reported from other countries. An earlier case-control study in West Germany of patients diagnosed in 1954–66 had apparently shown the risk in butchers (Doerken and Rehpenning, 1982). Proportional-mortality analysis of 223 deaths in butchers in Maryland in 1965–80 showed an excess of deaths from lung cancer, and also bladder, connective tissue, and haemopoietic/lymphatic neoplasms (Johnson and Fischman, 1982).

However, 2 negative studies have been reported from the US. Use of the file of data from Roswell Park inpatients treated in 1957–66 showed no evidence of increased relative risk for lung cancer in males who had ever been employed in the meat industry. The basic RR was 1.1, which reduced to 1.0 after adjustment for smoking. The authors accepted that the work environment may have changed since their data were collected (Vena *et al.*, 1982). Proportional-mortality analysis of deaths in Washington State in 1950–79 showed no evidence of such a hazard in butchers or meat cutters, whether or not they had worked in slaughterhouses (Milham, 1982a).

3.5.1 Conclusions

These results show a degree of consistency, but do not rule out confounding factors. In particular, it is important to clarify the long-term smoking habits of those apparently having an increased risk of death from lung cancer.

3.6 Car manufacture

Hoover *et al.* (1975) used the US cancer maps for bladder cancer in 1950–69 to examine the occupations in those countries with excess mortality. There was an increased risk (2.5) for manufacture of motor vehicles.

Chiazze, Ference and Woff (1984) identified 3379 deaths occurring in active and retired workers from 10 automobile assembly plants in the US in 1970–76, and carried out a proportional-mortality analysis using US and state rates as standards. There was no consistency across plants and cities involved in the study and thus no hard evidence of an industry-wide hazard. Though it is stated that the aim was to study any hazard in paint sprayers, these results relate to the total workforce involved in car assembly, and it was not stated what the proportion of paint sprayers was.

3.6.1 Conclusion

The above reports do not provide adequate evidence to evaluate the cancer levels in this industry.

3.7 Carpet manufacture

Vobecky *et al.* (1978) followed up a clinical lead in Canada, when 5 patients were treated in a short space of time with large bowel cancer—all were under 50, and had worked in one unit of a local carpet factory. This was checked in 2 ways; occupational histories were obtained from the last 1000 patients treated with large bowel cancer (by questioning the patients or their next of kin). Thirty patients reported working in the carpet factory out of the 1000 patients treated in 1965–75. Comparison with occupations recorded for the patients treated in 1971–75 suggested the risk was raised ten-fold. Also an attempt was made to quantify the incidence of large bowel cancer in workers from the carpet factory, in comparison with previous registration rates. The incidence of this cancer was reported to be raised 11.4-fold in 1974–75. However, Wen and Tsai (1979) have criticized the statistics of the above work; they suggested that the elevation in risk could not have been as great as reported, because of erroneous calculation of expected figures.

In the preliminary enquiries into the cause of the high risk of oesophageal cancer in northern Iran, the local carpet weaving had been considered as a possible factor. However, a detailed case-control study provided no support for this hypothesis (Cook-Mozaffari *et al.*, 1979).

3.7.1 Conclusion

There is inadequate evidence to evaluate the cancer levels in this industry.

3.8 Cement manufacture

McDowall (1984) identified 607 men recorded in the 1939 census in England and Wales as working in cement manufacture and traced deaths in the period 1948–81. There was a significant excess of stomach cancer deaths in comparison with E based on national rates (O = 22, E = 12.6, O/E = 1.75, 95% CL = 1.1–2.6). It was not clear how much this was a reflection of social class, or possible dust exposure.

3.8.1 Conclusion

Replication of these results is required, before analytical studies are carried out on the possible aetiology. At least some indication of a dose–response to dust levels would be an important point.

3.9 Chemical industry

Where possible, sections refer to more specific exposures than the broad label 'chemicals'. However, a number of studies have used this broad term and they are briefly described in the following notes. There is overlap with some of the other sections, most particularly with that on the petrochemical industry, which includes studies on workers in petrochemical plants (*see* 3.23).

The section begins with results from mortality statistics (both occupational and area analyses). Only one study is reviewed where a cohort of workers have been followed up; this deals with a subgroup of the industry in pharmaceutical manufacture. There follow comments about case-control studies on specific sites of malignancy.

3.9.1 Mortality statistics

Although routine occupational mortality statistics have not highlighted the chemical industry as having excess mortality from cancer, a wide range of positives were obtained in a US study of geographical mortality. Analysis of US cancer mortality in 1950–69 revealed significant excess of: liver, lung, and bladder cancer, but not leukaemia, in those 139 counties with highly concentrated chemical industry (Hoover and Fraumeni, 1975). In addition, screening of 30 other sites showed significant variation from the US national rates for a number of sites: in males a 10% difference for nasal, larynx, skin, bone, and melanoma; a 20% difference for mouth and throat, and other endocrine neoplasms; for females,

a 10% difference for nasopharynx, cervix, other uterus, and melanoma; a 20% difference for nasal sinus cancer.

3.9.2 Prospective study: pharmaceutical workers

Thomas and Decoufle (1979) obtained the cause of death in 1954–76 of 826 white pharmaceutical plant employees and 249 sales representatives. The proportional distribution was compared with the US national age, sex, calendar period mortality. There was an excess of respiratory cancer in male maintenance and female production workers. An increased relative frequency of melanoma in males (O = 4; E = 0.8; O/E = 5.0; 95% CL = 1.3–12.8) and leukaemia in female production workers was noted.

3.9.3 Case-control studies

Nasopharynx

One hundred and fifty-six patients diagnosed in Los Angeles in 1971–74 and 267 controls showed an increased risk for exposure to chemicals: RR = 2.4 (Henderson *et al.*, 1976).

Nasal cancer

Comparison of occupations of patients registered with nasal cancer in England and Wales in 1963–67 with census figures suggested that there was an increased risk in gas, coke, and chemical workers: O = 12; E = 6.5; O/E = 1.85; 95% CL = 0.9–3.2 (Acheson, Cowdell and Rang, 1981).

A case-control study of 160 patients treated in North Carolina and Virginia in 1970–80 showed a significant risk for those employed in chemical manufacturing: RR = 2.99; 95% CL = 1.0–9.0 (Brinton *et al.*, 1984).

Lung

Comparison of occupations recorded at death certification for 858 white males dying in coastal Georgia in 1961–74 and that for controls showed an excess reported work in the chemical industry: RR = 1.46; 95% CL = 1.0–2.2 (Harrington *et al.*, 1978).

Melanoma

Cancer surveillance of employees in Du Pont in 1956–74 showed a significantly increased risk of melanoma, in comparison with national incidence data for the US. However, despite greater potential exposure to chemicals, the wage earners had no higher risks than the salaried staff (Pell, O'Berg and Karrh, 1978). (*See also* Prospective studies, 3.10.1, US:2, in the next section.)

Skin cancer—non-melanoma

Detailed occupational histories were obtained for 598 patients with skin cancer in north-west England, with more limited information for 148 patients treated in 1967–69. Compared to the census results for 1931 and 1951, an excess of males had worked in the chemical industry (Whitaker, Lee and Downes, 1979).

Bladder

Of the case-control studies reviewed in 4.23.1, 7 reported results for exposure to 'chemical nos'. All the RRs were greater than 1.0, and 3 significantly raised.

Prostate

Occupations recorded at death certification for men dying from prostate cancer in 2 Californian counties were compared with those for controls matched for age and race (Ernster *et al.*, 1979). A non-significant elevated risk was found for exposure to chemicals (2.3 in one county and 2.0 in the other).

Hodgkin's disease

The occupations were abstracted from case notes for 88 patients treated for Hodgkin's disease in Lund, Sweden in 1973–78. These were compared with occupations for 3 different control groups (Olsson and Brandt, 1979). An excess of the cases had handled various chemicals compared with controls (RR = 8.78; 95% CL = 3.6–21.2). However, no support for this was found by Benn, Mangood and Smith (1979) using routine registration data for the north-west of England, or Fonte *et al.* (1982) in a case-control study of patients treated at Pavia Hospital, Italy.

3.9.4 Hazard to the next generation

Cultured lymphocytes from 73 workers in chemical laboratories and the printing industry (with solvent exposure) showed a significant increase in chromatid breaks in comparison with controls. Similar changes were also found in a small group of children whose mothers had worked in the laboratories during their pregnancies (Funes-Cravioto *et al.*, 1977).

3.9.5 Conclusion

There is very little consistency in the results. Because of the indefinite nature of the potential work exposure in these studies of the chemical industry, the reports can only be used as a base for considering the need for further studies.

3.10 Chemists

Four different groups of professional chemists have been studied—2 in the US, 1 each in Sweden and the UK. The design of these studies is described and the results are brought together in *Table 3.1*. In addition, brief reference is made to case-control studies on 2 sites of malignancy that have referred to risk in chemists.

3.10.1 Prospective studies

Sweden

Olin (1976) identified 530 men who graduated from the School of Chemical Engineering in Stockholm in 1930–50. Follow-up to 1974 was complete for 97.5%. Expected mortality was based on national rates. A senior member of the teaching staff attempted to identify those graduates who had subsequently worked in chemical laboratories (about 400); all but 1 of the malignant disease deaths occurred in this group. The study was extended to those graduating from an equivalent institute in Gothenberg (Olin, 1978); this added a further 335 men, all but 4 of whom were traced to 1974. A further extension involved those graduating up to 1959, all being traced to 1979. In addition to using national rates, a comparison was made with 657 architects followed over the same period (Olin and Ahlbom, 1980).

UK

McGinty (1978) described a study in the UK of members of the Royal Institute of Chemistry; he reported that the mortality from intestinal cancer was 'over-represented' compared with some other malignancies, but gave no specific details. In a further brief mention of this study, Searle *et al.* (1978) presented limited data on a proportional-mortality analysis of 291 deaths amongst members in 1965–75. Burrows (1980) gave further details of 1326 deaths that had occurred in 1965–75. National rates were used to provide the expected figures.

US: 1

Publications of the American Chemical Society were used to identify 4644 deaths in members in the period 1948–67; death certificates were only obtained for 3637 (78%). A proportional-mortality analysis was performed for 2152 male deaths, using national rates for 'all professional men' dying in the US in 1950 aged 20–64. For those over 64, expected deaths were based on national data for all males dying in 1959 (Li *et al.*, 1969).

Table 3.1 Mortality from various sites of malignancy for 4 groups of chemists*

Site	Sweden		UK		US: 1		US: 2†		Total		O/E	95% CL
	O	E	O	E	O	E	O	E	O	E		
Stomach					31	47	2	2.4	35	49.4	0.71	0.5–1.0
Colorectal			159‡	86.2	115	94	10	16.0	284	196.2	1.45	1.3–1.6
Liver biliary pass					25	19	1	0.9	26	19.9	1.31	0.8–1.9
Pancreas	2	1.6			56	35	2	1.1	60	37.6	1.60	1.2–2.0
Lung	3	4.0	314	551.6	109	108	8	20.0	434	683.6	0.63	0.6–0.7
Melanoma							8	8.3	8	8.3	0.96	0.4–1.9
Prostate	3	1.5					7	4.5	10	6.0	1.67	0.8–3.1
Bladder					26	21	3	2.0	29	23.0	1.26	0.8–1.8
Kidney							4	3.7	4	3.7	1.08	0.3–2.8
Brain	5	1.2	54	21.2			2	3.0	61	25.4	2.40	1.8–3.1
RES	7	3.2	146	74.3	127	76	12	10.0	292	163.5	1.79	1.6–2.0
Lymphoma	3§	0.7			78	42	6	5.2	87	47.9	1.82	1.4–2.2
Leukaemia					49	34	3	.3.5	52	37.5	1.39	1.0–1.8

*See text for description of method.
†Incidence data.
‡Colon only.
§Hodgkin's disease only.

US: 2

Hoar and Pell (1981) followed 3686 white males and 75 white females employed as 'professional' chemists by Du Pont in 1959–77. The company records for all those developing cancer were matched against the file of individuals whilst company and Social Security records were used to identify deaths. Expected events were calculated from incidence in a cohort of 'non-chemists', and national incidence and mortality rates.

Other related studies

Two reports of mortality in British pathologists and laboratory technicians have some aspects in common with the above studies (Harrington and Shannon, 1975; Harrington and Oakes, 1983). However, the working environment is rather different to that of industrial chemists; because of the possible exposure to formaldehyde, these studies were discussed in 2.36.

3.10.2 Case-control studies

Melanoma

In order to check on an observed high frequency of chemists registered with malignant melanoma in Los Angeles, interviews (by telephone) were conducted for chemists with melanoma and other malignancies. Those with melanoma reported an excess of exposure to multiple chemicals, solvents, plastics, pesticides, benzoyl peroxide, and ionizing radiation (Wright, Peters and Mack, 1983).

Hodgkin's disease

Comparison of the occupations from hospital notes of 88 men with Hodgkin's disease treated at one Swedish hospital in 1973–78, with 3 control groups, indicated an excess reporting exposure to chemicals, but no excess of chemists *per se* (Olsson and Brandt, 1979).

3.10.3 Hazard to the next generation

Records of pregnancy were obtained for about 70% of children registered with cancer in Finland in 1959–75 and control subjects. An increased risk was identified in children whose mothers had worked as pharmacists, although no RR is quoted (Hemminki, Sorsa and Vaino, 1979).

3.10.4 Conclusions

The pooled data from the 4 studies on chemists is heavily weighted by the results from 2 of these (England and Wales and US:2), which 'swamp' the contribution from the other two. There does seem to be a consistent excess of RES neoplasms—both lymphoma and leukaemia; also *Table 3.1* shows significant excesses in the pooled data for brain tumours, colorectal and pancreatic cancers. The RES excess had also occurred in the studies on English pathologists (*see* 2.36). The deficiency in deaths from lung cancer may reflect lower smoking consumption than in the general population.

3.11 Cleaners

Two reports have mentioned an increase of cancer.

Henry, Kennaway and Kennaway (1931) examined the occupations recorded at death certification for 5808 males dying from prostate cancer in England and Wales in 1921–28. Calculating rates from the census estimates of numbers in occupations, cleaners were identified as having an increased risk for this cancer.

In a case-control study of 265 patients with liver cancer treated in New Jersey, there was an increased risk for women employed in cleaning services: RR = 4.33; 95% CL = 1.2–15.7 (Stemhagen *et al.*, 1983).

3.11.1 Conclusion

These 2 reports are an inadequate basis to consider that there is an increased risk of cancer in this occupational group.

3.12 Electrical workers

Wertheimer and Leeper (1979) observed an association between childhood leukaemia and residence near high current electrical wiring configurations in Colorado. Though this was not found in a study in Rhode Island (Fulton *et al.*, 1980), an extension of the original study showed adult cancer was associated with the distribution of electric wiring (Wertheimer and Leeper, 1982). A variety of studies have recently explored the possible hazard to workers; this is also one of the factors for which hazard to the next generation has been investigated.

3.12.1 Occupational mortality and incidence

In the occupational mortality analysis of England and Wales for 1970–72 (Registrar General, 1978), there was an increased risk of brain cancer in electrical engineers. A further exploration of these data and a case-control study of occupations recorded at death registration in 1973 indicated raised values for leukaemia and particularly acute myeloid leukaemia for 'electrical occupations', with highest risks for telecommunication engineers (McDowall, 1983). Similar results were obtained by Coleman, Bell and Skeet (1983), on analysis of occupation recorded for patients registered with malignant disease in south-east England.

Milham (1982b) examined the occupations recorded at death certification in Washington State in 1950–79 in relation to cause. Ten of 11 jobs having exposure to electrical and magnetic fields had an increased PMR for leukaemia. Cross-check of these findings in the Los Angeles cancer register for 1972–79 again showed an excess of leukaemia in men whose job involved exposure to electric or magnetic fields. The PMRs were significantly raised for all electrical jobs for acute leukaemia and AML (Wright, Peters and Mack, 1982).

In an analysis of liver angiosarcoma registrations in Britain in 1963–77, Baxter *et al.* (1980) noted that 6 subjects worked in the electrical industry out of 35 cases. No expected figure was given, but the tumour is extremely rare.

3.12.2 Case-control studies

Oral and pharyngeal cancer

A case-control study of 232 women with oral and pharyngeal cancer treated in 1975–78 and matched for controls was carried out in North Carolina. There was an association with work in the electronic industry, with 6 cases and 1 control so employed: RR = 6.0; 95% CL = 0.9–38.5 (Winn *et al.*, 1982).

Pancreas

Data from the Los Angeles cancer register for 1972–77 showed men and women in electrical equipment manufacture were at increased risk of pancreas cancer O = 33, E = 18.9, O/E = 1.75, 95% CL = 1.2–2.4. However, this result was found after examination of many associations in their material and the significant level has to be treated with caution (Mack and Paganini-Hill, 1981).

Pharynx and respiratory

Data from the Swedish cancer environment registry for 1961–73 indicated a slightly increased incidence of cancer, especially for pharynx and respiratory system of cancers of workers in the electronics and electrical manufacturing industry (Vagero and Olin, 1983).

Bladder

The case-control studies reviewed in 4.23.1 revealed an increased risk for electrical workers in 2 of the 15 studies, neither of which was significant. The other 13 studies had not tabulated results for this occupation.

3.12.3 Hazard to the next generation

Kallen, Malmqvist and Moritz (1982) obtained detailed information on 2043 infants born to 2018 female physiotherapists in Sweden in 1973–78. There was no evidence of atypical perinatal mortality, birth weight, or congenital malformation in the total group. There was a suggestion of higher exposure to short-wave equipment in mothers having a dead or malformed infant, compared with controls.

A questionnaire was answered on reproductive hazards by 89% of 542 employees in Swedish power plants in 1979 (Nordstrom, Birke and Gustavsson,

1983). Men working as high-voltage switchyard workers appeared to report an excess of children with congenital malformations, though this was based on few events.

3.12.4 Conclusions

Bonnell (1982) reviewed this topic and argued that electrical fields up to 400 kV, (and possibly 800 kV) were harmless. Since this was published there have been a number of positive results reported. Though the recent reports may point to an environmental hazard, the range of sites involved in these positives shows little consistency and may merely reflect the publication of positive findings that have occurred by chance. There does seem to be greater consistency in relation to leukaemia, and this requires further study.

3.13 Electroplating

Electroplating involves caustic acids/alkalis, organic solvents, and metal fumes (e.g. nickel and chromium). There is thus overlap with this entry and other sections, particularly those on metals (2.42), chromium (2.19), and nickel (2.44).

Blair and Mason (1980) identified 126 counties in the US with at least 0.1% of the population employed in electroplating, and 2 control counties in the same geographical region with comparable demographic characteristics. For men, the age-adjusted mortality for index counties for 1950–69 was higher for cancers of: mouth and throat, oesophagus, larynx, bladder, and eye. For women there were raised risks for: oral cavity and pharynx, nasopharynx, stomach, lung, kidney and brain, and non-Hodgkin's lymphoma. The authors warned that these results must be interpreted with caution. The proportion of persons involved directly in electroplating was very low and there may have been many other unidentified differences between index and control counties.

3.13.1 Conclusion

The above study can only be used as a base to consider the need for further investigation bearing in mind the imprecise nature of this occupational category.

3.14 Farming

This section begins with brief comments on some analyses of occupational mortality and incidence statistics; these are in order of date of publication, and are more extensive than for many other sections. The bulk of the literature on case-control or prospective studies on farmers relates to a wide range of sites of cancer; the review is therefore set out in ICD order. Some of the material relates to associated occupations, such as veterinarians, but it was felt best to combine these because of the common theme of contact with farm animals. Reference should be made to the section on herbicides and pesticides (2.37).

3.14.1 Occupational mortality and incidence

The US cancer mortality data by county for 1950–69 was examined in relation to size of poultry population in the counties. Cervix and ovarian cancer, and myeloma were directly associated with poultry population. There was no relationship with Hodgkin's disease, other lymphoma, or leukaemia. The significant association for uterine cervix was thought to reflect social differences in the counties (Priester and Mason, 1974).

Routine occupational histories from about 14 000 patients admitted to Roswell Park in 1956–65 suggested that there was a risk of over 2.0 for prostate and kidney cancer in dairy farmers, though only the former was statistically significant (Decouflé *et al.*, 1977).

Williams, Stegens and Horm (1977) presented analyses for the US Third National Cancer Survey on occupation and industry reported by patients with different malignancies. Farmers were noted to have excess cancer risk of: oral cavity (2.02), prostate (1.52), testis (2.0), nervous system (1.73), Hodgkin's disease (1.50), and other lymphomas (2.15).

The occupational mortality analysis for England and Wales for 1970–72 (Registrar General, 1978) showed no SMR, for those aged 15–64, or PMR, for those aged 65–74, that was over 199 for farmers for any site of malignancy. However, this occupational unit had shown significantly increased registrations of brain tumours in 1966–67 and 1968–69; the mortality was also raised for this site in 1970–72.

Burmeister (1981) presented age-adjusted mortality rates, SMRs, and PMRs for farmers in Iowa in 1971–78. There was a deficiency of smoking-related cancers, but an excess from: lip, stomach, prostate, lymphoma, leukaemia, and multiple myeloma. It was not apparent that these findings were due to biases in the study, but no specific environmental agent was identified as an explanation.

Proportional mortality of veterinarians in 1947–77 showed significant increases in colon, skin, brain cancer and leukaemia. Blair and Hayes (1982) suggested that this excess of skin cancer and leukaemia was due to actinic rays and irradiation associated with work. This was an extension of the study reported by Blair and Hayes (1980).

Examination of mortality of farmers and labourers in the US in 1971–78 for broad groups of disease showed no excess from neoplasms; the age-adjusted mortality was 77% of that for non-farmers aged 20–64 in the same state (Burmeister and Morgan, 1982).

The occupations recorded on death certificates were used in a case-control study of 4 cancers in Iowa for 1964–78 (Burmeister *et al.*, 1983). Farmers showed a significant excess risk for: stomach cancer (1.32), prostate (1.19), non-Hodgkin's lymphoma (1.26), and multiple myeloma (1.48). The variety of farming involved varied with the different malignancies.

Merging the 1960 census records with 1961–73 cancer registration in Sweden permitted examination of the risks of malignancy in agricultural workers (Wiklund, 1983). For the majority of cancer sites the ratio of O/E was <1.0; this was statistically significant for lung cancer (O = 934, E = 2375, O/E = 0.39, 95% CL = 0.37–0.42), and for larynx (O = 94, E = 248, O/E = 0.38, 95% CL = 0.3–0.5). Lip registrations were significantly increased (O = 508, E = 278, O/E = 1.83, 95% CL = 1.7–2.0).

Buesching and Wollstadt (1984) examined the risk of cancer mortality in farmers in the north-west of Illinois in 1978–80. Significantly raised SMRs were found for non-Hodgkin's lymphoma (265), prostate cancer (195). There was a non-significant increase in leukaemia (200), and a non-significant reduction in lung cancer (82).

Proportional-mortality analysis was carried out for 28032 deaths in farmers in British Columbia in 1950–78 (Gallagher *et al.*, 1984). There were significantly raised PMRs for: lip (191), stomach (119), and prostate (113). Leukaemia risk was not significantly increased (122).

3.14.2 Studies on specific malignancies

The following notes deal with the various sites of malignancy in ICD order, indicating where studies have reported on the risk of different cancers in farmers or related occupations.

Lip

In a review of lip cancer in Finland, based on 3169 male and 303 female patients notified to the national registry in 1952–73, it was observed that the incidence was higher in the north-east and rural areas of Finland. There appeared to be an increase inversely related to solar radiation, and Lindquist and Teppo (1978) suggested that there might be synergism between occupation and UV exposure. No specific information was available on occupation, but the rural areas would have particularly involved farmers.

Stomach

In a large case-control study of patients dying from cancer in North Wales and Cheshire in 1952–56, there was an excess risk of stomach cancer in men occupied in farming in the high incidence part of the region (Stocks, 1961).

In a study of 360 stomach patients and controls in Santiago, increased risk was observed for those who had worked in agriculture. It was not possible to determine whether this represented confounding with some rural risk factor (Armijo *et al.*, 1981).

Digestive organs

Fasal, Jackson and Klauber (1966) used the state licensing system to identify all white male practising vets in California in 1950–62; the 1725 were all followed up and details obtained for the 148 males who had died. Expected figures were based on state mortality rates. Five cancer sites were originally selected for examination; there was no significant excess for cancer of the digestive system.

Liver

A case-control study of patients with liver cancer in New Jersey showed an increased risk in male farm labourers: RR = 1.89, 95% CL = 1.19–3.0 (Stemhagen *et al.*, 1983).

Larynx

Mapping of cancer indicated a high risk of laryngeal cancer in Richmond County, USA in 1950–69. Subsequently, a case-control study of 42 patients showed an increased risk of laryngeal cancer in grain farmers: RR = 3.3, 95% CL = 1.2–9.2 (Flanders *et al.*, 1984).

Lung

Fasal, Jackson and Klauber (1966) found no increased risk of lung cancer in vets in California (*see under* Digestive organs).

Melanoma

Fasal, Jackson and Klauber (1966) identified an increased mortality from melanoma in California male vets in 1950–62, though it was not clear if this was a chance finding (*see* Digestive organs for description).

Skin—non-melanoma

Detailed occupational histories from 598 patients in the north-west of England were compared with earlier census data (Whitaker *et al.*, 1979). This suggested there was an excess of skin cancers in farmers.

Prostate

Examination of occupations recorded for 5808 deaths from prostate cancer in England and Wales in 1921–28 showed an excess of gardeners, farm bailiffs, agricultural workers, shepherds, and farmers (Henry, Kennaway amd Kennaway, 1931). A more limited study in Texas also suggested an increased risk in farmers (MacDonald, 1956).

Ernster *et al.* (1979) used death certificates for men dying from prostate cancer and age/race matched controls in 2 Californian counties to compare the recorded occupations. An elevated risk in both counties was found for those involved in horticultural services (2.8 in one and 2.0 in the other).

Bladder and kidney

Fasal, Jackson and Klauber (1966) found no increased risk for these sites of malignancy (*see* Digestive organs for description).

Testis

A case-control study involved 347 patients with germ-cell tumours of the testis diagnosed in a Texas hospital in 1977–80. The clinical notes were abstracted and used to study occupation. There was a significantly raised risk for farming: RR = 6.27; 95% CL = 1.83–21.49 (Mills, Newell and Johnson, 1984). To check the findings from the US, McDowell and Balarajan (1984) examined occupations for 1384 deaths from testicular cancer and controls in England and Wales. There was an increased risk for farmers, that verged on the significant (RR = 1.89; 95% CL = 0.99–3.60). Registrations of 174 germ-cell testis cancers in Denmark in 1979–81 were used to compare occupations against a large number of controls. There was no difference in the proportion in farming occupations (Jensen, Olsen and Østerlind, 1984). The above prompted an analysis from a case-control study of 271 males with testicular cancer aged 18–42, diagnosed in 1976–81 in the Washington DC area (Brown and Pottern, 1984). There was an increased risk for work on a farm or rural residence as a child.

Penis

A high proportion of agricultural workers was reported by Kennaway and Kennaway (1946) in their study of all deaths occurring in England and Wales from penis cancer in 1911–40.

Brain

Buell, Dunn and Breslow (1960) found a reduced risk from brain cancer in farm labourers in California in 1949–51. In contrast, the occupational mortality for England and Wales (Registrar General, 1978) showed increased risk for farmers, farm managers, and market gardeners.

Examination of demographic details of 886 deaths from brain tumours in Minnesota in 1958–62 showed an excess in rural farm residents, but no occupation was reported more frequently than expected (Choi, Schuman and Gullen, 1970). In a study of children with brain cancers in Baltimore, an increased proportion had been exposed to insecticides or farm animals (Gold *et al.*, 1979). However, a case-control study in Los Angeles in 1972–75 showed no association with farm residence (Preston-Martin, Henderson and Pike, 1980).

Lymphosarcoma

In a follow-up of the cancer maps prepared for the US in 1950–69, examination of deaths from lymphosarcoma in California in 1971–72 suggested an increased risk in farm managers and labourers: O = 36, E = 14.6, O/E = 2.47, 95% CL = 1.7–3.4 (Goldsmith and Guidotti, 1977).

Hodgkin's disease

Priester, Oleinick and Connor (1970) suggested that there was an excess of patients with Hodgkin's disease on farms where bovine leucosis had appeared. However, the mortality from Hodgkin's disease was not appreciably different in farm and non-farm residents in California in 1959–61 (Fasal, Jackson and Klauber, 1968). Fasal, Jackson and Klauber (1966) had found no excess for lymphoma in general in Californian vets (*see* Digestive organs).

Non-Hodgkin's lymphoma

The occupations for 774 people dying from non-Hodgkin's lymphoma in Wisconsin in 1968–76 were compared with matched deaths from other causes. Farming was more frequently reported among the cases (RR = 1.22), especially those under 65: RR = 1.7; 95% CL = 1.1–2.5 (Cantor, 1982).

Multiple myeloma

There was an excess of deaths from multiple myeloma which reported farming occupations (especially contact with chickens) in Oregon and Washington in 1950–67 (Milham, 1971). A case-control study of 84 multiple myeloma patients showed significant excess risk for (*a*) prior allergies (RR = 3.1), (*b*) history of agricultural work (RR = 2.2), (*c*) prior myxoedema (RR = 5.0). There was no detailed information on type of farming (Gallagher *et al.*, 1983).

Leukaemia

Fasal, Jackson and Klauber (1966) found no evidence for increased risk of leukaemia in Calfornian vets (*see* Digestive organs for description). The mortality from leukaemia was not appreciably different in farm and non-farm residents in California in 1959–61 (Fasal, Jackson and Klauber, 1968).

A case-control study was carried out on mortality records for Oregon and Washington States for the period 1950–67. An excess of leukaemia deaths was associated with farming occupations, especially chicken farmers. It was accepted that the use of occupation recorded on death records was of questionable validity (Milham, 1971).

Blair and Thomas (1979) used death certificates issued for leukaemia in white males over 30 dying in Nebraska in 1957–74. Two age, sex, race, county, and year of death matched controls were selected. Comparisons were made of the reported occupations, and known information of types of farming in different counties. The risk of leukaemia was 1.25 in farmers, being greatest in those born after 1900 and working in heavy corn production localities. There was no indication of an association with pesticide or insecticide usage by county.

Examination of occupation recorded on death certification for 1499 persons dying from leukaemia and matched controls in Wisconsin in 1968–76 showed a non-significant increase in farmers with leukaemia. This appeared to be particularly for counties with dairy produce or fertilizer use (Blair and White, 1981).

Iowa has leukaemia rates, particularly for lymphoid leukaemia, above the average in the US. Examination of the distribution showed a correlation of lymphoid leukaemia and cattle density, with an excess in locations with herds affected by bovine lymphosarcoma (Donham, Berg and Sawin, 1980).

Analysis of death certificates of 1675 white males dying from leukaemia in Iowa in 1964–78 and matched controls showed a significant leukaemia risk in farmers. Various agricultural factors (high soybean and corn production, egg laying, herbicide use, number of milk cows) were related to various cytological types of leukaemia, though the number of comparisons made interpretation difficult (Burmeister, Van Lier and Isacson, 1982). However, there was no increased risk for farming occupations in all leukaemia patients diagnosed in Olmsted County, Minnesota in 1955–74 (Linos *et al.*, 1980), nor in 3441 veterinary surgeons followed from 1949–53 until 1975 in England and Wales (Kinlen, 1983).

3.14.3 Laboratory studies

Schneider and Riggs (1973) tested the serum of 626 volunteer veterinarians by an indirect immunofluorescent test for cell surface viral antigens (feline leukaemia virus—FLV). One sample was seropositive, but negative on subsequent testing 8 months later. Most of the subjects had ample opportunity for contact with cats, and about 5–10 might in their lifetime develop leukaemia or lymphoma. There was thus no evidence that FLV was associated with development of these malignancies in man.

A sero-epidemiological study tested for antibodies to bovine leukaemia virus (BLV) in farm employees and veterinarians in contact with cattle having lymphosarcoma. No positive sera were found in 45 subjects (Donham *et al.*, 1977).

Sera were tested for 192 persons in contact with herds positive for BLV, and 47 in contact with negative herds. No specimen was positive for BLV (Caldwell *et al.*, 1976).

In a review of bovine leukaemia (lymphosarcoma), Olson (1974) concluded that there was no evidence of transmission to man—BLV was not found in: 10 laboratory personnel working with affected animal material, 80 veterinarians with extensive dairy cattle practice, dairymen handling infected cattle, or 100 patients with leukaemia. Commercial pasteurization also destroyed BLV in milk.

Caldwell (1983) pointed out that the isolation of BLV and discovery of virus particles in cows' milk added to the interest of studies of the association of cancer in cattle and humans, but had not led to any confirmatory findings.

3.14.4 Hazards to the next generation

Pregnancy records were traced for mothers of about 70% of children registered with cancer in Finland in 1959–75 (Hemminki, Sorsa and Vaino, 1979). Non-significant increased risks were detected for both mothers and fathers who had worked in agriculture, gardening, and forestry.

3.14.5 Conclusions

The results from examination of mortality data show a wide range of sites with positive results. However, there does seem to be a recurrent mention of some RES neoplasms showing excess risk in association with farming. In 7 of 10 reports there was mention of either Hodgkin's disease, non-Hodgkin's lymphoma, leukaemia, or multiple myeloma; not all the excesses noted were statistically significant. The *ad hoc* studies also show positives for the main sites of malignancy, with no appreciable preponderance for any one site.

This pattern is atypical for most known carcinogens, which tend to show a more sharply defined site-specific picture. However, the range of environmental factors is wide, and the results are compatible with subsets of the broad occupational group being exposed to different potential carcinogens.

3.15 Fishermen

Little has been published on the development of chronic disease in professional fishermen—the major interest in the past has been the very high mortality from accidents that was emphasized by Moore (1969) and Schilling (1971). Two studies have investigated skin cancer in this occupational group.

It has long been suggested that exposure to sunlight might be a risk factor in lip cancer. This agreed with the known variation in incidence or mortality from this cancer, which was high for Canada as a whole, very high for Newfoundland, and markedly high for the coastal region of this island. To explore this issue, case-control and cohort studies were undertaken (Spitzer *et al.*, 1975). Having taken account of the influence of pipe smoking and working outdoors, together with adjustment for age, it was found that fishermen had an independently increased risk of this cancer (RR = 1.4 and 4.4 from the case-control and cohort studies). It was not possible to attribute the higher risk to a particular aspect of the work of the fishermen, nor was a specific carcinogen identified.

Whitaker, Lee and Downes (1979) obtained detailed occupational histories from 598 patients with skin cancer in north-west England, with more restricted information from 148. Comparing the results with the distribution from the censuses of 1931 and 1951, there was an excess risk in fishermen (RR = 3.40; 95% CL = 0.4–12.2).

3.15.1 Conclusion

The above two reports are compatible with an increased risk of skin cancer in fishermen, but are an inadequate base to determine the risk, or confirm that this is solely due to exposure to UV light.

3.16 Foundry workers

A number of studies have been carried out in foundries. These suffer from lack of clear definition of job terms and hence of work environment. Steel foundries can be divided into the foundry proper (where the furnace is, with work on sand preparation and moulding, and casting); the fettling shop (with fettling, blasting, burning, welding, and heat treatment); pattern making, machining, and miscellaneous tasks. The following notes deal predominantly with the risk of lung cancer; they cover the contribution from routine statistics, geographical studies, and historical prospective studies. Key results are given in *Table 3.2*.

Major steel plants also contain discrete coke plants; as these can also exist independently of steel works, they are covered in a section of their own.

3.16.1 Lung cancer: occupational mortality

Using death certificates for men dying in Sheffield in 1926–35 and census estimates of workers by occupation, Turner and Grace (1938) compared observed cancer deaths against expected. The expected figures were based on rates for the 3 healthiest occupations in the total group they studied. Significant excesses were found for foundry workers for upper alimentary, rectal, respiratory, and skin cancer. Analysis of autopsy data for 85 foundry workers in the Sheffield area dying in 1949–54 suggested an excess of lung cancer (13 out of the 85), but no expected figure was provided (McLaughlin and Harding, 1956).

More recent data for England and Wales (Registrar General, 1978) showed significantly raised lung cancer SMRs for foundry workers aged 15–64, and PMRs for men aged 65–74 in 1970–72, and PRRs for 1966–67 and 1968–70. These were especially raised in moulders and core makers. Similar results have been found for metal moulders dying in California in 1959–61 (Petersen and Milham, 1980) and in Washington State in 1950–71 (Milham, 1976), and foundry workers dying in Denmark in 1968–70 (Frost, 1972).

3.16.2 Geographical studies

Mortality over a 14-year period (1961–74) in 2 parishes adjacent to a Swedish metallurgical smelter showed significant excess of lung cancer, but this was not significant when those who had worked in the smelter were excluded (Pershagen, Elinder and Bolander, 1977).

Lloyd (1978) noted that there was a significant excess of deaths from respiratory cancer in the community downwind from a Scottish steel foundry. In a further report, Lloyd *et al.* (1982) described how evidence of metallic air pollution coincided with the location of the cancers. He used mapping and plotting of deaths from cancer by radial clustering from the foundry and a number of other foci in the town. These geographical statistics were compared with male deaths from heart disease. The author concluded that the relationship with environmental pollution from the foundry was not proved, but did appear closely associated. He pointed out that the work atmosphere may be different from the pollution of the neighbourhood due to physicochemical changes in the pollutants.

3.16.3 Historical prospective studies of steel workers

Austria

Neuberger *et al.* (1982) followed 1630 male workers exposed to silica and other dusts in Vienna from the 1950s until 1980, with matched controls. In foundry workers the SMR (173) was higher than in the total groups exposed to dusts (135).

Canada

All men who had worked for at least 5 years at a Hamilton integrated steel mill in 1967 and were aged 45 and over were identified, distinguishing those who had worked in the foundry for at least 5 years. Deaths up to 1976 were compared with an expected figure based on the Toronto age/sex mortality rates for 1971. The foundry workers had a significant excess of lung cancer deaths: O = 21, E = 8.4, O/E = 2.5, 95% CL = 1.5–3.8; this seem to be marked in certain jobs within the foundry, although the specific agent responsible could not be identified (Gibson, Martin and Lockington, 1977). Identical results were published by Gibson, Lockington and Martin (1979).

England and Wales: 1

Cochrane and Moore (1980) followed 91 foundrymen aged 25–34 and 65 aged 55–64. There were too few deaths to present results for cancer by site.

England and Wales: 2

Fletcher and Ades (1984) examined the mortality of 10 250 employees in 9 foundries in England who began work in 1946–65, and were employed for at least 1 year; 97.75% were followed until 1978. National rates were used to calculate expected deaths. There appeared to be an increased risk of lung cancer in the foundry and fettling shop, with weak evidence of increased risk with longer employment.

Finland: 1

Koskela *et al.* (1976) followed 3876 men who had worked for at least 3 months in 20 iron, steel, and non-ferrous foundries in Finland in 1950–73. The average follow-up was 12.2 years. National mortality rates were used to obtain expected deaths. There was an excess of lung cancer deaths, which was concentrated in the iron foundry workers with dusty jobs especially moulders working for 5 or more years.

Finland:2

Study of 3425 men who had worked for at least 1 year in 13 iron foundries in Finland in 1918–72 and who were followed up until 1976 identified 51 lung cancer deaths with an expected of only 35.3 from proportional mortality. It appeared that the moulders and casters were at highest risk, and it was suggested thast exposure to polycyclic hydrocarbons might be a factor (Tola *et al.*, 1979).

US: 1

A major study was carried out by Lloyd and his colleagues on steelworkers, which resulted in 7 publications (Lloyd and Ciocco, 1969; Redmond, Smith and Lloyd, 1969; Robinson, 1969; Lloyd *et al.*, 1970; Lloyd, 1971; Redmond *et al.*, 1972; Lerer *et al.*, 1974). All men employed in 7 steel plants in Allegheny County in 1953 were traced to 1962; only 97 were lost to follow-up. The cohort of 59 072 men

Table 3.2 Risk of lung cancer in foundry workers*

Occupation	Country	Data–years	Sex	No. subj.	O	E	O/E	Author
Foundry workers	Austria	1950–80	M	1630	175	101.2	1.7	Neuberger *et al.* (1982)
	Canada	1967–76	M	439	21	8.4	2.5	Gibson, Martin and Lockington (1977)
	England: 2	1946–78	M	10019	181	119.0	1.5	Fletcher and Ades (1984)
	Finland: 1	1950–73	M	3876	21	13.9	1.5	Koskela *et al.* (1976)
	Finland: 2	1972–76	M		51	35.3†	1.4	Tola *et al.* (1979)
	US: 1	1953–70	M	2167	20	17.7	1.1	Breslin (1979)
	US: 2	1973–74	M		44	29.6†	1.5	Radford (1976)
	US: 3	1938–67	M	2861	29‡	23.1	1.3	Decoufle and Wood (1979)
	US: 4	1971–75	M	2990	263	177.3†	1.5	Egan-Baum, Miller and Waxweiler (1981)
Total					805	525.5	1.5	
95% CL							1.4–1.6	

*See text for description of method. †PMR. ‡ICD 190–165.

represented 62% of all employed in iron and steel production in the county at that time. The initial reports (Lloyd and Ciocco, 1969; Robinson, 1969) compared mortality with national rates by age and race, but did not present mortality for specific neoplasms. Subsequent analyses used the pooled industry rates as a comparison for men working on particular plants.

Lloyd *et al.* (1970) presented data for all malignant neoplasms, but not for lung cancer on its own. As part of the study, mortality of crane operators was compared with that in the industry as a whole. The crane operators were divided into categories of work exposure (Lerer *et al.*, 1974). Lung cancer showed no significant excess in the 5 categories examined.

Two papers in this series described a marked excess of lung cancer in coke oven workers, that was not present in the other categories of steel worker. These are discussed in 2.50.5 on coke workers.

The 2167 men who had worked in the foundry in 1953 (including those with a number of years in the job) were followed to 1970. (The trace rate was not specified.) Expected mortality was calculated from the rates for the entire steelworker population. Though there was no appreciable excess for lung cancer in the entire group of 2167 men, Breslin (1979) suggested that there was an excess in those with longer service on the plant.

US: 2

Another US steel mill showed a proportional excess of deaths from lung cancer in 1973–74 in the general workers (Radford, 1976). There were possible differences in the work conditions, including use of chromium salts, compared with the 7 plants studied by Lloyd and his colleagues; these points may account for the excess noted in workers other than in the coke ovens.

US: 3

Two thousand, eight hundred and sixty-one men who had worked in a foundry in a northern US city for at least a month were identified and followed in the period 1935–69. Expected deaths were calculated from national rates (Decoufle and Wood, 1979). Those who had worked for more than 5 years prior to 1938 had an increased risk of lung cancer.

US: 4

Union records were used to identify 3013 deaths in foundry workers in the US in 1971–75; the subjects had been union members for at least 11 years, but it was not known how many workers were not paid-up members of the death benefit fund. A proportional-mortality analysis was performed, using US national rates for expected values (Egan *et al.*, 1979a). Exactly the same results were published by Egan *et al.* (1979b).

Union records were subsequently used to trace the cause of death of 2990 male foundry workers, who had been employed prior to 1961 and who had been identified as dead in 1971–75. US mortality was used to calculate PMRs (Egan-Baum, Miller and Waxweiler, 1981). There was a significant excess of lung cancer: O = 263, E = 177.3, O/E = 1.48, 95% CL = 1.3–1.7. Internal case-control analysis showed an excess for iron foundry workers when compared with those from steel and non-ferrous foundries.

3.16.4 Other studies of the risk of lung cancer

In a case-control study of 325 men who had died of lung cancer in eastern Pennsylvania, an increased risk was shown in steel workers. Adjusted for smoking the risk was 1.8 (95% CL = 1.2–2.8), and it was higher in those who had worked in foundry operations and been long-term employees (Blot *et al.*, 1983). The risk was greatest for small cell tumours compared with all forms of histology.

In an attempt to clarify the epidemiological evidence of an excess of lung cancer in workers in ferrous foundries, Gibson *et al.* (1983) carried out mutagenicity studies of particulate matter in a foundry. This identified mutagenicity levels higher than in urban air, with distribution of levels within the foundry consistent with the epidemiological evidence of variation in risk.

Simard *et al.* (1983) examined the sputum cytology of 677 male foundry workers. Though prevalence of atypia varied with smoking level, there was no apparent variation in workers from different departments in the foundry.

3.16.5 Other sites of malignancy

Nose

Occupational histories obtained for patients registered with nasal cancer in England and Wales in 1963–67 suggested an excess risk in steel foundry furnacement (Acheson, Cowdell and Rang, 1981).

Laryngeal cancer

A case-control study of 204 patients with laryngeal cancer diagnosed in 1977–79 in Ontario used individually matched neighbourhood controls. All subjects were interviewed by trained interviewers at home (Burch *et al.*, 1981). There was an increased risk for moulder and core makers: RR = ∞, 95% CL = 3.5–∞; those exposed to foundry fumes: RR = 5.0, 95% CL = 2.1–11.9.

Bone

Mapping of bone tumour patients in Gavleborg County, Sweden showed aggregations in localities with iron works and marked air pollution. In these localities there was a five-fold excess of these cancers, which was significantly greater than the national rate (Lindahl, 1972).

Leukaemia

The Registrar General (1978) indicated an increased SMR for myeloid leukaemia in furnace, forge, and foundry workers. In a preliminary report on chromosome aberrations in Swedish smelter workers, Beckman, Beckman and Nordson (1977) reported excess aberrations compared with control subjects. The smelter workers had been exposed to arsenic and other agents; it was not clear what the responsible factor was, and no comment is made of a risk from leukaemia in the workers.

3.16.6 Conclusions

It seems clear that there is an increased risk of lung cancer in 'foundry workers'. There is no clear agreement as to the specific jobs at highest risk, nor the responsible agent. In a review of the topic, Palmer and Scott (1981) suggested that although silica was the predominant airborne substance in foundries, PAH from a variety of sources was the most likely carcinogen. The role of silica is discussed in Chapter 2, 2.51.

An important issue is whether the smoking habits of these workers is different from the general population. Lloyd Davies (1971) surveyed 1997 foundrymen aged 35–64 and 1777 workers in engineering factories in Great Britain in 1964–65. A slightly higher proportion of the foundrymen smoked than the controls (73.9% and 70.4%); no details were given of the number of cigarettes smoked. This is unlikely to account for the above results.

The results for other cancer sites are not sufficiently clearcut to consider that there is an increased risk in foundry workers.

3.17 Hairdressers

3.17.1 Background

There has been considerable interest in the possible hazard to man of various permanent and semi-permanent hair dyes (*see* IARC, 1978a and 1982a for reviews). This has been associated with a number of studies on the development of cancer in those using such dyes; these studies are not reviewed here. The present section covers occupational mortality and the analysis of risks from routine data

systems including occupation as one of the items. Four studies have been done on groups of hairdressers, following them for a number of years; each of these is reviewed. The next subsection deals with a number of case-control studies on bladder cancer, which have included data on risk in hairdressers.

3.17.2 Occupational mortality/incidence

Occupational mortality for male barbers or single women employed as hairdressers in England and Wales in 1970–72 showed no significant excess of malignancy for a specific site (Registrar General, 1978).

Cancer registrations in Denmark in 1943–72 showed lower cancer in male hairdressers for all major sites compared with expected. There were about twice the expected in females: digestive organs: O = 205, E = 92.0; respiratory: O = 34, E = 14.7; breast: O = 168, E = 101.0; uterus: O = 206, E = 108.8; urinary tract: O = 38, E = 14.3; skin: O = 53, E = 34.8; RES: O = 43, E = 26.5. However, Clemmesen (1977a) expressed reservations about the estimate of the number of women employed, which was used to calculate the expected values from national incidence rates. This may have accounted for the discrepancy between the observed and expected numbers.

Analysis of occupations recorded for 6434 white males and 7515 white females admitted to Roswell Park in 1956–65 were examined for 22 sites of malignancy (National Institute for Occupational Health and Safety, 1977). Male barbers showed a significant excess of laryngeal cancer (O = 10, E = 3.53, O/E = 2.83, 95% CL = 1.4–5.2), whilst female hairdressers and beauticians showed significant increases for cancer of corpus uteri (O = 6, E = 2.0, O/E = 3.0, 95% CL = 1.1–6.5) and ovary (O = 10, E = 3.36, O/E = 2.98, 95% CL = 1.4–5.5).

Garfinkel, Selvin and Brown (1977) used 3460 death certificates for females in Alameda County, California in 1958–62 dying of cancer and control deaths from other causes. There was a non-significant increased risk of cancer among beauticians (RR = 1.73); the excess was much greater for lung cancer (RR = 6.0), than other sites. Menck *et al.* (1977) used cancer registrations for females in Los Angeles in 1972–75. A proportional incidence analysis suggested a significantly raised risk for lung cancer (O = 20, E = 11.4, O/E = 1.76, 95% CL = 1.1–2.7).

A preliminary report of sickness absence from work indicated significantly raised proportional certification for cancer of various sites in cosmetologists in the US in 1969–72; digestive organs: O/E = 1.46; respiratory organs: O/E = 1.59; breast: O/E = 1.54; genital organs: O/E = 1.35. The numbers of subjects on which this was based were not given (Kennedy and Spirtas, 1977).

3.17.3 Prospective studies

Hammond (1977) examined the mortality of 5117 beauticians aged over 30 at entry to the 1 million subject American Cancer Society study, who were followed for 13 years. This was a major prospective study coordinated by the American Cancer Society, which used local representatives to recruit volunteers, who completed detailed questionnaires and were then followed up. The prime focus of the study was to investigate the influence of smoking on cancer. Compared with matched controls there were 113 deaths from cancer, with 115 expected. There was not a single site of cancer with significantly more deaths in beauticians than controls (the actual figures were not provided).

A sample of 1831 hairdressers was identified in the 1961 census in England and Wales, and followed to 1978. Expected mortality was based on national rates. Five sites were investigated, which had been noted as increased in other studies: cancer of the oesophagus, larynx, lung, bladder, and leukaemia. There was no appreciable or significant excess for any of these malignancies (Alderson, 1980b).

An historical prospective study of 7736 female beauticians in Japan over the period 1953–77 showed a significant excess from stomach cancer (O/E = 1.34), with no other excess for any other site (Kono *et al.*, 1983).

The cancer incidence in 11 845 female and 1805 male cosmetologists working in Connecticut, who began work prior to 1966 was compared with the expected based on state rates. All had been licensed for work for over 5 years in the period 1935–78 (Teta *et al.*, 1984). Results were provided for 15 sites of malignancy, but only respiratory tract showed a significant excess. The risk was not evident in those who had begun work after 1935; no information was available on smoking in the subjects.

3.17.4 Bladder case-control studies

A number of studies of bladder cancer have indicated an increased risk for hairdressers and associated work. These studies are all reviewed in the section on bladder cancer (*see* 4.23.1). The relative risks are: ∞ for US hairdressers (Wynder, Onderdonk and Mantel, 1963); 2.8 for US barbers (Dunham *et al.*, 1968); ∞ and 4.0 for hairdressers in England with 2 different sources of controls (Anthony and Thomas, 1970); 0.6 for US barbers (Cole, Hoover and Friedell, 1972); ∞ in Canadian barbers (Howe *et al.*, 1977); 0.9 for English hairdressers (Cartwright, 1982); 1.27 for US hairdressers (Schoenberg *et al.*, 1984).

Though 2 of these studies failed to show an increased risk of bladder cancer, the weight of evidence points to such an association in hairdressers.

3.17.5 Multiple myeloma

Cancer registrations in Los Angeles in 1972–78 identified 286 patients with multiple myeloma. A proportional analysis suggested that there was an excess risk in cosmetologists and hairdressers: O = 8, E = 1.7, O/E = 4.67, 95% CL = 2.0–9.2. This was not due to the proportion of whites or sex differences (Guidotti, Wright and Peters, 1982).

3.17.6 Conclusions

It must be remembered that some of the occupational studies relate to employment before the introduction of suspect hair dyes. There is also the possible exposure to other chemicals (e.g. propellants with fluorocarbons or vinyl chloride).

IARC (1978a) concluded that there was an elevated risk of cancer in those with occupational exposure to certain hair dyes (i.e. barbers and hairdressers). However, IARC (1982a) suggested that the evidence relating bladder cancer or any other cancer to hairdressing was inconclusive and further studies were required.

3.18 Health professionals

Those working in the health field may have specific exposures, which are considered elsewhere: anaesthetics (2.4), and formaldehyde (2.36). This section provides a brief note on the pattern of cancer mortality in doctors, the possible hazard from bladder cancer in nurses, and of RES neoplasms in doctors and nurses. Mention is made of a few studies of hazard to the next generation.

3.18.1 Prospective study of doctors

Doll and Peto (1977) followed, until 1977, 20 540 male doctors in the UK who had completed a questionnaire in 1951 when aged 35 and over. They demonstrated slight variation in risk of cancers other than lung, mouth, and oesophagus by specialty recorded in 1952, none of which were significantly different. Unfortunately, no comparison with an external standard was made.

3.18.2 Studies of particular neoplasms

Bladder cancer

There was a suggestion from the case-control study of Anthony and Thomas (*see* England and Wales: 1 (a) and (b) in 4.21.1) that nurses were at increased risk of bladder cancer. This is not reflected in the general review of these studies, with the study from Canada: 2 showing a non-significant risk in health professionals, whilst no other results refer to this group of workers.

RES—leukaemia

In a study of all patients developing leukaemia in Olmsted County, Minnesota in 1955–74, there was no evidence of increased risk in those reporting work in the health professions (Linos *et al.*, 1980).

Hodgkin's disease

It had been suggested that contact with patients developing Hodgkin's disease might place doctors at risk. Vianna *et al.* (1974) examined the mortality in New York from 1960 to 1972 amongst physicians and suggested that there appeared to be a relative risk of 1.8 in the mortality of this group. Smith, Kinlen and Doll (1974) examined the observed and expected mortality from Hodgkin's disease, using follow-up data available from the study of British doctors and their smoking habits. They found no evidence for an excess of Hodgkin's disease over the expected, and no subcategory by occupational group appeared to have an exceptional risk of this condition. Matanoski, Sartwell and Elliott (1975) used records from 3 medical specialty associations in the US to identify enrollees in 1920–49, who were followed until 1969. There was no evidence of an atypical mortality from Hodgkin's disease: O = 13, E = 13.7, O/E = 0.99, 95% CL = 0.5–1.7.

3.18.3 Nurses injecting anti-neoplastic agents

Knowles and Virden (1980) reviewed the hazards from handling injectable anti-neoplastic agents. Mutagenic activity was identified in the urine of nurses administering these drugs, although the specific cause or portal of entry was not identified. Norpa *et al.* (1980) found an increased sister chromatid exchange rate in exposed nurses. However, Staiano *et al.* (1981) found no evidence of mutagenicity in pharmaceutical workers, whilst Bos *et al.* (1982) only observed this activity in nurses who smoked. In a study of hospital staff handling cytotoxic drugs, Venitt *et al.* (1984) found that unexposed staff gave positive results in a high proportion of urine mutagenicity assays, as well as staff exposed to a variety of drugs (6 of 9 control subjects and 5 of 10 exposed staff). Hirst *et al.* (1984) found cyclophosphamide in the urine of nurses giving this drug to patients. It was not clear if this was absorbed from the skin or via inhaled aerosols of the drug.

A recent review (*Lancet*, 1984a) indicated the difficulty at present in quantifying the extent of the hazard from reported studies.

3.18.4 Hazards to the next generation

Strandberg *et al.* (1978) questioned 56 women working in a hospital laboratory about pregnancy history. Of the 71 pregnancies reported, 8/24 ended in spontaneous abortion when the mother had been working in her pregnancy, whilst 9/47 when the mother was not working in the laboratory. After adjustment for confounding factors, RR = 1.9, 95% CL = 1.0–3.6.

Interviews of 77 women working in a virology laboratory suggested a significantly increased perinatal mortality amongst conceptions of the staff, with 4 perinatal deaths in 69 pregnancies (Axelson *et al.*, 1980).

A postal questionnaire completed by sterilizing staff in hospitals in Finland in 1980 and checked against hospital discharge records, suggested an increase in spontaneous abortions in those exposed to ethylene oxide but not to other agents including formaldehyde (Hemminki *et al.*, 1982).

3.18.5 Conclusions

The range of studies, variation in the work environment and inconsistent results fail to provide a clear picture of increased risk of cancer. The topics of (*a*) staff handling anti-neoplastic agents, and (*b*) outcome of pregnancy in laboratory staff warrant further study.

3.19 Jewelry workers

Proportional-mortality analysis of 931 deaths of jewelry workers dying in Massachusetts in 1956–76 indicated an excess of stomach cancer in the subgroup involved in polishing (O = 5, E = 1.14, O/E = 4.4, 95% CL = 1.4–10.2). This was using the remainder of the group to calculate an expected value (Sparks and Wegman, 1980).

There was no indication if there was some particular occupational or environmental factor involved.

3.19.1 Conclusion

There was insufficient human data available for this occupational group to evaluate the level of cancer.

3.20 Leather workers

Following the initial papers on adenocarcinoma of the nose in furniture workers (*see* 3.38), a number of studies identified a possible hazard in leather workers. However, prior to this period, some analyses of occupational mortality had already suggested that there might be increased risk of cancer in leather workers. General case-control studies of occupation in bladder cancer had also recorded positive results.

The following notes provide a brief guide to the method used in the various studies; occupational mortality and incidence studies are dealt with first, including those mounted to study the specific association with leather work. A few case reports are briefly noted. A number of studies have compared occupations reported by patients, with expected values based on census statistics. Many case-control studies have been carried out that are at least partly relevant to the risks in the leather industry; the key ones are reviewed. Preliminary results only are available from one prospective study. In this section the text concentrates on the method used in different studies, whilst the results are in *Table 3.3*.

Some of the studies have contrasted the occupations for patients with adenocarcinoma of the nasal passages against those with other histology of the same site. The estimates of risk from such a comparison need to be treated with great caution. If the occupation under study only causes adenocarcinoma, and the occupations of the patients with other histology are an unbiased reflection of the occupations in the catchment area for the study, the results are not distorted (apart from a small number effect, or the validity of the data recording). If the occupation causes adenocarcinoma and other forms of nasal cancer, or there is a powerful association between the non-adenocarcinoma malignancies and another occupation, the relative risks may be appreciably distorted.

3.20.1 Occupational mortality and incidence

Examination of the occupation recorded for male deaths from bladder cancer in England and Wales in 1921–28 indicated an excess for leather and tannery workers (Henry, Kennaway and Kennaway, 1931).

Examination of occupation recorded for male lung cancer deaths in England and Wales in 1921–38 showed an excess in leather tannery workers (Kennaway and Kennaway, 1947).

In a general examination of occupational mortality for the Netherlands in 1931–35 (Versluys, 1949), data are provided on cancers in 'shoemakers and shoehands'.

The occupations of 2161 white males dying from lung cancer aged 20–64 in Los Angeles in 1968–70 and 1771 incident cases diagnosed in 1972–73 were compared with census estimates (Menck and Henderson, 1976).

The decennial supplement on occupational mortality for England and Wales for 1970–72 (Registrar General, 1978) showed a raised SMR for myeloid leukaemia for leather workers.

The distribution of mortality from oral and pharyngeal cancer in counties of the US in 1950–69 was compared with the proportion of the population employed in 18 different industries, including leather processing (Blot and Fraumeni, 1977).

Use of the Swedish Cancer Environment file (*see* the Appendix, Chapter 1) permitted examination of the cancer incidence in shoemakers in 1961–73 (Englund, 1980). Though there were excesses for oesophageal, liver, and biliary tract cancer, and leukaemia, none were significant. The same file was used to identify 1629 leather tanners and 4504 shoe workers in 1960, who were followed to 1973. Cancers of the kidney, renal pelvis, and bladder were reported to be increased (Malker *et al.*, 1984).

3.20.2 Case reports

A review of occupational histories for 149 patients with multiple myeloma diagnosed in Hamburg in 1935–65 suggested that excess risk was associated, *inter alia*, with leather dressing (Dorken and Vollmer, 1968). The expected distribution by occupation was not given and many subjects had several jobs.

Occupational histories were studied for 30 male patients with nasal cancer treated in one Belgian hospital in 1958–68 (Debois, 1969); 20 of the patients had an adenocarcinoma. The proportion of leather workers was thought to be raised.

Occupations recorded for 144 deaths from bladder cancer in the Stoke area in 1965–70 were examined by Veys (1974). Two shoe repairers were included in the 36 males thought to have exposure to various occupational risks.

3.20.2 Comparison of occupational histories from cases and expected distribution based on the census

In an expension of the studies of nasal cancer in furniture workers in the Oxford region, the regional registry identified 46 patients with nasal cancer resident in Northamptonshire diagnosed in 1953–67 (Acheson, Cowdell and Jolles, 1970). The occupation was obtained by postal questionnaire, or interview of patient or relative. Census estimates of 1961 for males by occupation and age were used to calculate approximate incidence rates. The histology was reviewed by a pathologist, when specimens were available. In addition, several sources of information were used to identify patients who had worked in the boot and shoe industry and suffered from nasal cancer outside the period 1953–67 (the regional cancer registry, union records, and the death register for Northampton County Borough). This study was extended to cover nasal cancer patients diagnosed in the period 1950–79 in Northamptonshire, again using the 3 different sources of information. A postal questionnaire was sent to the patients or their relatives to obtain information on occupation, smoking and use of snuff (Acheson,

Table 3.3 Risk of various cancers in leather workers*

Site	Method	Country	Data–years	O	RR	Comment	Author
Oral, pharyngeal	Occupational mortality	Netherlands	1931–35	5	2.63		Versluys (1949]
	Mortality × country	US	1950–69			Excess in counties with leather industries	Blot and Fraumeni (1977)
	Case-control	US	1956–65	18	3.22		Decoufle (1979)
Nasal	Case reports	Belgium	1958–68			Excess in leather workers	Debois (1969)
	Case vs census	England and Wales	1953–67	17	7.3		Acheson, Cowdell and Jolles (1970)
	Case vs census	England and Wales	1950–69	70	4.8	Males only	Acheson et al. (1982)
	Case vs census	England and Wales	1961–66	7	14.0	Adenocarcinoma	Acheson, Cowdell and Rang (1972)
	Case vs census	England and Wales	1963–67	26	4.36		Acheson, Cowdell and Rang (1981)
	Case vs census	Sweden	1961–71	3		Possible excess in females	Engzell, Englund and Westerholm (1978)
	Case-control	Netherlands	1944–67	2	∞		Delemarre and Themans (1971)
	Case-control	Germany	1931–77	1	2.26		Lobe and Erhardt (1978)
	Case-control	Italy	1963–77	7	∞		Cecchi et al. (1980)
	Case-control	Italy	1969–79	3	3.38		Merler et al. (1982)
Larynx	Case-control	US	1956–65	7	3.31		Decoufle (1979)
Lung	Occupational mortality	England and Wales	1921–38	51	1.41		Kennaway and Kennaway (1947)
	Occupational mortality and incidence	US	1968–73	7	2.33		Menck and Henderson (1976)
Bladder	Occupational mortality	England and Wales	1921–28	17	1.68		Henry, Kennaway and Kennaway (1931)
	Occupational mortality	Netherlands	1931–35	14	1.73		Versluys (1949)
	Occupational incidence	Sweden	1961–73	29	1.49		Malker et al. (1984)
	Case reports	England and Wales	1965–70	2		Excess shoe repairers	Veys (1974)
	Case-control	US	1957–61	12	∞		Wynder, Onderdonk and Mantel (1963)
	Case-control	US	1967–68	79	2.0		Cole, Hoover and Friedell (1972)
	Case-control	US	1956–65	11	6.30		Decoufle (1979)
	Case-control	Italy	1970s	5	5.0		Vineis et al. (1982)
	Case-control	US	1981–82	19	1.78		Schoenberg et al. (1984)
Kidney	Occupational incidence	Sweden	1961–73	8	2.35		Malker et al. (1984)
Lymphosarcoma	Case-control	US	1956–65	15	2.16		Decoufle (1979)
Multiple myeloma	Case reports	Germany	1935–65			Excess in leather dressers	Dorken and Vollmer (1968)
Leukaemia	Occupational mortality	England and Wales	1970–72	8	1.06		Registrar General (1978)
	Occupational incidence	Sweden	1961–73	21	1.56		Englund (1980)

(see also Benzene review, 2.8)

*See text for description of method.

Pippard and Winter, 1982). Census estimates for 1931, 1951, 1961, and 1971 were used to calculate incidence rates.

(Note: these two studies may have differentially inflated the proportion of boot and shoe workers due to the use of union records, and the incidence rates are only approximate due to the use of census estimates.)

Patients with adenocarcinoma of the nose were identified from all regions of England and Wales excluding Oxford, for 1961–66. For each such patient a control with nasal cancer of other histology was selected. The histology was reviewed and an occupational history obtained by postal questionnaire to the patients or their relatives. The observed distribution for 27 occupational groups was compared with the expected, based on the proportions from the 1961 census (Acheson, Cowdell and Rang, 1972). This study was extended to all patients with any histology of nasal cancer known to the national registry of England and Wales in 1963–67 (Acheson, Cowdell and Rang, 1981). Histology was verified and questionnaires sent to patients or their relatives to record occupational history, smoking, and use of snuff. The last occupation was available for 875 males (94.6% of those in the study). The patients were separated into 27 occupational groups and an expected figure calculated. (The details of this are not provided, but the 1961 census estimates were presumably used.)

Cancer registry records were used in Sweden to identify (*a*) 36 men and 10 women with adenocarcinoma of the nose diagnosed in 1961–71 and (*b*) 177 men and 85 women with squamous or poorly differentiated cancers diagnosed in 1965–71. Information on prior occupation was obtained from hospital records, questionnaires to the patients or their relatives, or church records. Approximate relative risks were based on union and census statistics of the exposed population (Engzell, Englund and Westerholm, 1978).

3.20.4 Case-control studies

Nose

Delemarre and Themans (1971) compared the occupations of 16 patients with nasal cancer adenocarcinoma treated in 1944–67 and 33 patients with other histology treated in 1956–68 in one hospital in the Netherlands.

A questionnaire was answered on occupational history by 179 (43%) patients with nasal cancer treated in 1931–77 in West Germany (Lobe and Ehrhardt, 1978). A comparison of occupation was made between those with adenocarcinoma and other histology, and also against estimates of the proportion of the population who were woodworkers.

A case-control study of 64 patients with nasal cancer (including 11 with adenocarcinoma) treated in Florence in 1963–77, involved interview of the patients or their relatives, and non-cancer hospital controls (Cecchi *et al.*, 1980).

A small case-control study of 19 patients from northern Italy explored the occupational histories, particularly considering leather and wood exposure (Merler *et al.*, 1982). However, the confidence limits of the results are very wide.

Larynx

A general case-control study of 258 men with laryngeal cancer treated in 5 cities in the US in 1970–73 had provided limited information about occupation and did not mention results for leather workers (Wynder *et al.*, 1976).

Mesothelioma

Decoufle (1980) reported 3 patients with mesothelioma who had worked as shoemakers. In conjunction with the report of Vianna and Polan (1978) of a married couple who were shoemakers, this suggested there may be a slight risk in the industry perhaps from asbestos filler in rubber soles and heels.

Bladder

Sixteen case-control studies of bladder cancer have examined the association with occupation. Increased risks for leather workers was noted by Wynder, Onderdonk and Mantel (1963), Cole, Hoover and Friedell (1972), Vineis *et al.* (1982), Schoenberg *et al.* (1984). Three other studies did not find a significant increase, whilst the remaining 9 studies did not present results for leather workers. These studies are reviewed in 4.23.1.

Additional analysis of the bladder cancer study from Yorkshire (*see* Cartwright *et al.*, 1983 in 4.23.1) examined the risk of this tumour in leather workers amongst the 923 male patients. Though there was an apparent increase in risk in tanners and boot and shoe repairers, this was not significant (Cartwright and Boyko, 1984).

Leukaemia

Benzene had been used as a solvent in shoe making and a number of studies have been reported of the risk of haemopathies and leukaemia in exposed workers. These are reviewed in the section on benzene (*see* 2.8).

Multisite studies

Occupations recorded for patients admitted to Roswell Park in 1956–65 were used to examine the risks of various cancers in comparison with clerical workers and control patients. Limited results were quoted by Viadana, Bross and Houten (1976), whilst a general report of this work has been published by Decoufle *et al.* (1977) (*see* 1.4.3). A more detailed probe of this material examined the risk for workers in the leather industry for 4 specific cancers (Decoufle, 1979). Additional data were collected for those bladder cancer patients treated in 1966–71, who had worked at one shoe manufacturing company.

3.20.5 Prospective studies

A follow-up study of 5108 boot and shoe workers, and 848 tanners in England from 1939 until 1982 did not find an excess of kidney or bladder cancer (Acheson and Pippard, 1984).

3.20.6 Hazard to the next generation

In a study of spontaneous abortion in the rubber and leather industries in Finland, Hemminki *et al.* (1983a) found evidence of higher frequencies in women who had been employed for less than 2 years. It was suggested that there might be selection bias for those having longer employment.

3.20.7 Conclusions

IARC (1981) considered that there was no evidence to suggest an association between leather tanning and nasal cancer.

Employment in the boot and shoe industry is causally related to nasal adenocarcinoma, and it is most likely that leather dust plays a part. There may also be a risk for other histological types of nasal cancer.

Although there was evidence of an increased risk of bladder cancer in the industry, it is not possible to determine whether this relates to boot and shoe manufacture in particular.

Benzene exposure in shoemakers leads to aplastic anaemia and leukaemia (*see* 2.8).

It was not possible to review the positive findings in relation to cancer of the oral cavity, pharynx, stomach, larynx, lung, kidney or lymphoma because of lack of adequate data.

3.21 Masons

Using occupational histories collected from inpatients at Roswell Park hospital in 1956–65, Bross, Viadana and Houten (1978) found a statistically significant risk of kidney cancer in brick masons. This has not been replicated elsewhere and is difficult to interpret.

3.21.1 Conclusion

The above is an inadequate base to consider that there is a risk of cancer in these workers.

3.22 Miners

This section covers two categories of miner: (*a*) coal miners, and (*b*) other metal miners. There is an important category of miner covered elsewhere—iron-ore, uranium, and other miners known to be exposed to irradiation; these are discussed with the other sources of radiation (*see* 2.39.4). Miners are one group exposed to silica; the hazards from this are discussed in 2.51. *Table 3.4* shows the results for stomach and lung cancer in coal miners.

3.22.1 Coal miners

This section begins with analyses of mortality statistics, and then describes a number of studies with *ad hoc* data collection.

3.22.1.1 Occupational mortality statistics

Kennaway and Kennaway (1953) used all death certificates from lung cancer in England and Wales in 1937–46 to examine the death rates in miners. The mortality was lower than in the general population, though it had increased over time (as in other groups). The risk was higher in face workers than others (though the latter could smoke at work) and was also higher in the South Wales fields, where there was a higher prevalence of pneumoconiosis.

Using death certificates from South Wales, Doll (1958) examined the risk of lung cancer in steel and colliery workers; a PMR was calculated with expected based on 'all other occupations in the locality'. He noted a reduced risk of lung cancer in miners in 1948–56 (O = 73, E = 152, O/E = 0.48, 95% CL = 0.4–0.6).

Stocks (1962) used the Registrar General's data to examine the mortality rate from stomach cancer amongst coal miners in 1949–53 in 9 areas in England and Wales. He compared the age-adjusted mortality with that amongst non-miners living in the same counties, taking account of urbanization of place of residence. He suggested that the data showed an occupational hazard for stomach cancer which was greater in South Wales, intermediate in northern England, and least in the Midlands.

Enterline (1964) used the 1950 data on deaths by occupation and population estimates by age for miners in the US, to calculate SMRs for those aged 20–64. This showed a significantly raised SMR for stomach (O = 146; E = 53; O/E = 2.75; 95% CL = 2.3–3.2); lung (O = 161; E = 84; O/E = 1.92; 95% CL = 1.7–2.3) and a number of other sites.

Ashley (1969) used mortality and environmental data for 53 towns in England and Wales, to study factors associated with gastric cancer. There was a significant regression coefficient for those living in towns with excess exposure to coal and textile industries.

A special enquiry checked the occupations for 5362 men dying in 1961 in England and Wales and recorded as having worked in coal mines (Liddell, 1973). This showed an indication of raised mortality for stomach cancer in underground workers and a low SMR for lung cancer in underground and surface workers.

Crofton (1969) defined localities in Scotland associated with coal mining from the 1961 census. She then calculated expected age-adjusted mortality for bronchitis and lung cancer in these and comparison localities. There was an increase in the deaths in males, but a decrease in females from lung cancer in the coal mining localities. She also reported surveys showing lower weekly cigarette consumption in miners compared with the general population in England and Wales, and Scotland.

Matolo *et al.* (1972) examined the gastric cancer incidence in coal mining locations in Utah; there are only 2 coal mining counties in this state, and after adjusting for age and sex, they appeared to have four-fold the gastric cancer incidence of the state. The records of patients developing stomach cancer were examined; it was suggested that there was an increased risk of this cancer in miners three-fold that

of other males in the same counties and eight-fold that of men in other counties in Utah.

Klauber and Lyon (1978) examined the incidence of stomach cancer in the same coal mining counties in Utah for 1970–75. Indirect SRRs were based on data from the whole of the state; these were 110 and 129 for the 2 counties, showing less excess than the previous report. Review of data for the entire period 1965–75 suggested that registration in 1965 may have been atypical as it was the first year of the state registry.

Creagan, Hoover and Fraumeni (1974) used data for gastric cancer mortality in 23 coal mining counties in 7 states in the US for 1950–69 and compared this with other counties matched on educational level, but with no coal mining. Observed stomach cancer mortality was 20–30% greater than expected in the coal mining counties (*P*<0.01), but a similar excess was noted for other cancers associated with low social class (lung and cervix).

3.22.1.2 Prospective studies

Australia

Armstrong *et al.* (1979) followed 213 coal miners in Western Australia from 1961 to 1975. Expected deaths were based on state mortality rates. The results, based on few deaths, were compatible with an excess risk of stomach cancer and decreased risk for lung cancer. There was an excess of deaths from melanoma: O = 3, E = 0.2, O/E = 15.0, 95% CL = 3.0–43.8.

Table 3.4 Risk of stomach cancer and lung cancer in coal miners*

Study		Stomach		Lung		Author
		O	E	O	E	
Occupational mortality						
US, 1950		146	53.0	161	84.0	Enterline (1964)
Washington State, 1950–79		79	63.0	197†	148.0	Milham (1983)
England and Wales, 1970–72, aged 15–64		252	147.4	843	735.3	Registrar General (1978)
Ad hoc studies						
Australia	213 miners, 1961–75	2	0.9	1	4.0	Armstrong *et al.* (1979)
Canada	Silicotic miners, 1940–59	20‡	18.8	38	15.3	Finkelstein, Kusiak and Suryani (1982)
Canada	Silicotic miners, 1960–75	4‡	7.0	7	7.4	Finkelstein, Kusiak and Suryani (1982)
US: 1	553 miners, 1938–66	8‡	3.8	4	3.6	Enterline (1972)
US: 2	3726 miners, 1963–71			24	36.0	Costello, Ortmeyer and Morgan (1974)
US: 3	23 232 miners, 1959–71	129	92.4	352	310.9	Rockette (1977)
Total		640	386.3	1627	1344.5	
O/E		1.66		1.21		
95% CL		1.5–1.8		1.1–1.3		

*See text for description of method.
†ICD 160–165.
‡ICD 150–154.

Canada

Using compensation records, Finkelstein, Kusiak and Suranyi (1982) identified 1190 miners with silicosis in 1940–75 in Ontario, who were followed until 1978. Expected deaths were based on province mortality rates. There was a two-fold excess of lung cancer deaths in those awarded compensation in 1940–59, but no increase in those diagnosed after this period.

Great Britain: 1

Goldman (1965) presented several sets of data. Material from the National Coal Board for men aged 20–65 showed a reduced SMR for lung cancer in 1955, that was more marked in underground workers (O = 216, E = 308, O/E = 0.70, 95% CL = 0.6–0.8) than surface workers (O = 54, E = 59, O/E = 0.91, 95% CL = 0.7–1.2). The SMR was not reduced for miners in the south-west. Follow-up of 5096 miners and ex-miners in 1951–56 showed variation in risk of lung cancer in relation to initial X-ray findings, with those having intermediate changes of pneumoconiosis having a lower risk of cancer than those with no changes or with progressive massive fibrosis. Goldman emphasized that numerous investigators had found no evidence of difference in smoking habits of miners and other men.

Great Britain: 2

Jacobsen (1976), in a follow-up of a large number of men employed in the UK by the National Coal Board, was able to relate measurement of dust exposure to subsequent mortality and had demonstrated a dose–response relationship to risk of stomach cancer. An extension of this study of nearly 30 000 men indicated an increased mortality from stomach cancer with increasing duration since first exposure to dust, after allowing for radiological evidence of pneumoconiosis. It was not clear from the available data whether dust directly 'causes' the gastric cancer or only by way of initial pneumoconiosis (Miller, Jacobsen and Steele, 1981).

US: 1

Enterline (1972) reported a small prospective study of 553 miners followed in the US in the period 1938–66. There was an excess of deaths from digestive cancers and a negligible excess of lung cancer deaths.

US: 2

A prevalence study of pneumoconiosis was carried out in 1963–64 on 2549 miners and 1177 ex-miners from Appalachia. These men were then followed up until 1971 (Ortmeyer *et al.*, 1974). Expected deaths were calculated from US mortality rates in 1968. No data were presented on malignant disease. However, a second report (Costello, Ortmeyer and Morgan, 1974) identified a decrease in lung cancer deaths: O = 24, E = 36, O/E = 0.67, 95% CL = 0.4–1.0. Though data were collected on smoking, no comment was made about the prevalence of this in the miners compared with the general population.

US: 3

A 10% sample of men in the United Mine Workers Health and Retirement Funds (23 323) identified in 1959 were followed until 1971. Expected deaths were calculated from US mortality rates. The SMR was higher for stomach cancer in pensioners than those still at work (Rockette, 1977).

US: 4

Four cohort studies of US white male coal miners were used to identify 317 deaths from lung cancer in the period 1959–75. Controls were (*a*) living miners, and (*b*) those dying from neither cancer nor accidents (Ames *et al.*, 1983). Information on smoking was available. There was no evidence of risk of lung cancer in the miners, independently of smoking, nor appreciable difference from either group of controls.

US: 5

Using the same 4 cohorts of miners, Ames *et al.* (1983) identified 46 men who had died from stomach cancer and age-matched controls from the same cohorts. There was an increased risk from (*a*) prolonged exposure to coal dust, and (*b*) smoking; there was no effect from prior evidence of pneumoconiosis.

3.22.1.3 Case-control studies

Nasal cancer

A general survey of patients registered with nasal cancer in England and Wales in 1963–67 obtained information on occupation from hospitals, patients, or next-of-kin (Acheson, Cowdell and Rang, 1981). A significant excess risk was shown for coal miners.

Prostate cancer

Williams, Stegens and Goldsmith (1977) presented analyses from the US Third National Cancer Survey on occupation reported by patients with different malignancies. Miners had an increased risk of prostate cancer.

3.22.2 Other miners

A few studies have examined the risk in other miners than coal (*see* 2.39 on hazard from irradiation in certain categories of miners).

Australia

A study of 1974 gold miners in Western Australia followed in 1961–75 documented a relatively high mortality from lung cancer: O = 59, E = 40.8, O/E = 1.4, 95% CL = 1.1–1.9. However, this was inconclusively related to underground miners experience and might possibly be due to excess smoking reported in these mines (Armstrong *et al.*, 1979). The level of radon in the mines was much lower than in some of the other studies where this was thought to be a factor; the level of arsenic was also low, with no evidence of arsenicism in the miners. No results were presented for stomach cancer.

Canada

Miners with pneumoconiosis who had worked in metal mines (copper, gold, iron, lead, tin, and zinc) in Quebec were followed in the period 1967–77. One of 85 with advanced silicosis had died of lung cancer, but 10 out of 118 milder cases. Though no expected deaths were presented, it was suggested that this excluded a silicosis predisposition to lung cancer (Enzenwa, 1982).

Sweden

A case-control study of 29 lead and zinc miners with lung cancer in Sweden in 1956–76 showed a marked increase in risk in the miners in comparison with population controls (Axelson and Sundell, 1978). Surprisingly, the relative risk appeared to be higher in non-smokers, though the smokers developed lung cancer at a younger age. These findings were based on small numbers.

US

Wagoner *et al.* (1963) identified 930 deaths in 1759 metal miners who had worked underground at least 15 years in the US in 1937–59. Using state mortality rates a person-years mortality analysis showed an increased risk for both digestive and respiratory cancers. There was no evidence of increased radioactivity in the mines; the general demographic characteristics and smoking habits of the miners did not explain the findings.

3.22.3 Conclusions

There appears to be consistent evidence of a hazard from stomach cancer in coal miners. It is not clear whether these findings are due to confounding with other environmental factors, though the dose–response found with dust levels is persuasive evidence (Miller *et al.*, 1981). A number of authors have found a relationship between risk of stomach cancer and a variety of dust exposures (Kraus, Levin and Gerhardt, 1957; Registrar General, 1978), or atmospheric pollution (Winkelstein and Kantor, 1969). This issue of general dust exposure is discussed in 2.25. Stukonis and Doll (1969) demonstrated an increased risk of stomach cancer in occupations involving physical activity, which was independent of social class. They suggested this might be a reflection of increased intake of food and thus exposure to a greater quantity of dietary carcinogens.

These findings are not quite so clearcut for lung cancer. Some of the earlier studies on coal miners showed a reduced risk of lung cancer. However, 6 of the 9 reports in *Table 3.4* show an increased risk of death from lung cancer; this is particularly noticeable for the 4 largest studies. It appears from the more recent data that there is consistent evidence of an increased risk of lung cancer.

3.23 Petrochemical industry

This sections begins with a brief note on some early background studies; this is followed by comments on occupational mortality. A number of case-control studies have identified associations with potential exposure to petrochemicals. There have been 11 prospective studies of workers at refineries and petrochemical plants published in recent years; these are briefly described and the results presented in *Table 3.5*.

A number of specific chemicals have been reviewed in other sections that overlap with the present topic: benzene (2.8), isopropyl alcohol (2.40), polynuclear aromatic hydrocarbons (2.50), vinyl chloride (2.58).

3.23.1 Background

Gafafer and Sitgreaves (1940) studied the incidence and mortality from cancer in workers in an oil refining company in the US in 1933–38. It was not clear from the material presented whether there was any specific excess. Baird (1967) found no association between cancer and occupational exposure in the petrochemical industry. A more specific study in one refinery in the US (Hendricks *et al.*, 1959) found no overall increase in cancer, but an appreciable risk of scrotal cancer in wax pressmen who had been employed for more than 10 years. Study of workers in 3 large refineries in the US in 1949–61 showed no evidence of increase in skin cancer in those exposed to a high-boiling-point aromatic petroleum fraction

Table 3.5 Mortality in 11 historical cohort studies of workers in oil refineries

		I^a		II		$III^{b,c}$		IV		V	
		O	E	O	E	O	E	O	E	O	E
Buccal cav. phar.	140–149							6	7.0		
Oesophagus	150							37	32.4		
Stomach	151					47	25.9^d	167	160.9	6	7.7
Colon	153							84	78.9	14	18.0
Rectum	154							58	56.4	6	4.6
Gastrointestinal tract	150–154	57	41.6	12	10.2	174	158.9	346	328.6	26	30.3
Liver	155–156					12	7.0	24	22.8^e		
Pancreas	157					29	16.9	50	51.5	11	11.4
Nose	160							7	3.1		
Larynx	161							13	13.4		
Lung	162	67	35.4					416	532.7	57	83.6
Respiratory system	160–163	67	35.4	3	8.5	223	175.7	436	549.2	57	83.6
Bone	170										
Melanoma	172							14	6.5	5	4.4
Skin	172–173			1	0.4	21	11.3				
Prostate	185	18	21.4					47	45.9	5	6.7
Testis	186										
Bladder	188							34	44.2	3	4.2
Kidney	189					12	8.7^d	22	21.7		
CNS	191–192			3	0.8	32	22.7	36	44.8	8	6.4
Lymphoreticulosarcoma	200							16	16.3		
Hodgkin's disease	201							12	16.8	2	2.2
Multiple myeloma	203					6	3.6^d	11	10.2		
Leukaemia	204–207					21	13.9^d	30	32.0	4	7.8
RES	200–209	13	14.8	3	2.4	70	60.7	69	75.3	6	10.0

		VI		VII^b		$VIII^{b,f}$		IX		X		XI	
		O	E	O	E	O	E	O	E	O	E	O	E
Buccal. cav. phar.	140–149	2	7.6							13	21.5	20	29.5
Oesophagus	150	7	7.3							11	15.2	12	27.0
Stomach	151	11	13.7	1	2.4	48	31.6			30	28.5	68	69.8
Colon	153	24	25.1			44	40.6	11	14.2	42	53.2	65	77.2
Rectum	154	3	7.8			8	16.1			19	18.8	19	31.6
Gastrointestinal tract	150–154	45	53.9	1	2.4	108	88.3	11	14.2	102	115.7	164	205.6
Liver	155–156	3	4.5	3	0.6	8	10.9	5	3.1	13	10.8^g	8	22.6
Pancreas	157	23	15.1	2	1.7	37	26.0	10	9.3	33	35.0	53	48.5
Nose	160												
Larynx	161					4	7.4			3	10.1		
Lung	162–163	78	85.3	16	14.0	157	137.6	48	56.6	173	216.9	239	241.8
Respiratory system	160–163	79	89.9	16	14.0	161	145.0	48	56.6	176	227.0	250	258.8
Bone	170									1	2.9	11	5.4
Melanoma	172			4	0.5								
Skin (all)	172–173			5	0.6	13	7.2					16	13.1
Prostate	185	19	28.9			46	33.4	2	6.2	30	31.5	78	72.3
Testis	186	2	0.9							3	3.1	5	5.8
Bladder	188	9	9.2	1	0.8	2	14.4	2	4.0	7	17.3	13	28.0
Kidney	189	9	5.8	2	0.8	15	11.0	5	4.7	11	16.0	22	19.7
CNS	191–192	5	4.9	3	1.2	33	15.7	12	7.4	17	19.3	30	30.4
Lymphoreticulosarcoma	200	5	4.2							15	14.1	4	16.4
Hodgkin's disease	201	3	1.6			8	5.9			6	7.1	16	11.0
Multiple myeloma	203					9	4.6						
Leukaemia	204–207	9	9.3	1	0.5	33	18.0	9	7.7	20	22.7	38	33.3
RES	200–209	25	23.0	7	4.6	71	44.0	9	7.7	65	58.5	80	78.7

continued

Table 3.5 Continued

	Pooled data for 11 studies			
	O	E	O/E	95% CL
Buccal cav. phar.	41	65.5	0.62	0.5–0.8
Oesophagus	67	81.9	0.82	0.6–1.0
Stomach	374	340.5	1.11	1.0–1.2
Colon	284	307.2	0.92	0.8–1.0
Rectum	113	135.3	0.84	0.7–1.0
Gastrointestinal tract	1046	1049.7	1.00	0.9–1.1
Liver	76	82.3	0.92	0.7–1.2
Pancreas	248	215.4	1.15	1.0–1.3
Nose	7	3.1	2.26	0.9–4.6
Larynx	20	30.9	0.65	0.4–1.0
Lung	1241	1403.9	0.88	0.8–0.9
Respiratory system	1516	1643.7	0.92	0.9–1.0
Bone	12	8.3	1.45	0.7–2.5
Melanoma	23	11.4	2.02	1.3–3.0
Skin	56	32.6	1.72	1.3–2.2
Prostate	245	246.3	0.99	1.0–1.1
Testis	10	9.8	1.02	0.5–1.9
Bladder	71	122.1	0.58	0.4–0.7
Kidney	98	88.4	1.11	0.9–1.3
CNS	179	153.6	1.16	1.0–1.3
Lymphoreticulosarcoma	40	51.0	0.78	0.6–1.1
Hodgkin's disease	47	44.6	1.05	0.8–1.4
Multiple myeloma	26	18.4	1.41	0.9–2.1
Leukaemia	165	145.2	1.14	1.0–1.3
RES	418	379.7	1.10	1.0–1.2

I   = Hanis, Stavraky and Fowler (1979)
II   = Theriault and Goulet (1979)
III   = Thomas, Decoufle and Moure-Evaso (1980)
IV   = Rushton and Alderson (1981a)
V   = Schottenfeld *et al.* (1981)
VI   = Hanis *et al.* (1982)
VII   = Reeve *et al.* (1982)
VIII = Thomas, T.L. *et al.* (1982)
IX   = Austin and Schatter (1983)
X   = Kaplan (1983)
XI   = Wen *et al.* (1983)

[a]Hanis, Stavraky and Fowler (1979) present only O and RR from which E has been calculated.
[b]E for these studies is based on PMRs.
[c]Results refer to whites except for larynx, which includes non-whites.
[d]Restricted to men in petroleum refineries and production of petrochemicals.
[e]Liver plus gallbladder.
[f]Results are for white plus non-white except for brain which is whites only.
[g]Primary plus secondary.

(Wade, 1963). Baylor and Weaver (1968) identified 462 men working on asphalt (bitumen) plants in 25 refineries and 379 control men. There was no evidence of a cancer risk in the group exposed to bitumen for a minimum of 5 years.

3.23.2 Occupational mortality

The Registrar General's decennial supplement does not identify mortality for oil refinery workers as a separate subgroup. Initial use of the cancer maps in the US suggested that there was increased mortality from kidney cancer in the locations of the petroleum industry (Mason, 1976). Further analyses indicated excess deaths from cancer of the stomach, nasal cavities, rectum, lung, skin (melanoma), and testis in counties with at least 100 persons and 1% of the workforce employed in the petroleum industry compared with 'matched' counties (Blot *et al.*, 1977). Such crude statistics must be interpreted with great caution and at best can only be used as a guide

to further studies. Hearey *et al.* (1980) found no evidence of increased mortality from cancers in the vicinity of petrochemical installations in the San Francisco Bay area in 1971–77.

3.23.3 Case-control studies

Liver

A case-control study in New Jersey of 265 patients with liver cancer and matched controls found an increased risk in males working in gasoline service stations: RR = 2.88, 95% CL = 1.2–6.9 (Stemhagen *et al.*, 1983).

Pancreas

To follow-up the descriptive suggestion of an excess of pancreatic cancer in Louisiana (Blot, Fraumeni and Stone, 1978), deaths from pancreatic cancer were matched with deaths from other causes by age, sex, race, year of death, and locality for 876 pairs of deaths in 1960–75. The occupation recorded at death registration was examined (Pickle and Gottlieb, 1980). There was a two-fold risk for workers in oil refineries: 95% CL = 0.9–5.2, whilst residents near oil refineries had a slight elevation in risk.

A multihospital multisite case-control study was used to probe the occupational associations of pancreas cancer (Lin and Kessler, 1981). There was a significantly raised risk for exposure to solvents and gasoline.

Lung

Tsuchiya (1965) obtained numbers of deaths and numbers of employees in Japan by questionnaire from 200 large organizations in 1957–79. He reported an excess of lung cancer in those exposed to kerosene and petroleum products, but no expected figure was provided.

Gottlieb (1980) compared the occupation recorded on the death certificate for persons dying from lung cancer and non-cancer control deaths matched for age, sex, race, residence, year of death, in Louisiana in 1960–75. There was an increased risk of lung cancer in refinery process workers, craftsmen, and oilfield workers.

Testis

A case-control study of 347 patients with germ-cell tumours of the testis in Texas in 1977–80 showed an excess with reported work in the petroleum and natural gas industry: RR = 2.29, 95% CL = 1.0–5.1 (Mills, Newell and Johnson, 1984).

Bladder

Sixteen case-control studies are reviewed in 4.23.1. Of those referring to exposure to petroleum, there were 7 with RR > 1.0, but only 3 of these were significant. Others gave RR = 1.0, and 0.5; no reference to this occupation was made by the other reports.

Brain

In 1978 the US Occupational Safety and Health Administration (OSHA) was approached by a worker from a Texas plant, where there appeared to be several men who had developed brain tumours (Robbins, 1982). This 'cluster' of brain tumours was reinforced by the excess noted in a historical study in Canada (Theriault and Goulet, 1979) and a PMR study of Union workers in Texas (Thomas, Decoufle and Moure-Evaso, 1980). A conference held by the New York Academy of Sciences reviewed the topic (Selikoff and Hammond, 1982). There appeared to be fairly consistent findings from the general

mortality studies (*see* next subsection); 7 of the 9 studies showed an excess of deaths from CNS tumours and the pooled results a significant excess O = 179, E = 153.6, O/E = 1.16, 95% CL = 1.0–1.3). A retrospective study of over 7000 men employed in a petrochemical plant in Texas in 1941–77 showed an excess of brain tumours (Waxweiler *et al.*, 1983). Follow-up of these findings failed to identify any clearcut factors associated with risk of brain cancer, other than employment prior to 1945 (Bond *et al.*, 1983; Reeve *et al.*, 1983).

Multiple myeloma

Blattner, Blair and Mason (1981) noted that areas of petroleum and paper production in the US in 1950–75 had increased SMRs from multiple myeloma.

3.23.4 Prospective studies

There have been 11 studies of the patterns of mortality in the industry recently reported. Each is now briefly described in chronological order of publication and the key results are collated in *Table 3.5*. It must be remembered that the studies cover groups of workers whose particular environment during working hours may have been very different from one study to another, the potential exposures will have differed very greatly in subgroups of the workforces doing different jobs, and some of the men will have been initially employed many years ago. At the same time, the way of life of the different groups of men may vary considerably and expose them to a range of quite different non-occupational hazards.

(I) Hanis, Stavraky and Fowler (1979) followed 21 732 male employees from a Canadian oil company in the period 1964–73. Those exposed to crude petroleum and its products had an increase in oesophageal, stomach, and lung cancer; the excess increased with duration of employment. The refinery workers also had an excess of intestinal cancer.

(II) The mortality of 1205 men who had worked for at least 5 years in the period 1928–76 in an oil refinery in east Montreal was compared with the death rates of Quebec. It was thought that the 3 deaths from brain tumours required further detailed investigation and also the non-significant increase in digestive tract cancers (Theriault and Goulet, 1979).

(III) Thomas, Decoufle and Moure-Evaso (1980) examined 3105 deaths occurring in 1947–77 in union members in Texas employed in petroleum refineries, petrochemical plants, and related industries. A PMR was calculated, based on US mortality from various cancers. There was an excess of deaths from digestive system neoplasms and some other sites, but no clear relationship of excess risk to length of service. The findings were thought to need further investigation.

(IV) Rushton and Alderson (1981) examined the mortality of nearly 35 000 employees who had worked for at least one year in 8 oil refineries in Great Britain in 1950–75. Amongst the 4400 deaths there were excesses of melanoma, nasal cancer, and cancers of the gastrointestinal tract.

(V) Schottenfeld *et al.* (1981) followed 76 336 white and Hispanic males employed in 144 petroleum and petrochemical plants in the US in 1977–79. Expected mortality was based on national rates.

(VI) Follow-up of 8666 employees, working at least one month in a refinery and chemical plant in Louisiana in 1970–77, showed non-significant increased SMRs for certain cancers (kidney, testis, brain, pancreas, lymphoreticular system). Further study was recommended (Hanis *et al.*, 1982).

(VII) Reeve *et al.* (1982) carried out a proportional-mortality analysis of 264 petroleum union members working in 2 refineries and resident in Texas City who had died in 1947–79. An excess of deaths from malignant melanoma was observed and some other increases over expected, but the nature of the study limited the weight that could be placed upon these.

(VIII) Thomas, T.L. *et al.* (1982) calculated PMRs for union members working at 3 refineries in the Beaumont/Port Arthur area of Texas, who had died in 1943–79. There were excess deaths from stomach cancer, brain tumours, leukaemia, other lymphomas, and multiple myeloma. It was suggested these findings indicate the need for analytical studies. Thomas *et al.* (1984) carried out a within refinery case-control study; detailed job histories were obtained for 52 men dying of stomach cancer, 37 from brain tumours, and 36 from leukaemia, together with data for controls. There was no clear association for brain or leukaemia subjects; an association of stomach cancer with lubricating oils and paraffin wax processing was recorded.

(IX) Mortality of a cohort of 6588 white male employees in a Texas petrochemical plant showed fewer deaths from all neoplasms than expected, and no statistically significant excess of brain tumours (O = 12, E = 7.42). There was no other significant excess in any site (Austin and Schnatter, 1983).

(X) Kaplan (1983) extended the earlier study of Tabershaw and Cooper (1974) of 20 131 workers in 17 refineries in the US in the period 1962–76. All workers were included except those on petrochemical plants. There was an unexplained excess of deaths from other lymphatic tissue neoplasms.

(XI) A study of mortality at Gulf Oil Refinery in Port Arthur, Texas involved 16 880 employees in the period 1937–78 with average follow-up of 24.1 years. There were significant deficits of oesophageal, liver, and bladder cancer. The excess of bone cancer (O = 11, E = 5.37, $P < 0.05$) was thought to reflect errors in the data rather than a real hazard. This was the only significant excess (Wen *et al.*, 1983). Further analyses of this material (Wen *et al.*, 1984) have looked at the relationship of risk of malignancy to length of service, latent interval, and type of work exposure.

3.23.5 Conclusions

When the results of the 11 studies are pooled in *Table 3.5* (remembering the general caveats about this) there are a number of sites showing a statistically significant excess: stomach (O/E = 1.11), pancreas (1.15), melanoma (2.02), and central nervous system (1.16). The results for stomach cancer are based on 7 studies, though 2 of these are very small; the data for pancreas comes from the same 7 and a further small one. In neither site is the increase very marked. The results for nasal cancer are based on only one study, and small numbers of deaths due to the rarity of this cancer. Brain tumours (which are the predominant neoplasm of the CNS) have already been discussed.

The result for melanoma is based on only 2 studies; unfortunately 4 other studies do not split melanoma from other skin cancers. The geographical study of Blot *et al.* (1977) had identified melanoma as a possible hazard, whilst Pell, O'Berg and Karrh (1978) had identified a significant excess in a large petrochemical company.

The risk for leukaemia is significantly raised (O/E = 1.14). Though no other specific lymphatic or haematopoietic malignancy shows a significant excess mortality, the pooled statistics for all neoplasms of the reticulo-endothelial system (RES) show a statistically significant excess (O/E = 1.11).

These results are an indication for further study; none can be taken as confirming a specific hazard and they must be considered in relation to the significant deficits from other sites of malignancy and the major non-malignant causes of death (which have been reported in the 11 studies reviewed above).

3.24 Photographic work

Brief comments are provided on studies of (*a*) processors, (*b*) photographers.

3.24.1 Photographic processors

Follow-up of a 1964 cohort of 478 photographic processors in the US showed no evidence of excess mortality, cancer incidence, or sickness absence after 16 years (Friedlander, Hearne and Newman, 1982).

3.24.2 Photographers

Proportional-mortality analysis of deaths in 1965–79 in the US union of press photographers suggested an excess of pancreas cancer: O = 6, E = 2.3, O/E = 2.61, 95% CL = 0.9–5.7 (Miller, 1983).

Three of the 15 bladder case-control studies reviewed in 4.23.1 indicated raised risks in those involved in photography. However, none were significant, and the other 12 studies failed to distinguish this occupation.

3.24.3 Conclusion

The above reports are an inadequate base on which to evaluate any cancer hazard.

3.25 Physical activity

Stukonis and Doll (1969) graded the various occupations identified in the Registrar General's statistics in relation to activity involved in different jobs. SMRs for stomach cancer were then related to social class and physical activity. Within social class 3, gastric cancer showed a marked trend with physical activity, whilst other cancers and other alimentary diseases provided only minor evidence of such a relationship.

3.25.1 Conclusion

It was impossible to tell whether this was due to: (*a*) the direct work environment, (*b*) an indirect effect of the physical activity, such as through an effect on diet, (*c*) confounding with non-occupationally induced effects, (*d*) chance. No adequate studies have been done to resolve this.

3.26 Pilots

Three bush pilots in Ontario were found to have nasopharyngeal cancer. With the small (but unspecified) number of such pilots, it was suggested that this was not a chance finding (Andrews and Michaels, 1968).

3.26.1 Conclusion

This appears to be the sole resort of such a finding. Such case reports can be no more than a possible indication for further study, and would usually require former information before mounting any hypothesis testing study.

3.27 Policemen

Two studies have reported on the risk of specific cancers in policemen or security staff.

MacDonald (1956) reported a relative excess of prostate cancer in guards and policemen in Texas, in contrast to the census distribution of workers in the State.

In the review of bladder cancer (*see* 4.23.1), one study was found to have identified a statistically significant risk in security guards. None of the other studies presented results for this specific occupation: these therefore cannot be counted as 14 negative results.

3.27.1 Conclusion

The above reports are an inadequate base to consider there is an increased risk of cancer in policemen.

3.28 Quarrying

Men working in quarries have not been separated from surface miners in occupational mortality statistics; the epidemiological studies on this group of workers have concentrated on the respiratory hazard of men working in slate mines/quarries (e.g. *see* Glover *et al.*, 1980).

In a large case-control study of patients dying from cancer in North Wales and Cheshire in 1952–56, there was an excess risk of stomach and lung cancer in men working in slate and igneous rock quarries (Stocks, 1961).

3.28.1 Conclusion

The above report is an insufficient basis for evaluation of the cancer levels in men employed in quarrying. However, the lung cancer increase is compatible with the general hazard noted for exposure to silica (*see* 2.51).

3.29 Road transport drivers

Recent studies have reported a range of positive findings for various categories of road transport drivers. The following notes deal with: nasal, lung, and bladder cancer, leukaemia, and the hazard to the next generation. The methods used for these studies have included occupational mortality, case-control and prospective studies.

3.29.1 Studies on specific neoplasms

Nasal cancer

Using data from the Los Angeles cancer registry in 1972–76, Preston-Martin, Henderson and Pike (1982) found an increased risk for men aged 25–64 reporting occupation in transport: $O = 35$, $E = 22.58$, $O/E = 1.55$, 95% $CL = 1.1$–2.2.

Lung cancer

Blot and Fraumeni (1976) examined lung cancer mortality at county level in the US in 1950–69 against indices of distribution of occupation. A significant excess rate occurred in those counties with more than 1% of the population employed in transportation.

Williams, Stegens and Goldsmith (1977) also found an increased risk for drivers, using the data from the US Third National Cancer Survey for a case-control study. Examination of union records of the mortality of truck drivers in central and southern US in 1976, in comparison with expected deaths based on national rates, showed a non-significant excess of deaths from respiratory cancer: $O = 34$, $E = 28.2$, $O/E = 1.21$, 95% $CL = 0.8$–1.7 (Leupker and Smith, 1978). Two prospective studies of drivers in London Transport in the period 1950–74 both showed a deficiency of lung cancer in comparison with national or local mortality (Waller, 1981; Rushton, Alderson and Nagarajah, 1983).

Bladder cancer

Proportional-mortality analysis of deaths in Washington State in 1950–79 by occupation showed an increased risk of bladder cancer in transport drivers: $O = 74$, $E = 61$, $O/E = 1.21$, 95% $CL = 0.9$–1.5 (Milham, 1983).

Of the 16 case-control studies on bladder cancer reviewed in 4.23.1, 2 reported a raised risk and 2 a lowered risk for transport workers: in 1 of the 2 with a raised risk this was significantly different from 1.0 and there was a relationship with duration of work. There were 5 which reported a risk > 1.0 for those exposed to engine fumes, but none of these differences were significant.

Analysis of the occupational data for patients admitted to Roswell Park hospital in 1956–65 showed an increased risk for bladder cancer in drivers (Decoufle *et al.*, 1977).

There was an apparent deficiency of bladder cancer amongst 23306 men working at oil distribution centres in Great Britain in 1950–74. Nearly half these men would have been drivers (Rushton and Alderson, 1983). In contrast, there was a non-significant increase in maintenance staff at London Transport garages (Rushton, Alderson and Nagarajah, 1983).

RES neoplasms

Mortality on follow-up of 10% of the Canadian labour force in 1965–73 showed a significant excess of leukaemia in truck drivers, though this was only based on 5 deaths (Howe and Lindsay, 1983).

Analysis of mortality of 23306 men employed at oil distribution centres in Great Britain in 1950–74 showed a slight excess of deaths from RES neoplasms. Forty-three per cent of the men were drivers and there was a non-significant excess of Hodgkin's disease in these men: $O = 9$, $E = 4.96$, $O/E = 1.81$, 95% $CL = 0.8$–3.4. The numbers of deaths for specific cancers were small, making interpretation difficult (Rushton and Alderson, 1983).

Using cancer registration data for England and Wales, Balarajan (1983) found a non-significant increase of malignant lymphoma in road transport workers. Examining the data for Hodgkin's disease and non-Hodgkin's lymphoma showed variable results for 5 categories of such workers. Increased SMRs were also observed in the occupational mortality for England and Wales in 1970–72 (Balarajan and McDowall, 1983).

3.29.2 Hazards to the next generation

Fabia and Thuy (1974) examined the occupations reported for fathers at the time of birth of children who subsequently died of malignant disease in Quebec province in 1965–70. The occupations were compared with those reported for a control group of birth registrations. These authors identified an excess of fathers in hydrocarbon-related occupations with $RR=2$. Using a different technique, Hakulinen, Salonen and Teppo (1976) failed to find any excess of fathers reporting hydrocarbon-related occupations in children registered with malignant disease in Finland. An extension of this study to 2659 children registered with cancer in Finland in 1959–75 identified an excess of fathers with occupations of motor vehicle driving (Hemminki *et al.*, 1981). A case-control study of children with Wilm's tumour found an association with parental occupation involving exposure to lead, including drivers (Kantor *et al.*, 1979). Zack *et al.* (1980) compared the occupations of parents of 296 children with cancer with histories for control children: (*a*) other patients at hospital, (*b*) sibs of parents, (*c*) neighbourhood controls. They particularly probed hydrocarbon exposure, but found no difference in comparison with any of the control groups.

3.29.3 Conclusion

In a review of 12 occupational mortality and incidence studies, Dubrow and Wegman (1983) noted the consistently increased lung cancer in motor vehicle drivers. They indicated this might be from exposure to diesel and petrol fumes, cigarette smoking, or a combination of these 2 factors.

3.30 Rubber industry

The initial hazard in the rubber industry was identified by Case and Hosker (1954); this and the study by Davies (1965) of the cable industry have already been discussed in the section on aromatic amines (*see* 2.6). These studies led to a series of cohort studies in Great Britain and the US, which are discussed below, together with smaller cohort studies in Finland and Switzerland. A number of case-control studies have also been published which are dealt with in ICD order by site involved.

3.30.1 Prospective studies

The results for 8 studies are given in *Table 3.6*.

Finland

A historical prospective study was reported by Kilpikari *et al.* (1982), who followed 1331 males who worked in the rubber industry in Finland in 1953–76. Observed cancers were compared with expected from national registration statistics. The results are given in *Table 3.6*.

Great Britain: 1

A more detailed probe of past risk in bladder cancer was initiated in one large tyre factory in the Midlands (Veys, 1969), whilst at the same time two major studies were being initiated—Great Britain: 2 and 3. Follow-up of 5948 men potentially exposed to antioxidants containing 1-naphthylamine in 1945–49 showed a significant excess had developed bladder tumours by 1970 (O = 49, E = 23.5, O/E = 2.09, 95% CL = 1.5–2.8). However, there was little difference in the incidence in bladder tumours (O = 6, E = 4.5, O/E = 1.33, 95% CL = 0.5–2.9), in those only employed after 1950 and cessation of use of the suspect antioxidants (Veys, 1981). This factory is included in the larger study reported by Parkes *et al.* (1982) and discussed below.

Great Britain: 2 (Health and Safety Executive Study)

A census was used to identify 40 867 men aged 35 and over employed for at least 1 year in the rubber and cable industry in Great Britain in 1967. Fox, Lindars and Owen (1974) presented mortality up until 1971; Fox and Collier (1976a) extended the analyses to 1974. As the results depend upon the validity of the death certificates, Fox and White

(1976) checked this; they found no evidence that screening or doctors' awareness of the industrial hazard had influenced the statistics.

Baxter and Werner (1980) provided a more detailed analysis for the period 1967–76. The factory of employment (381 were involved) was known, and whether antioxidants which contained naphthylamines were used prior to 1950. The expected deaths were based on national rates, with regional correction and also adjustment for social class. The results were examined for 13 sectors in the industry handling different products. A significant excess of bladder cancer was found in men who had worked prior to 1950 in factories using the suspect antioxidant, but not in other workers. There was a highly significant excess of lung cancer, which occurred particularly in sectors handling: adhesives; rubber solutions; belting; hose, and rubber with asbestos flooring; ebonite and vulcanite. It was thought that the excess was associated with exposure to rubber fumes. There was also a significant excess of stomach cancer, concentrated in the tyre sector. The overall results are shown in *Table 3.6*. It should be noted that 18% of the men in this study were included in the next study discussed.

Great Britain: 3 (British Rubber Manufacturers Association Study)

Nearly 34 000 men who first started work in 6 large rubber factories in Great Britain in 1946–60 were followed until 1975. National mortality rates were used to calculate expected values. There was no excess of bladder cancer in those entering after 1950, but there was a statistically significant excess of lung cancer and stomach mortality (Parkes *et al.*, 1982). About 22% of the men in this study were also included in the previous one. Earlier results were published by Waterhouse (1979).

Parkes (1984), in a preliminary report of an extension to this study, noted a relative increase in lung cancer and to a lesser extent bladder cancer, on follow-up of the cohort of the whole industry to 1980.

Switzerland

The mortality of rubber workers in Switzerland followed from 1955 to 1975 was compared with expected figures based on national rates (Bovet and Lob, 1980).

US

Three large companies involved in tyre and rubber manufacture in Akron, Ohio have been carefully investigated in a coordinated series of epidemiological and hygiene studies.

Table 3.6 Risk of various cancers in different groups of rubber workers*

Country	Buc cav., phar		Oesoph.		Stomach		Large int.		Rectum		Liver		Pancreas	
	O	E	O	E	O	E	O	E	O	E	O	E	O	E
Finland														
GB: 2	21	22.4	35	44.0	216	176.4	107	93.2	75	70.6	9	8.6	66	70.8
GB: 3			40	31.8	183	141.8	67	73.7	50	54.1				
Switzerland					8	4.6								
US: 1					39	20.9	39	31.8	7	11.7			17	19.8
US: 2			8	10.5	34	27.6	53	45.7	14	16.9	3	3.6	34	27.9
US: 3 (*a*)	19	36.1	24	26.4	98	93.9	104	103.1	42	47.2	30	33.8	53	60.3
US: 3 (*b*)			4	4.9	5 ·	7.6	4	4.9			4	2.4	7	4.4
US: 4	4	1.7			3	3.0	9	4.6	0	1.8			6	2.8
Total O&E	44	60.2	111	117.6	586	475.8	383	357.0	188	202.3	46	48.4	183	186.0
O/E	0.73		0.94		1.23		1.07		0.93		0.95		0.98	
95% CL	0.5–1.0		0.8–1.1		1.1–1.3		1.0–1.2		0.8–1.1		0.7–1.3		1.8–1.1	

*See text for description of method.
†ICD 160–163.
‡ICD 200.
§ICD 200–203.

US: 1 (Akron Company A)

In this company, 6678 male production workers were identified on 1/1/64 as over 40 and either active or retired. They were followed until the end of 1972 and observed mortality compared with expected based on national rates (McMichael, Spirtas and Kupper, 1974). Subsequent analyses extended the follow-up until 1973 (McMichael, Haynes and Tyroler, 1975) and probed the risk of 7 cancers by category of job (McMichael *et al.*, 1976). Other studies of these workers have examined risk for particular cancers (*see* Stomach, Prostate, and Leukaemia in next section).

US: 2 (Akron Company B)

In the second company, 8418 white male production workers were identified on 1/1/64 as over 40 and either active or retired. They were followed until the end of 1973, and observed mortality compared with expected based on national rates (Andjelkovic, Taulbee and Symmons, 1976). Further analyses probed mortality by category of job (Andjelkovic *et al.*, 1977). A further study examined the mortality of female workers at the same plant over the same period (Andjelkovic, Taulbee and Blum, 1978). Data pooled for the 2 companies were examined by Tyroler *et al.* (1976). Studies of specific neoplasms have also been based on material for these 2 companies (*see* Stomach, Lung, Prostate, Brain, and Leukaemia in next subsection).

US: 3 (Akron Company C)

Initially 13571 white male production workers employed at a rubber plant in Akron who had

worked for at least 5 years in the period 1940–71 were followed to 1974. The first phase of the study only examined mortality (Monson and Nakano, 1976a, b). In the second phase, the mortality was recorded up to 1976 and cancer morbidity was identified from the hospital tumour registries for 1964–74 (Monson and Fine, 1978). Multiple cause coding of death certificates was utilized. Comparisons were initially made against US mortality, but then extended by comparing selected departments using all incident cancers. Excess cases occurred of: stomach and intestine in rubber making; lung in tyre curing, fuel cells, and de-icers; bladder in chemical plant and tyre assembly; brain cancer in tyre assembly; lymphatic cancer in tyre building; leukaemia in calendering, tyre curing, tyre building, elevators, tubes and rubber fabrics.

Analysis of mortality of rubber workers exposed to acrylonitrile showed 9 deaths from lung cancer with 5.9 expected (based on national rates). The excess was greatest in those who worked 5–14 years; few men had worked for longer than this (Delzell and Monson, 1982b).

US: 4 (Connecticut Company)

A smaller study (Delzell *et al.*, 1981) followed 1792 white males who had worked for at least 2 years in a tyre factory in the period 1954–72. Expected values were based on US mortality rates and state cancer registrations.

The general results from all the above studies are shown in *Table 3.6*. Deaths from brain tumours in these workers have been used for case-control studies (*see* next subsection).

Lung		Prostate		Bladder		Kidney		Brain		Lymphoma		Leukaemia	
O	E	O	E	O	E	O	E	O	E	O	E	O	E
3	2.0			2	0.3								
822	716.5	55	55.8	73	57.6	25	28.4	21	34.8			33	33.8
638	517.4	30	45.4	36	43.0			35	41.1			31	28.1
5	10.6			4	1.1			2	0.9				
91	109.3†	49	34.4	9	12.3			4	5.9	14	6.2‡	16	12.5
116	139.8	50	45.9	21	18.1			8	8.7			25	18.1
234	253.1	82	89.0	48	39.5	19	24.8	20	25.1	51	50.4§	55	43.0
16	22.2			1	1.8					6	3.5§		
15	15.2	.2	3.5	1	1.6	4	1.3	0	1.7			1	2.2
1940	1786.1	268	274.0	195	175.3	48	54.5	90	118.2	71	60.1	161	137.7
1.09		0.98		1.11		0.88		0.76		1.18		1.17	
1.0–1.1		0.9–1.1		1.0–1.3		0.6–1.2		0.6–0.9		0.9–1.5		1.0–1.4	

3.30.2 Case-control and other studies

The following notes cover the case-control studies that have stemmed from the above prospective studies. These are interleaved, in ICD site order, with other studies on workers in the rubber industry. Brief comments are then made about the general case-control studies that have recorded information on occupation and noted an association with work in the rubber industry.

Salivary glands

Amongst 5735 deaths for males in 8 rubber plants (unspecified location) there were 10 salivary gland tumours. It was suggested, without presentation of an expected figure, that this represented an increase (Mancuso and Brennan, 1970).

Oesophagus

Record linkage between the 1960 census and cancer registration in Sweden suggested that in vulcanizers there was a ten-fold increase of oesophageal cancer: O = 8, E = 0.79, O/E = 10.1, 95% CL = 4.4–19.9 (Norell *et al.*, 1983).

Stomach

Blum *et al.* (1979) identified 100 workers from the Akron Company A who had died from stomach cancer and controls matched for year of entry to the firm. There appeared to be an excess risk for work involving exposure to talc (RR = 2.5 in one location and 1.3 in the second). The authors point out that the talc may have been contaminated with asbestos.

Biliary tract

Data from 8 rubber plants (not identified) revealed 21 deaths in males from cancer of the biliary tract amongst 6505 deaths from all causes. No expected figure was provided, but it was suggested that this is an increased proportion (Mancuso and Brennan, 1970).

Larynx

Record linkage between the 1960 census and cancer registrations in Sweden suggested that vulcanizers had an increased risk of laryngeal cancer: O = 4, E = 1.04, O/E = 3.8, 95% CL = 1.0–9.8 (Norell *et al.*, 1983).

Lung

Delzell, Andjelkovic and Tyroler (1982) identified all the lung cancer deaths from the prospective study in Akron Company B. the occupational details for the 121 deaths were compared with 448 controls matched for age and year of entry. There was evidence of an increased risk for those working for 5 years in rubber reclaim operations (RR = 2.2) and making special products (RR = 1.7).

Prostate

Goldsmith, Smith and McMichael (1980) identified 88 deaths from prostate cancer in 1964–75 in men who had worked in the Akron Company A; 258 controls were matched for age, race, and date of entry to the plant. There was a statistically significant risk for men who had worked in 'batch preparation' and to a lesser extent some of the other functions.

Bladder

Job histories were compared for 220 men in Akron Company B with bladder cancer against age, sex, race, and plant-matched controls. There appeared to be about a two-fold risk for those who had worked in milling and calender operations (Checkoway *et al.*, 1981). No specific agent was implicated.

Some of the general case-control studies (*see* Bladder review) have shown an association with work in the rubber industry. However, only one was of borderline significance.

Brain

Initial examination of 5036 cancer deaths in Ohio in 1947 showed an excess of brain tumours in the rubber industry. To check these findings, Mancuso (1963) followed workers from a rubber plant manufacturing tyres and employed in 1920–30 until 1955. There were 2 deaths from CNS tumours with only 0.25 expected. More recently Lamperth-Seiler (1974) observed increased risk of brain tumours in German rubber manufacturing industries.

The principal job held was examined for 22 employees in Akron Companies A, B, and C dying from brain and CNS neoplasms in 1951–71 and controls matched on year of birth, sex, and race (Symons *et al.*, 1982). There was no evidence of association with work in tyre assembly or building (as had been previously suggested from analyses of Monson and Nakano, 1976a).

Using the linked 1960 census and registration data for 1961–73 in Sweden, Englund, Ekman and Zabrielski (1982) noted a significant excess of CNS tumours in those who had worked in the rubber and plastics industry (O = 22, E = 12.6, O/E = 1.75, 95% CL = 1.1–2.6).

Leukaemia

Wolf *et al.* (1981) identified 72 employees from 4 companies (chiefly Akron A and B) who had died from leukaemia in 1964–73. There was an increased risk of leukaemia in those exposed to solvents (which would have included benzene), but this was less than had been suggested by the earlier reports (*see* 2.8).

Lymphosarcoma

In a follow-up of the US cancer mortality maps, Goldsmith and Guidotti (1977) examined death certificates for one county in Ohio for deaths from lymphosarcoma. There were 35% reporting employment in the rubber industry, with only 20% expected (the number of deaths or the years involved are not stated). These authors also examined 484 death certificates from California in 1971–72; these showed no excess in comparison with the census estimates of rubber workers.

3.30.3 Conclusions

There was about a two-fold risk of bladder cancer in the studies of workers employed in Great Britain in 1936–51. Subsequent follow-up of large numbers of workers indicated that the risk of excess bladder cancer was virtually confined to those employed prior to 1950. Equivalent work from the US indicated restriction to those employed before 1935.

This is in line with the original investigations of the extension of the hazard from workers exposed to aromatic amines in the chemical industries. It is important to bear in mind that (*a*) there were relatively few workers exposed in the chemical industry, but the level of exposure was high; (*b*) there were larger numbers exposed prior to 1950 in the rubber industry, but the level of exposure was lower (IARC, 1974a).

The more recent data reviewed above, particularly for those employed in specific sectors of the industry had indicated excess cancers of stomach, large intestine, lung, skin, prostate, brain, lymphoma, and leukaemia. IARC (1982b) also noted that oesophagus, liver, pancreas, cervix, and thyroid cancers have been increased in some studies; these results were based on small numbers and have not been consistently reported.

3.31 Retail trade

There have been limited references to risk of cancer amongst those in the retail trade, stemming from case-control 'fishing' studies.

The Third National Cancer Survey data from the US were used by Williams, Stegens and Goldsmith (1977) to explore the risks for various cancers. This suggested that sales personnel were at increased risk of colorectal cancer, leukaemia, and multiple myeloma.

In the review of bladder cancer (*see* 4.23.1), 3 studies present results from the retail trade, with RR = 6.0, 1.0 and 0.9. The first of these is statistically significant. This occupation was not identified in the other 12 reported case-control studies.

3.31.1 Hazard to the next generation

Children registered with cancer in Finland in 1959–75 were identified and about 80% of maternity records traced, with controls. There were 2659 pairs of parental occupations for analysis (Hemminki *et al.*, 1981). Children of mothers working as saleswomen had a non-significant increased risk: RR = 1.22, 95% CL = 0.9–1.6.

3.31.2 Conclusion

The above reports are inadequate for an evaluation

of the cancer levels in this rather broad occupational group.

3.32 Seamen

There have been limited studies on the mortality and morbidity of seamen.

The mortality of seafarers registered in Sweden in 1945–54 was compared with that from national data by age and sex (Otterland, 1960). For all neoplasms the SMR was 104. Out of 157 deaths, 12 were from pancreas cancer; it was suggested that this was raised, but no expected figure was given. There was no other site identified as having excess mortality.

The extensive morbidity data collected by Ellis (1969) for the UK Royal Navy may represent very different health hazards to that of merchant seamen. The material did not indicate a hazard from cancer. Other studies of acute illness are not relevant to consideration of cancer patients (e.g. Levy, 1972; Carter, 1976).

3.32.1 Conclusion

The above are inadequate as a basis for an evaluation.

3.33 Tailoring

The only specific site for which several results are available is bladder cancer (*see* review, 4.23.1). For different jobs within the general field of tailoring, there was a scatter of results from 8 of the 16 studies. In 6 of the 8, RR > 1.0, but none was significantly raised; no results were available for the other 8 studies for this occupation.

3.33.1 Conclusion

There is insufficient information from which to draw firm conclusions.

3.34 Teaching

Analysis of occupations recorded in the US Third National Cancer Survey (Williams, Stegens and Goldsmith, 1977) suggested that there was an excess risk of melanoma in school teachers.

Four students at a high school in New York developed Hodgkin's disease in a relatively short time. Enquiry then suggested there was a network of contact in a larger number of cases (Vianna, Greenwald and Davies, 1971). This initial report did not identify an excess of teachers, but a further study suggested that there was an excess of

secondary cases involving both teachers and students in other schools (Vianna and Polan, 1973). However, a study in the Oxford area using a carefully controlled approach failed to find any excess person-to-person contact in Hodgkin's disease (Smith *et al.*, 1977). Milham (1974a) used proportional-mortality analysis of Hodgkin's disease in school teachers in Washington State over the period 1950–71; he suggested that the relative risk of Hodgkin's disease was 1.7. However, this finding was challenged by Bahn (1974) who suggested that the use of proportional-mortality analysis might have been misleading due to the overall lower mortality from all causes amongst teachers. Hoover (1974) tried to calculate observed and expected deaths on a reworking of Milham's data and from this suggested that the RR = 0.7 for all causes and 1.5 for Hodgkin's disease. He commented that this excess is compatible with the reported social class gradient that has been reported for this condition.

3.34.1 Conclusion

The above studies are insufficient grounds on which to accept that there is a hazard of cancer in teachers.

3.35 Textile industry

One of the first occupational cancers to be recognized was the mule spinners' scrotal cancer. This is discussed in the section on mineral oils (*see* 2.50.7). In the 1940s, the chief health concern of the industry was that of respiratory disease in workers in cotton mills (Schilling, 1956). However, some follow-up studies have been analysed which include hazard from cancer; these are discussed in the first subsection. A number of case-control studies investigating various sites of malignancy have identified risks in textile workers; these are discussed in ICD site order.

3.35.1 Proportional-mortality and prospective studies

In 1976–78 there were 4462 deaths in white women in North Carolina indicating previous work in the textile industry. Significantly raised PMRs were found for malignancy of: larynx (RR = 2.8, 95% CL = 1.0–7.3), connective tissue (RR = 2.6, 95% CL = 1.3–5.2), thyroid (RR = 2.2, 95% CL = 1.0–5.0), and non-Hodgkin's lymphoma (RR = 1.7, 95% CL = 1.2–2.3). There was no evidence of an increased risk of bladder cancer (Delzell and Grufferman, 1983).

Henderson and Enterline (1973) followed up (*a*) 5822 men who had worked in 1938–41 at 1 of 3 cotton textile mills in Georgia, and (*b*) 6316 men who had worked at the same mills in 1948–51. Of the total group, 1772 had been employed in both time periods in the mills. Deaths up to age 64 were identified, but only 87% of death certificates were traced; the other 13% of deaths were allocated in proportion to the distribution of the 87% known causes. Expected deaths were based on state mortality rates. There was a significant deficit of respiratory cancer (O = 28, E = 62.9, O/E = 0.45, 95% CL = 0.3–0.6), but no appreciable difference for digestive, urinary, or all other cancers.

Men and women who had worked at 2 cotton mills in North Carolina in 1937–40 were identified and followed to 1975; follow-up was complete for 1092 (97.4%) males and 391 (99.2%) females for whom a job history was available. National rates were used to obtain expected values. There was an overall deficit of neoplasms (O = 61, E = 91.0, O/E = 0.67, 95% CL = 0.5–0.9) and of lung cancer (O = 18, E = 24.3, O/E = 0.74, 95% CL = 0.4–1.2). There was a suggestion that those involved in dyeing might have a higher risk of cancer, but this was based on very small numbers (Merchant and Ortmeyer, 1981).

Beck, Schachter and Maunder (1981) followed 692 cotton workers from 4 mills in Columbia in 1973–79; no analysis of mortality by cause was provided.

Berry and Molyneux (1981) followed 1359 subjects from 14 Lancashire cotton mills in 1966–77; 6.4% of the women and 6.0% of the men could not be traced. Expected deaths were based on national rates adjusted for the local mortality differential. There was no evidence of increase in neoplasms (O = 30, E = 37.7, O/E = 0.80, 95% CL = 0.5–1.1), but results for individual sites were not given.

3.35.2 Studies on specific cancers

Oral and pharyngeal cancers

Analysis of US counties with high SMRs for oral and pharyngeal cancers in 1950–69 showed an excess with women employed in the textile industry (Blot and Fraumeni, 1977).

Occupational mortality statistics for England and Wales and cancer incidence had suggested that those working in textiles were at increased risk of oral cancers (Binnie et al., 1972). Moss and Lee (1974) considered that this lead warranted further exploration; Whitaker et al. (1979) carried out a case-control study in the two main textile regions of England, matching patients for age and sex with other cancer patients. No particualr type of textile work occurred more frequently in the cases than in the controls in all 4 subgroups examined; for males in the north-west, the proportions of textile workers amongst cancer patients with tongue, mouth, and

pharynx lesions was significantly greater than controls, but were not thought to confirm any association with a particular aspect of textile work.

Two hundred and fifty-five women in North Carolina developing oral and pharyngeal cancer in 1975–78 and 2 matched controls for each case were investigated (Winn et al., 1981). There was no evidence of increased risk in these workers in the textile industry, after taking into account snuff dipping. This habit was prevalent in the industry and itself associated with increased risk of these cancers. Very similar results were published by Winn et al. (1982): RR = 1.1, 95% CL = 0.7–1.7.

Nasal cancer

Acheson, Cowdell and Rang (1972, 1981) found an excess of textile workers in (a) patients with nasal adenocarcinoma registered in 1961–66 in England and Wales, and (b) nasal tumours of all histology registered in 1963–67, in comparison with expected figures based on census estimates of numbers by occupation.

Analysis of the reported occupations for 85 women registered with squamous cell and poorly differentiated nasal cancers in Sweden in 1961–70 showed 8 (9%) were textile workers, but no expected figure was provided (Engzell, Englund and Westerholm, 1978).

A small case-control study of 45 patients with nasal cancer diagnosed in Finland in 1970–73 recorded occupational and leisure exposure to various agents. In women there was a significant excess with leisure knitting and sewing: RR = 4.87; 95% CL = 1.2–19.9 (Tola et al., 1980a).

Thirty-seven deaths from nasal cancer in North Carolina in 1956–74 were matched with 73 control deaths and comparisons made of the occupations recorded for each decedent (Brinton et al., 1977). There was no increase in the proportion reporting textile work. In a subsequent study 160 patients with nasal cancer treated in 4 hospitals in North Carolina and Virginia in 1970–80 were matched to (a) hospital patients, (b) decedents on age, sex, race, county of residence, and year of death if the index patient was dead (Brinton et al., 1984). A non-significantly increased risk was found for the textile and clothing industry: RR = 1.28; 95% CL = 0.7–2.2.

Larynx

A case-control study of 314 persons with laryngeal cancer treated in 5 cities in the US in 1970–73 reported no evidence of increased risk in textile workers (Wynder et al., 1976).

A case-control study of 204 patients with laryngeal cancer diagnosed in 1977–79 in Ontario used individually matched neighbourhood controls.

All were interviewed at home by a trained interviewer (Burch *et al.*, 1981). There was an association with exposure to textile dust, based on small numbers (RR = ∞; 95% CL = 2.1–∞).

Due to high mortality from laryngeal cancer in Richmond County, US in 1950–69, a case-control study was carried out there. Forty-two cases and 85 matched controls were questioned about their occupations. Taking smoking and alcohol into account, there was a significant association with exposure to textile processes: RR = 3.2; 95% CL = 1.3–8.0 (Flanders *et al.*, 1984).

Lung cancer

A case-control study of 858 patients with lung cancer who died of lung cancer in coastal Georgia in 1961–74 showed no evidence of increased risk from textile work: RR = 0.88; 95% CL = 0.3–2.4 (Harrington *et al.*, 1978).

A case-control study of 134 lung cancer patients diagnosed in New York in 1971–80 showed an increased risk in women employed in textile work: RR = 3.10; 95% CL = 1.11–8.64. Kabat and Wynder (1984) pointed out that the influence of passive smoking was not clear in these subjects.

Death certificates in Prato, Italy were used to identify lung cancer subjects and relatives were then interviewed (Buatti *et al.*, 1979). This identified those who had worked for at least 12 months in textile processing when aged 14–60. Compared with census estimates there was excess risk, especially those selecting and sorting old fabrics and dyeing.

Skin—non-melanoma

Whitaker, Lee and Downes (1979) obtained detailed occupational histories from 598 patients with skin cancer in north-west England, with more restricted information from 148 patients. Comparing the histories with the distribution of workers by occupation from the 1931 and 1951 censuses, they found men and women had an excess of workers in the textile industry.

Cervix

The latest decennial supplement of the Registrar General (1978) showed, amongst 27 occupational orders, that women textile workers had the highest PMR: O = 9, E = 3.05, O/E = 2.95, 95% CL = 1.3–5.6. For the 223 occupational units, there was only one with a significant PMR at the 1% level—women working as spinners/doublers/twisters: O = 2, E = 0.29, O/E = 6.90, 95% CL = 0.8–24.9.

Bladder

The general case-control studies on the aetiology of bladder cancer (*see* 4.23.1) refer to risks in various categories of textile workers, including primary manufacture and tailoring. Of the 19 results, 15 had a RR > 1.0, one = 1.0, and 3 < 1.0; however, none were significant at the 5% level.

3.35.3 Conclusion

Though the reports reviewed above include a number with increased risk of cancer, some of which are significant, there is no consistency in the positives and the range of sites involved in isolated positives wide. The material does not measure up to evidence of cancer risk in this occupation.

3.36 Tobacco manufacture and retail

Analysis for occupations for all men dying from lung cancer in 1921–32 in England and Wales showed increased risks for tobacco manufacturers: O/E = 1.96, and tobacconists: O/E = 1.75 (Kennaway and Kennaway, 1936). Surveillance of all employees who had worked for at least 1 year for the American Tobacco Company in 1946–52 showed no increase in deaths from respiratory cancer: O = 6, E = 7, O/E = 0.86, 95% CL = 0.3–1.9 (Dorn and Baum, 1955). Extension of this study for 1957–60 again showed no increase in respiratory cancer (Cohen and Heimann, 1962).

Deaths in tobacco workers were identified from obituary listings of their union in the US in 1957–78 and a proportional-mortality analysis performed using national mortality rates (Blair *et al.*, 1983b). There was a non-significant excess of deaths from lung cancer: O = 129, E = 115.4, O/E = 1.12, 95% CL = 0.9–1.3. Results were presented for another 16 sites, of which 5 showed an excess over expected with that for colon cancer being the only significant difference.

3.36.1 Conclusion

The above results do not show any consistent excess of lung cancer and no information is available about the smoking habits of the workers.

3.37 Veterinary surgeons

A number of studies have been reported on the risks of cancer in vets. As these overlap with the contact with animals in farming, the studies are included in 3.14.

3.38 Woodworkers

Clinical observation of patients with adenocarcinoma of the nasal passages led to the confirmation of a high risk of this cancer in furniture workers. The early work in England that stemmed from the initial observation is described. A subsection then covers the use of occupational mortality and incidence data studied in various ways. Much of the subsequent literature concentrates on nasal cancer; a section reviews the case reports and case-control studies for this site. The association of woodwork with other sites of malignancy is then briefly reviewed. Compared with many other occupations, relatively limited results are available from follow-up studies; 2 studies are covered. The overall results from the studies reviewed are brought together in *Table 3.7*.

Lumberjacks and forestry workers are potentially exposed to herbicides, and studies on these workers are included in 2.37.

A review (IARC, 1981) pointed out that the separation of workers in the wood industry into different sections was not consistent in different sources of data. Technology might differ between countries and in one plant over time; there was particular difficulty in determining exposure due to: (*a*) many different chemicals being used; (*b*) raw materials and additives could change; (*c*) workers may handle a number of quite different types of wood; (*d*) new materials may be formed as byproducts of some chemical actions. This review provided an excellent description of the industry, including chemicals used in handling woods from initial stain control, seasoning, and other phases of production.

3.38.1 Nasal cancer in furniture workers in England and Wales

The first publication of the clinical observation of a new occupational association with nasal cancer was given in a lecture by Macbeth (1965): '...I am indebted to Miss Esme Hadfield of High Wycombe for drawing my attention to these patients. Out of 20 cases, 17 were male and 15 were woodworkers, whilst the local population had about 23.5% woodworkers ... I am uncertain to what extent these figures are statistically significant.' Preliminary examination of registration and hospital data supported this suggestion (Acheson, Hadfield and Macbeth, 1967). Further enquiry investigated all patients registered with nasal cancer in Oxfordshire, Berkshire, and Buckinghamshire within the Oxford Regional Health Authority in 1956–65. Comparison with census estimates for the nearest equivalent locality showed a substantially increased risk for adenocarcinoma of the nasal cavity and sinuses amongst those working in the manufacture of

general furniture in Buckinghamshire and Oxfordshire (Acheson *et al.*, 1968). Less complete data were available for persons diagnosed before 1955 or after 1965, with ascertainment of a few cases elsewhere in southern England.

Patients with adenocarcinomas of the nose were identified from all regions in England and Wales, excluding Oxford, for 1961–66. For each such patient a control with nasal cancer of other histology was selected. The histology was reviewed and an occupational history obtained by postal questionnaire to the patients or their relatives. The observed distribution for 27 occupational groups was compared with the expected, based on the proportion from the 1961 census (Acheson, Cowdell and Rang, 1972). This study was extended to all patients with any histology of nasal cancer known to the national register in 1963–67 (Acheson, Cowdell and Rang, 1981). Histology was verified and questionnaires sent to patients or their relatives to record occupational history, smoking, and use of snuff. The last occupation was available for 875 males (94.6%). The patients were separated into 27 occupational groups and an expected figure calculated. The details of this are not provided, but the 1961 census estimates were presumably used. These analyses indicated a general risk of nasal cancer for woodworkers elsewhere in the country, particularly following work in the furniture industry.

3.38.2 Occupational mortality and incidence data

Henry, Kennaway and Kennaway (1931) examined the occupations recorded for individuals dying in England and Wales between 1921 and 1928 from cancer of the bladder and prostate. They obtained death certificates for 5808 males with prostate cancer and age-adjusted rates were calculated for 47 different occupations, using the census data as a denominator. High SMRs were found for french-polishers.

Examination of the distribution of lung cancer in the US for 1950–69 showed that there was a significant excess of cancer in white males in eastern and southern counties where paper and pulp industries were located (Blot and Fraumeni, 1976). However, those counties in which lumber and furniture industries were concentrated showed lower lung cancer mortality rates than average.

Examination of the distribution of oral and pharyngeal mortality in the US in 1950–69 showed significantly raised rates among white males in counties in the eastern states where many paper industries were located (Blot and Fraumeni, 1977). Counties with more than 1% of the population employed in the furniture industry had significantly lower oral and pharyngeal mortality.

US counties with at least 1% of the total population employed in the furniture industry, were matched with control counties on region, population size, percentage non-whites, income, and educational level. Age-adjusted mortality rates for white males were compared for 30 cancer sites for the period 1950–69 (Brinton *et al.*, 1976). Unfortunately the confidence limits cannot be calculated from the results.

Deaths in males 35 years or older from nasal cancer in Connecticut in 1935–75 were identified and occupations recorded at death registration compared with those for control deaths from other causes. Occupational information was also obtained from earlier city directories in which the decedents were identified (Roush *et al.*, 1980).

Occupation recorded at death certification for 3327 patients with lung cancer dying in southern Louisiana in 1950–75 were compared with control deaths matched for age, sex, residence, and race (Gottlieb *et al.*, 1979); 103 had worked in the paper industry.

The occupations of 2161 white males dying from lung cancer aged 20–64 in Los Angeles in 1968–70 and 1771 incident cases diagnosed in 1972–73 were compared with census estimates (Menck and Henderson, 1976). There was a significant excess in those involved in paper manufacture and sales.

Cancer registry records in Sweden were used to identify (*a*) 36 men and 10 women with adenocarcinoma of the nose diagnosed in 1961–71 and (*b*) 127 men and 85 women with squamous or poorly differentiated cancers of the nose diagnosed in 1965–71. Information on prior occupation was obtained from hospital records, questionnaires to patients and relatives, and church records. Approximate relative risks were based on union and census statistics of the exposed population (Engzell, Englund and Westerholm, 1978).

3.38.3 Case reports of nasal cancer

Due to the apparently high relative risk of adenocarcinoma of the nose in workers exposed to hard wood dusts, case reports have provided more information than is usual. Some of the studies have also attempted to collect all known cases from a defined population and relate these to estimates of the workforce in the locality. These studies are described first and then the case-control studies of nasal cancer.

Australia

The index of patients treated at the Cancer Institute in Victoria was used to identify 69 with adenocarcinoma and 80 with other histological cancers of the nasal passages (Ironside and Matthews, 1975). The years spanned by the enquiry were not stated.

Routine questioning of patients by admission clerks provided occupational details.

Belgium

Amongst 30 patients diagnosed with nasal cancer in the Leuven hospital in 1958–68, 19 (63%) had worked in the furniture industry. Of the 20 with adenocarcinoma, 14 (70%) had been so employed (Debois, 1969). [The figures in the text do not agree exactly with the table.]

Denmark

Examination of all 123 deaths from nasal cancer in Denmark in 1956–66 identified 9 with an occupation involving woodworking. Of these 9, 4 had been employed in the furniture industry and all 4 had adenocarcinoma; the other 5 had more limited exposure to wood and none had an adenocarcinoma (Mosbech and Acheson, 1971).

All nasal cancers treated in Aarhus and derived from a population of about 2 million in Denmark in 1965–74 were identified. Out of 186, 116 were in males, of whom 17 had adenocarcinoma and 99 other histology. The occupations available from routine records were examined (Andersen, Andersen and Solgaard, 1977). The same material has been reported by Andersen (1975) and Andersen, Solgaard and Andersen (1976).

The Danish Cancer Registry was used to identify 839 patients with nasal cancer, and 2465 controls with other cancers in 1970–82. Linkage with pension fund records provided information on occupation back to 1960 (Olsen and Jensen, 1984). There was a significant risk from exposure to wood dust: RR = 2.5, 95% CL = 1.7–3.7.

France

Review of the medical notes of 35 patients with ethmoid and maxillary cancer presenting in 1952–67 in one Paris hospital showed 17 were woodworkers. Sixteen of these 17 had adenocarcinoma (Gignoux and Bernard, 1969).

Three furniture makers with nasal cancer presented at one clinic in Paris in 1966–77. Two had adenocarcinomas, and one had started work in 1941; this was later than any of the patients reported by Acheson and his colleagues (Fombeur, 1972).

Investigation of 29 patients treated at one clinic in Angers, France in 1966–72, identified the occupation of 7 with adenocarcinoma; 6 were woodworkers (Desnos and Martin, 1973).

Of 36 patients treated at Rennes in 1964–74 with carcinoma of the nasal sinuses, 14 had worked with wood. Of those with adenocarcinoma, 13 out of 19 had worked with wood (Curtes, Trotel and Bourdiniere, 1977).

There were 115 patients with carcinoma of the nasal sinuses treated at one French clinic; occupations were obtained from the medical histories, and these were compared for the different histologies (Haguenauer, 1972). Twenty-five of 58 patients with adenocarcinoma were furniture workers, but only 2 out of 57 with other histology. [The text and tables show minor discrepancies.]

Netherlands

Delemarre and Themans (1971) compared the occupations of 16 patients with adenocarcinoma of the nose treated in 1944–67 and 33 patients with nasal cancer of other histology treated in 1956–68 in one hospital in the Netherlands. A significant excess with adenocarcinoma had been woodworkers.

West Germany

A questionnaire on occupational history was answered by 179 (43%) of patients with nasal cancer treated in one hospital in 1931–77 in West Germany (Lobe and Ehrhardt, 1978). A comparison of occupations was made between those with adenocarcinoma and other histology, and also against estimates of the proportion of the population who were woodworkers.

3.38.4 Case-control studies

Canada: 1

Ball (1967) identified 340 male deaths from nasal cancer in Canada in 1956–65 and controls matched on province, age, and year of death. Occupation was

Table 3.7 Risks of various cancers in different categories of worker exposed to wood*

Site (histology)	Occupation	Method	Country	RR	95% CL	Author
Nose (Adeno vs other)	Furniture	C–C	England and Wales	4.98	1.9–14.1	Acheson, Cowdell and Rang (1972)
	Carpenters	C–C	England and Wales	2.56	0.6–11.0	Acheson, Cowdell and Rang (1972)
	Carpenters	C–C	Australia	7.31	0.8–64.9	Ironside and Matthews (1975)
	Carpenters	C–C	Sweden	27.27	10.8–68.7	Engzell, Englund and Westerholm (1978)
	Woodworkers	C–C	Netherlands	22.00	4.8–101.7	Delemarre and Themans (1971)
	Woodworkers	C–C	Denmark	31.20	11.4–85.0	Andersen, Andersen and Solgaard (1977)
(Adeno)	Furniture	C–C	US	5.7	n.a.	Brinton et al. (1984)
	Woodworkers	C–C	Italy	89.7	19.8–407.3	Battista et al. (1983)
	Woodworkers	C–C	Italy	3.75	0.2–80.4	Cecchi et al. (1980)
(All)	Furniture	C–C	Canada	2.00	0.2–21.0	Ball (1968)
	Furniture	Area mort.	US	1.19	n.a.	Brinton et al. (1976)
	Furniture	C–C	US	4.4	1.3–15.4	Brinton et al. (1977)
	Carpenter	Prospect.	US	0.50	0.2–1.0	Milham (1974b)
	Carpenters	Prospect.	Denmark	4.67	2.5–6.8	Olsen and Sabroe (1979)
	Woodworkers	C–C	Canada	1.17	0.7–2.0	Ball (1967)
	Woodworkers	C–C	US	1.5	0.4–4.3	Brinton et al. (1977)
	Woodworkers	C–C	US	4.0	1.5–10.8	Roush et al. (1980)
	Woodworkers	C–C	Finland	1.0	1.0–1.1	Tola et al. (1980a)
	Woodworkers	C vs census	England and Wales	2.84	2.2–3.7	Acheson, Cowdell and Rang (1981)
	Woodworkers	C–C	Canada	2.3	1.1–4.7	Elwood (1981)
	Woodworkers	C–C	Italy	∞	0.7–∞	Merler et al. (1982)
	Woodworkers	C–C	Italy	5.4	1.7–17.2	Battista et al. (1983)
	Wood soft & hard	C–C	Scandinavia	12.0	2.4–59.2	Hernberg et al. (1983a)
	Wood soft	C–C	Scandinavia	3.3	1.1–9.4	Hernberg et al. (1983a)
	Lumber	C–C	US	1.4	0.7–2.6	Brinton et al. (1984)
Larynx	Furniture	Area mort.	US	0.87	n.a.	Brinton et al. (1976)
	Furniture	C vs census	Germany	7.81	2.5–18.2	Wolf (1978)
	Paper industry	C–C	US	4.37	1.4–10.2	Bross, Viadana and Houten (1978)
	Woodworker	C–C	US	23.6	5.1–107.8	Wynder et al. (1978)

Table 3.7 Continued

Site (histology)	Occupation	Method	Country	RR	95% CL	Author
Lung	Carpenter	Prospect.	US	1.07	1.0–1.1	Milham (1974)
	Carpenter	C–C	US	1.22	n.a.	Decoufle *et al.* (1977)
	Furniture	Area mort.	US	low	n.a.	Blot and Fraumeni (1976)
	Furniture	Area mort.	US	0.87	n.a.	Brinton *et al.* (1976)
	Furniture	C–C	Sweden	6.0	n.a.	Esping and Axelson (1980)
	Lumber	Prospect.	US	<0.80	n.a.	Milham (1974)
	Lumber	Area mort.	US	low	n.a.	Blot and Fraumeni (1976)
	Lumber	C–C	US	3.4	1.9–6.1	Harrington *et al.* (1978)
	Paper manuf.	Area mort.	US	sign.xs	n.a.	Blot and Fraumeni (1976)
	Paper manuf.	Occup. mort./ inc.	US	1.71	1.1–2.5	Menck and Henderson (1976)
	Paper manuf.	C–C	US	1.0	n.a.	Blot *et al.* (1978)
	Paper manuf.	Occup. mort.	US	1.05	0.8–1.4	Gottlieb *et al.* (1979)
	Woodwork	C–C	US	1.28	0.8–1.8	Harrington *et al.* (1978)
	Woodwork	Prospect.	Denmark	1.04	0.9–1.2	Olsen and Sabroe (1979)
	Woodwork	C–C	Sweden	4.1	1.6–10.6	Esping and Axelson (1980)
Hodgkin's disease	Carpenter	C–C	US	1.48	0.9–2.5	Milham and Hesser (1967)
	Carpenter	Prospect.	US	1.77	1.1–2.6	Milham (1974b)
(Mixed cellul.)	Carpenter	C–C	Israel	5.25	2.0–13.7	Abramson *et al.* (1978)
	Furniture	C–C	US	∞	0.1–∞	Milham and Hesser (1967)
	Furniture	Area mort.	US	0.98	n.a.	Brinton *et al.* (1976)
	Lumber	C–C	US	2.80	1.0–7.4	Milham and Hesser (1967)
(Mixed cellul.)	Lumber	C–C	Israel	2.33	0.6–8.7	Abramson *et al.* (1978)
	Paper manuf.	C–C	US	4.00	1.2–12.9	Milham and Hesser (1967)
	Paper manuf.	C–C	US	2.45	n.a.	Decoufle *et al.* (1977)
	Woodworker	C–C	US	2.30	1.5–3.5	Milham and Hesser (1967)
	Woodworker	C vs census	England and Wales	0.75	0.1–2.2	Acheson (1967)
	Woodworkers	Area mort.	US	sign xs	n.a.	Spiers (1969)
	Woodworkers	Occup. mort.	US	1.63	1.2–2.1	Petersen and Milham (1974)
	Woodworker	C–C	US	1.75	1.1–2.7	Petersen and Milham (1974)
	Woodworker	C vs census	US	1.6	0.9–2.6	Grufferman, Duong and Cole (1976)
	Woodworker	C–C	Israel	1.09	0.7–1.7	Abramson *et al.* (1978)

*See text for description of method.

C–C = case-control studies.

n.a. = cannot be calculated.

obtained from the registration particulars. There were 28 woodworkers in the cases and 24 in the controls. Subsequent analysis (Ball, 1968) showed no clear difference in type of wood exposure. However, the controls were the next age/sex matched deaths in the registry and this may have led to overmatching on occupation.

Canada: 2

Medical records identified 121 men with nasal cancer treated in British Columbia in 1939–77, and matched controls. Data were also available on smoking and this appeared to be a risk factor, in addition to wood dust exposure (Elwood, 1981).

Finland

A case-control study of 45 patients with nasal cancer diagnosed in central and southern Finland in 1970–73 identified no specific occupation at significantly high risk. There were 2 adenocarcinoma, of which 1 was a joiner. No patients had been exposed to nickel or chromium (Tola *et al.*, 1980a).

Italy

A case-control study of 64 patients with cancer of the nose and nasal sinuses (including 11 with adenocarcinoma) treated in Florence in 1963–77 involved interview with the patients or their relatives, and non-cancer hospital controls (Cecchi *et al.*, 1980).

A small case-control study of 19 patients with nasal cancer in northern Italy identified 5 with exposure to wood dust, but none in the controls (Merler *et al.*, 1982). [It is impossible to align the text with the tables.]

A case-control study of 36 male patients with nasal cancer in Sienna diagnosed in 1963–81 showed a relative risk of 5.4 for all forms of histology and 89.7 for adenocarcinomas (Battista *et al.*, 1983).

Scandinavia

A collaborative case-control study of 169 patients with nasal cancer in Denmark, Finland, and Sweden diagnosed in 1977–80 used controls with colorectal cancer, matched for age and sex (Hernberg *et al.*, 1983a, b).

US

A case-control study compared the occupation recorded at death registration for 37 nasal cancer patients and 73 control deaths in North Carolina (Brinton *et al.*, 1977).

One hundred and sixty patients with nasal cancer treated in 4 hospitals in North Carolina and Virginia in 1970–80 were matched to (*a*) hospital patients, (*b*) decedents on age, sex, race, county of residence, and year of death, if the index patient was dead (Brinton *et al.*, 1984).

3.38.5 Other sites of malignancy

Nasopharynx

Mould and Bakowski (1976) obtained particulars about patients with adenocarcinoma of the nasopharynx from hospital and regional cancer registries in the UK. Among 35 males, 6 were woodworkers. It was suggested that this greatly exceeded the proportion of such workers in the population.

Larynx

Routine occupational histories for patients admitted to Roswell Park in 1956–65 permitted examination of association of various cancers with work as carpenters or in the paper industry (Bross, Viadana and Houten, 1978).

There were 46 patients with laryngeal cancer treated in 3 districts of East Germany in 1969–76. Occupation was obtained from the patients and compared with the general distribution in the population (Wolf, 1978).

A case-control study compared 258 men and 56 women with laryngeal cancer treated in 5 US cities in 1970–73 with patients matched for age, sex, hospital status, and year of admission (Wynder *et al.*, 1976). In males, it was stated that there was a significant excess exposed to wood dust, but the basic data are not provided in the paper.

Lung

One study from Sweden and 2 from the US have provided information on the association with potential exposure to wood or paper manufacture.

Sweden

Death registers for 1963–77 in a small Swedish town with a furniture industry were used to identify 25 deaths in males from respiratory cancer, 70 from gastrointestinal cancer, and control deaths from other causes. Occupation was obtained from the particulars recorded at death registration. Although there were no deaths from nasal cancer, the material was used to examine the risk from laryngeal and lung cancer (Esping and Axelson, 1980).

US: 1

Eight hundred and fifty-eight white male deaths from lung cancer in the coastal area of Georgia were identified in 1961–74 and matched with deaths excluding lung and bladder cancer and chronic respiratory disease. The statements on occupation were used to examine risks of this cancer (Harrington *et al.*, 1978). Though there was only a small increase in the risk for workers in the paper industry, the counties in the part of the area where the lumber industry was located had an increased risk to workers in this industry.

US: 2

To follow-up the mapping of mortality in the US, a case-control study of 458 males with lung cancer in coastal Georgia diagnosed in 1970–76 focused on employment in shipyards. However, occupational histories obtained by interview with patients or relatives showed no risk from employment in the paper industry. This was an incidental finding, and the paper does not discuss the results of Harrington and his colleagues (Blot *et al.*, 1978).

Hodgkin's disease

Occupation recorded on death certification for 1549 white males aged 25 or over, dying from Hodgkin's disease in Upstate New York in 1940–53 and 1957–64 were compared with data for matched deaths (Milham and Hesser, 1967).

All patients diagnosed with Hodgkin's disease in the Oxford region in 1956–65 were identified from cancer registry records. There was no evidence of an appreciable increase of patients in the locality where the furniture industry was located, and no evidence of an increased proportion of woodworkers of any kind amongst the 140 male patients aged 15–64 in the region (Acheson, 1967).

Spiers (1969) used proportions of Hodgkin's disease deaths to other RES deaths to get an index of variation in Hodgkin's disease mortality by state and compared this with (*a*) an index of the percentage of white persons employed in wood, lumber, and furniture industries, and (*b*) the percentage of commercial forestland in the state covered by pine. Analysis suggested that there was a significant association of the index for Hodgkin's disease variation and the commercial statistics for male deaths east of the Rocky mountains, but not to the west.

Petersen and Milham (1974) used the file of death records for males in Washington State for the period 1950–71 to explore this issue. First, by selecting matched controls for the Hodgkin's patients, it was possible to look at the occupations recorded. Also a proportional-mortality ratio was calculated for the wood-related occupations.

Patients with Hodgkin's disease in Boston diagnosed in 1959–73 were identified from various hospital sources; the occupations in the notes were abstracted and the distribution compared with census results in the locality in 1961 and 1971 (Grufferman, Duong and Cole, 1976).

A general case-control study of patients diagnosed with Hodgkin's disease in 1960–70 in Israel showed a significant association with wood or trees in those with mixed cellularity tumours (Abramson *et al.*, 1978). It is not clear if this subdivision was planned before the analysis, or merely reflected the subgroup found to have the closest relationship.

Greene *et al.* (1978) reported a family of 21 members of whom 3 of the males and 1 female were known to have developed Hodgkin's disease. Two of the affected brothers had worked in a fence installing company; they had applied pentachlorophenol to the wood as a preservative.

3.38.6 Prospective studies

Union records were used to identify 16443 deaths in carpenters and joiners in the US in 1969–70. There were adequate data for the calculation of expected deaths by cause from the membership statistics and national rates of mortality (Milham, 1974b).

Ferris, Puleo and Chen (1979) followed 271 men working in a pulp and paper mill in New Hampshire from 1963 to 1973. There was no overall increased mortality compared with expected based on national rates. There were only 7 deaths from malignant disease and no expected figure was given for specific cancers.

Forty thousand, four hundred and twenty-eight men aged 20–84 in 1971 in the Danish Carpenter and Cabinet makers' trade union were followed until 1976. Olsen and Sabroe (1979) used union, insurance, and central records to identify all deaths

in the cohort. Expected values were based on national mortality rates.

3.38.7 Conclusions

The introduction to this section mentioned a number of specific problems of interpretation. In studying *Table 3.7*, it can be seen that the comparisons for nasal cancer have varied in different studies: (*a*) some have taken cases with adenocarcinoma and calculated an RR against nasal cancer of other histology; (*b*) others restrict the cases to those with adenocarcinoma, but compare the results with subjects not having nasal cancer, and (*c*) the third group includes all forms of histology in the cases, and uses non-nasal cancer subjects as controls. The calculated risks vary between these different approaches, particularly depending on whether the occupational hazard only influences the risk of adenocarcinoma, affects the risk of adenocarcinoma to a greater extent than other forms of histology, or increases the risk equally for any histological type.

IARC (1981) concluded that the epidemiological data were not sufficient to assess the carcinogenic risk in lumber and sawmill workers, carpenters and joiners, or the paper and pulp mill industries. It was agreed that employment in the furniture-making industry caused adenocarcinoma of the nasal passages. The evidence points to the highest risk being in those exposed to hardwood dusts.

The case reports contribute to the picture by confirming that the hazard of nasal cancer in furniture workers: (*a*) was not confined to one country; (*b*) involved use of more than one specific wood; (*c*) followed exposure predominantly in the 1920s and 1930s; (*d*) could occur after only a few months work; (*e*) usually developed after a latent interval of about 30 years.

Examination of *Table 3.7* does suggest that the nasal cancer risk is not restricted to furniture workers. This could only be quantified if detailed job histories of all workers permitted analyses restricted to those who had never worked in furniture manufacture, and appropriate controls were available.

There is also a slight but consistently raised risk for Hodgkin's disease. These results are based on 8 studies from different countries, using different methods; there is no obvious confounding factor that could account for this picture.

Recommended reading

See end of Chapter 2.

4

The aetiology of cancer

The following notes review the aetiology of cancer by specific sites, which are listed in order of the ICD. The intention of these comments on each site are to (a) indicate briefly the non-occupational factors that have been associated with each site of malignancy, and (b) indicate those occupational factors for which there is substantial evidence of an association with increased risk of cancer. This chapter therefore provides a cross-index to the more extensive series of occupational reviews in Chapters 2 and 3, and at the same time indicates those non-occupational factors which may contribute to the variation of risk of specific cancers in the population.

When a fresh association is observed, with apparently increased risk of a specific cancer in a group of workers, it is hoped that this chapter will facilitate consideration of (a) the likelihood that there is confounding with some non-occupational factor, which is the actual cause of the excess noticed in the workers, (b) the possibility that there is some (common) factor, responsible for the present new finding that is also responsible for an association already suggested or recognized in another occupation. As indicated in Chapter 1 (*see* 1.2.5 and 1.2.6) errors in the available data or chance may result in false positive associations.

4.1 Oral cavity (ICD 140–145)

Evidence strongly suggests that smoking, chewing tobacco, oral snuff usage, and alcoholic beverages were aetiological factors (Sanghvi, Rao and Khanolkar, 1955; Wynder and Bross, 1957; Brown, Suh and Scarborough, 1965; Larson, Sandstrom and Westling, 1975; Graham *et al.*, 1977). Chewing tobacco

includes the use of betel-nut and betel leaf and lime in some communities.

One of the factors associated with increased alcohol intake may be occupations involving manufacture or sale of beers, wines, and spirits. There is evidence that persons in these occupations have increased incidence of or mortality from cancer of the buccal cavity (*see* 3.1).

There is evidence that printing workers have an increased mortality from buccal cancer (*see* 2.50). The pooled results for 4 studies showed O/E = 1.42, 95% CL = 1.1–1.9 (*Table 2.20*).

4.2 Nasopharynx (ICD 147)

There appears to be a genetic component to this condition, with an increased frequency of HLA-2 in patients. It has been suggested that this may be linked to the ability to metabolize a potential carcinogen (Henderson *et al.*, 1976).

The main aetiological agent identified is the increased prevalence of Epstein–Barr infection (identified in cells from the tumours or in patients' sera). Hospital studies showed an increased prevalence of infection in staff nursing these cancer patients, which increased in relation to the proximity of patient and staff (Ho *et al.*, 1978). A case-control study investigated a number of carcinogens known to induce nasal or lung cancer; these showed no association with nasopharyngeal cancer (Ho, Huang and Fong, 1978). However, such patients were found to be more likely to eat traditional foods, such as salted fish. The significance of this was not clear.

4.3 Oesophagus (ICD 150)

Many authors have defined a high-risk zone involving parts of East Africa, the Middle East through northern Iran, southern portions of the USSR, Afghanistan into China. Evidence suggests that there are a number of different aetiological agents, not all of which are present in each high-risk zone.

Work in the UK and Iran suggests that there is a genetic component which can influence risk of the disease. It is only likely to be responsible for a small proportion of the total cases (Howel-Evans *et al.*, 1958; Pour and Ghadirian, 1974). Alcohol undoubtedly plays a part, for example in northern France (where distilled apple spirits are drunk), and an independent effect of smoking has been noted. Analysis of data on both factors indicates that there is a multiplicative effect in persons smoking and drinking (Tuyns, Pequignot and Jensen, 1977). Extensive studies in northern Iran and China have not yet identified specific causal factors — although alcohol is certainly not responsible. There is a strong suggestion that dietary deficiency is associated with high risk (Cook-Mozaffari *et al.*, 1979), whilst one paper has incriminated a particular usage of opium (Hewer *et al.*, 1978). Elsewhere dietary deficiency (in the form of the Plummer–Vinson syndrome) had also been identified as a risk factor (Wynder *et al.*, 1957).

Though no specific dietary carcinogen has been identified, consumption of food at high temperatures appears to increase the risk of this cancer (de Jong *et al.*, 1974). A specific but rare aetiological factor was lye burns (Imre and Kopp, 1972).

4.4 Stomach (ICD 151)

Genetic studies, despite their limitations, suggest that gastric cancer is concentrated in some families (Graham and Lilienfeld, 1958). There is also increased incidence in persons with blood group A (Aird *et al.*, 1954), ABH non-secretors (Doll, Drane and Newell, 1961), blacks compared with whites in the US (Wynder *et al.*, 1963), and those with pernicious anaemia (Mosbech and Videbaek, 1950) — although it was not clear whether this was due to changes resulting simply from the presence of the pernicious anaemia or some common aetiological factor.

Collation and case-control studies suggest that deficiency of fresh fruit, vegetables and salads is associated with increased risk; no specific carcinogen in the diet has been identified (Haenszel *et al.*, 1976). Endogenous and exogenous nitrosamines have been proposed as relevant on somewhat tenuous evidence (Alderson, 1980b).

Other work indicates that cigarette smoking (Hammond and Horn, 1958) and atmospheric pollution (Stocks, 1960) may be associated with increased incidence or mortality from stomach cancer. In contrast to the US study, there was no association with smoking in the UK doctors (Doll and Peto, 1976; Doll *et al.*, 1980). Specific studies have also incriminated poor dental hygiene or oral sepsis (Herbert and Bruske, 1936), and use of liquid paraffin as a purgative (Boyd and Doll, 1954); these findings have not been confirmed in other studies. Conflicting views also exist on whether the subsequent risk of stomach cancer following peptic ulcer is different from that in the general population (Hirohata, 1968; Nicholls, 1974).

There has been consistent evidence, from a variety of sources, of an increased risk of stomach cancer in coal miners (*see* 3.22). The pooled data in *Table 3.4* for 8 studies showed O/E = 1.66, 95% CL = 1.5–1.8.

When the results of 11 prospective studies of workers in petroleum refineries are pooled, there is an excess of stomach cancer of borderline significance: O/E = 1.11, 95% CL = 1.0–1.2 (*see 3.23* and *Table 3.5*).

Recent studies of workers in the rubber industry (*see* 3.30) have shown increased mortality from stomach cancer. The pooled data for 8 prospective studies indicated a borderline increase: O/E = 1.23, 95% CL = 1.1–1.3 (*Table 3.6*).

None of these positive findings for the 3 occupational groups have resulted in any clear pointers to the aetiological agent involved.

4.5 Colorectal (ICD 153–154)

Persons living in rural areas tend to have low rates (Clemmesen, 1977b). Mormons have a lower rate of these cancers than the general population (Enstrom, 1978), whilst a recent study suggests this is also so for Seventh Day Adventists (Phillips, 1975). Migrant studies show low rates for Japanese living in Japan, which rise in first and then second generation migrants into the US (Haenszel and Kurihara, 1968). Collation of national statistics has suggested that increased risk of colorectal cancer is associated with: diets containing excess fat and animal protein (Gregor, Toman and Prusova, 1969; Shrauzer, 1976), and those that are deficient in fibre, particularly the pentose fraction (Bingham *et al.*, 1979), and excess beer consumption (Enstrom, 1977).

A definite genetic component exists, although this is only directly responsible for a small proportion of the cancers that develop. In addition to familial polyposis coli (Bussey, 1975), there is increased incidence in (a) other syndromes with multiple colonic adenoma — such as Garner's and Turcot's syndromes, and (b) other hereditary large bowel disease — such as coeliac disease, Crohn's disease, and ulcerative colitis (Wennstrom, Pierce and McCusick, 1974). Quite apart from such hereditary disease it has been suggested that bowel cancers are more likely to follow appendicectomy (Hyams and Wynder, 1968; Hornbak and Astrup, 1970), schistosomiasis (Chen *et al.*, 1965) and ureterosigmoidostomy (Haney and McGarity, 1971).

The international data on diet have stimulated a search for an association with specific nutrients in case-control studies. There are very limited positive results; one study suggested that excess meat intake was a factor to consider (Haenszel *et al.*, 1973), whilst a small case-control study suggested that the cases had a diet that combined high saturated fat food with low fibre-containing foods (Dales *et al.*, 1979). Many other studies were negative for both fat and meat intake. International comparisons had suggested that the bacterial flora and faecal bile acids were different in high-and-low-risk populations (Aries *et al.*, 1969; Hill *et al.*, 1971). Support for this was obtained from a small case-control study of inpatients (Hill *et al.*, 1975). However, subsequent findings from this research team's work have generated some unexplained results (Bone, Drasar and Hill, 1975; IARC, 1977c); other groups carrying out comparable projects in metabolic epidemiology failed to confirm the work (Finegold, Attebery and Sutter, 1974; Mower *et al.*, 1979).

Case-control studies have shown no clear relation with alcohol intake. Three historical prospective studies have explored the subsequent incidence or mortality from colorectal cancer in those thought to consume above average quantities of alcohol (particularly beer) (Hakulinen *et al.*, 1974; Dean *et al.*, 1979; Jensen, 1979). Only one of these (Dean *et al.*, 1979) showed an appreciable excess of large bowel cancer (that was significant for rectum, but not for colon).

Other factors highlighted by one or more case-control studies have been constipation and the use of laxatives (Boyd and Doll, 1954), prior irradiation (Brinkley and Haybittle, 1969; Smith and Doll, 1976), and a raised risk in women having higher parity than control subjects (Bjelke, 1971; 1974).

Follow-up of 3 groups of professional chemists in the UK and the US identified an increased risk of colorectal cancer: O/E = 1.42, 95% CL = 1.3–1.6 (*see 3.10* and *Table 3.1*). Recent studies of workers in the rubber industry (*see 3.30*) have shown an increase in colon cancer mortality. The pooled data for 7 prospective studies showed a borderline significant increase: O/E = 1.07, 95% CL = 1.0–1.2 (*see Table 3.6*). Neither of these positive results have indicated any specific agent that might be responsible.

Follow-up of luminizers (exposed to irradiation from radium) has shown an increased mortality from colorectal cancer (*see 2.39.3*).

Workers exposed to asbestos fibres have an increased mortality from cancer of the gastrointestinal tract. The overall increase was significant for the studies reviewed in 2.31, with the most marked excess in insulators (*see Table* 2.8).

4.6 Liver (ICD 155)

This section is chiefly concerned with primary hepatocellular cancer of the liver; some comments are also made about angiosarcoma of the liver.

There are clusters of high mortality of liver cancer in (a) eastern South Asia, (b) south of the Sahara, and (c) in south and east Europe (Aoki, 1978). Many of the population so involved are not covered by adequate incidence or mortality statistics; where mortality statistics are available the distinction between primary and secondary cancers may vary in precision.

Glycogen-storage disorders and haemachromatosis, which have a genetic aetiology, are associated with an increased risk of such cancers (Mulvihill, 1975).

Studies in Africa, Asia, Australia, Greece, UK and the US have shown more frequent evidence of present or past infection with hepatitis B in cases compared with controls (Vogel *et al.*, 1970; Anthony *et al.*, 1972; Maupas *et al.*, 1975; Larouze *et al.*, 1976; Tabor *et al.*, 1977; Turbitt *et al.*, 1977; McCaughan, Parsons and Gallagher, 1979). That this was not so for patients with liver metastases suggests that it is not the presence of the cancer in the liver that is leading to the evidence of infection (Trichopoulos *et al.*, 1978). There is indication that prior infection with typhoid (Welton, Marr and Friedman, 1979) is more likely to be followed by liver cancer; this is only thought to be relevant to a small proportion of cases.

In Africa surveys have indicated an association between high incidence of the cancer in populations and the degree to which they eat aflatoxin-contaminated foods (Peers and Lindsell, 1973). There is some suggestion that prior infection with hepatitis or dietary deficiency may be an added risk factor in such populations (Shank, 1977).

The evidence on cirrhosis and alcohol is somewhat confusing. Patients with cancer of the liver have a higher prevalence of cirrhosis than controls (Mori, 1967). A case-control study of liver cancer found an association with alcohol intake (Williams and Horm, 1977). However, a number of prospective studies of individuals consuming an excess of alcohol have failed to find a raised mortality from liver cancer, e.g. Robinette, Hrubec and Fraumeni, 1979; others have suggested an excess (Hakulinen *et al.*, 1974).

A limited role has been suggested for various drug usage, such as anabolic steroids (Johnson *et al.*,

1972), immunosuppression (Kinlen *et al.*, 1979), and oral contraceptives (Baum *et al.*, 1973; Klatskin, 1977). The latter risk is thought to be very low in the UK (Vessey *et al.*, 1977).

It must be emphasized that angiosarcoma of the liver is a much less frequent tumour that is still predominantly of unexplained aetiology. However, increased risk occurs in individuals exposed to arsenic, anabolic steroid, thorotrast, and vinyl chloride monomer (Falk *et al.*, 1979).

There is clear evidence from a number of countries of the markedly raised hazard of angiosarcoma of the liver in workers exposed to VCM (*see* 3.37). This is also reflected in an increase in overall deaths from liver neoplasms identified in prospective studies of exposed workers: O/E = 4.68, 95% CL = 3.3–6.5 (*see Table 2.22*).

Occupations involving manufacture or retail of beers, wines, and spirits are associated with an increased risk of death from liver cancer (*see* 3.1).

4.7 Gallbladder and biliary tract (ICD 156)

Biliary tract cancer is much less common than primary liver cancer. In a US study, patients with cancer of the gallbladder had a significantly higher prevalence of gall stones than would be expected from the population incidence of this condition (Maram, Ludwig and Kurlano, 1979).

Autopsy studies in the Far East have shown that biliary tract cancer may be associated with parasite infestations, such as *Clonorchis sinensis* (Hou, 1956) or opisthorchiasis (Bhamarapravati and Viranuvatti, 1966; Sonakul *et al.*, 1978).

4.8 Pancreas (ICD 157)

Japanese migrants to the US appear to have higher mortality from pancreas cancer than Japanese in Japan or whites in the US (Haenszel and Kurihara, 1968), whilst rates rise for migrants from a number of European countries going to the US (Haenszel, 1961).

Collation studies have shown associations with consumption of coffee (Stocks, 1970), sugar or sweets (Shennan and Bishop, 1974), alcohol (Breslow and Enstrom, 1974), egg and animal protein (Armstrong and Doll, 1975). Dietary studies of patients have not confirmed any of these suggestions.

Case-control studies of alcohol consumption have given conflicting results (Burch and Ansari, 1968; Wynder *et al.*, 1973), whilst follow-up of these known to take alcohol show virtually the same observed and expected deaths when pooling 6 studies (*see* Alderson, 1982).

Three case-control studies showed an excess of diabetics (Clark and Mitchell, 1961; Karmody and Kyle, 1969; Wynder *et al.*, 1973), whilst follow-up of a large cohort of diabetics confirmed that a significant excess developed pancreatic cancer (Kessler, 1970). There have also been case reports (Bartholomew, Gross and Comfort, 1958; Gambill, 1971) and case-control studies indicating an association with pancreatitis (Wynder *et al.*, 1973), but it is not clear if this is due to confounding with alcohol consumption. One case-control study showed an association with prior cholecystectomy (Wynder *et al.*, 1973).

Case-control studies (Wynder *et al.*, 1973) and prospective studies (e.g. Doll and Peto, 1976) have clearly shown an increased risk with cigarette smoking, which is compatible with the trends in mortality for this cancer.

Follow-up of 3 groups of professional chemists in Sweden and the US identified an increased mortality from pancreas cancer: O/E = 1.60, 95% CL = 1.2–2.0 (*see* 3.10 and *Table 3.1*). Follow-up of 11 groups of workers from petroleum refineries showed a borderline significant increase in pancreatic cancer mortality: O/E = 1.15, 95% CL = 1.0–1.3 (*see* 3.23 and *Table 3.5*). In neither of these occupational groups was there any indication of the aetiological factors involved.

Follow-up of British medical staff potentially exposed to ionizing irradiation showed an increase in deaths from pancreas cancer: O/E = 3.2, 95% CL = 1.1–6.9 (*see* 2.39.1). This excess was restricted to those entering the profession before 1920.

4.9 Nasal cancer (ICD 160)

No non-occupational aetiological factor has been identified.

A number of quite different, but specific occupational hazards have been recognized. Chapters 2 and 3 review the publications that have confirmed the increased risk from the following compounds.

Chemicals

Isopropyl alcohol manufacture (*see* 2.40). The evidence indicates that the risk is associated with the strong acid process and may be due to exposure to alkyl sulphate produced in this process.

Metals

(a) Chromium

Production of chromate from ore and handling of chrome pigments appear to increase the risk of nasal cancer. It has been suggested that the hexavalent salts of chromium are the compounds with greater carcinogenicity, rather than the trivalent compounds (*see* 2.19).

(b) Nickel

There is consistent evidence of an increased risk of nasal cancer from nickel refining, but not from subsequent use of nickel (*see* 2.44).

Vegetable dusts

(a) Leather

The review (*see* 3.21 and *Table 3.3*) provided evidence from 8 countries of increased risk of nasal cancer in leather workers. The risk appeared to be greatest for those exposed to the dusty processes in boot and shoe manufacture.

(b) Wood

Section 3.38 and *Table* 3.7 present data from 9 countries showing an increased risk of nasal cancer (especially adenocarcinoma) for those exposed to hardwood dust.

Though the specific carcinogen has not been identified, the evidence shows the closest relationship to dust exposure for both leather workers and woodworkers. There is no indication that chemical additives used in the various manufacturing processes are responsible.

4.10 Larynx (ICD 161)

This is not a site for which an appreciable genetic component is usually suggested, but Trell *et al.* (1976) have found that an excess proportion of male patients possess the appropriate enzymes for aryl hydrocarbon hydroxylase inducibility.

Smoking and alcohol consumption have both been indicated as associated with increased risk of the disease, in case-control (Wynder, Bross and Day, 1956; Hinds, Thomas and O'Reilly, 1979) and prospective studies (Jensen, 1979; Robinette, Hrubec and Fraumeni, 1979). There was also a suggestion from a Swedish case-control study that sideropenic dysphagia was more frequent in the cases with extrinsic cancer (Wynder, Bross and Day, 1956); this was not found in the associated American study.

Irradiation, which has clearly been shown to cause cancer at other sites, has been noted in one larynx study as associated with the cases — especially more frequent dental X-ray (Hinds, Thomas and O'Reilly, 1979).

Prospective studies of asbestos workers showed excess deaths from laryngeal cancer in those exposed in: mining/milling, manufacturing, insulating, shipyard work (*see Table 2.9*). Though a case-control study in north England had shown a very high risk from prior exposure to asbestos, this finding has not been replicated in a number of other case-control studies (*see* 2.31.7 and *Table 2.14*).

4.11 Lung (ICD 162)

Familial clustering had been reported (Tokuhata and Lilienfeld, 1963); a possible explanation was the genetically transmitted ability to induce aryl hydrocarbon hydroxylase (Kellermann, Shaw and Luyten-Kellermann, 1973). The early work was not confirmed by other groups until recently (Emery *et al.*, 1978).

Smoking has been indicated as the main causal agent; this is on the basis of collation (Waller, 1967), case-control (e.g. Doll and Hill, 1950), and prospective studies (e.g. Doll and Peto, 1976; Doll *et al.*, 1980). A powerful point in the argument is the lower risk of cancer in those who give up smoking compared with those who continue; this has been indicated in broad subgroups of the population and confirmed in prospective studies. Some authors have questioned the causal relationships, suggesting that genetic liability to lung cancer might be associated with a desire for smoking. Some of the arguments against the generally accepted hypothesis have been set out by Burch (1980).

Atmospheric pollution has been associated with increased risk of lung cancer (Gardner, Crawford and Morris, 1969); in a number of countries there is evidence that persons living in towns smoke more than rural dwellers. There appears to be about a two-fold increase in lung cancer after adjusting for this (Wicken, 1966). Both smoking and air pollution increase the incidence of chronic bronchitis; it is thus not straightforward to determine whether the presence of chronic bronchitis *per se* adds to the risk of lung cancer developing, but several studies suggest that this is so (Finke, 1956; Rimington, 1968, 1971).

Recent work has indicated that persons with an adequate intake of vitamin A are at reduced risk of developing cancer in general and lung cancer in particular (Bjelke, 1975; Wald *et al.*, 1980).

The literature on occupational associations with risk of lung cancer is extensive. It is not clear whether: (*a*) the relative frequency of this cancer permits identification of significant associations, by virtue of the numbers of cases or deaths available in many studies, (*b*) the variation in smoking habits in different occupational groups results in confounding with this powerful factor influencing risk of lung cancer, (*c*) there are multiplicative effects of occupational exposure and smoking, (*d*) the opportunity for lung cancer to be initiated is due to the ease of exposure of bronchial epithelium to inhaled agents.

The following lists in alphabetical order the agents and occupations which have been found to have a significant association with lung cancer: acrylonitrile (2.1 and *Table 2.1*); aluminium industry (3.2); arsenic (2.7); beryllium (2.11 and *Table 2.5*); butchers (3.5); cadmium (2.13); chromates (2.19); fibres: asbestos (2.31 and *Table 2.10*); fibres: man-made mineral fibres (2.32 and *Table 2.15*); foundry workers (3.16 and *Table 3.2*); irradiation — health professionals (2.39.1), miners (2.39.4); miners — coal (3.22.1 and *Table 3.4*); mustard gas (2.43); nickel (2.44); polynuclear aromatic hydrocarbons — coke plants (2.50.5 and *Table 3.4*); oil mists (2.50.8 and *Table 2.19*); printing (2.50.12 and *Table 2.20*); road transport drivers (3.29); rubber industry (3.30 and *Table 3.6*); silica exposure (2.51 and *Table 2.21*); vinyl chloride (2.58 and *Table 2.22*).

In addition to the above associations with lung cancer, there is a very greatly increased risk of mesothelioma of the pleura in those exposed to asbestos (*see* 2.31.9 and *Table 2.12*).

4.12 Bone (ICD 170)

There is a genetic component to one variety of bone neoplasm: patients with retinoblastoma, or their relatives, are at increased risk of bone sarcoma (Sagerman *et al.*, 1969; Mutsunaga, 1980).

Rather different is the definite association between Paget's disease and oesteogenic sarcoma occurring in the deformed bones (Price, 1962).

An increase in oesteogenic sarcoma was observed in luminizers by Martland (1929). Long-term follow-up of those employed in the US in 1915–29 showed a significant excess of deaths from this malignancy: O/E = 73.3, 95% CL = 45.9–111.0 (*see* 2.39.3).

4.13 Melanoma (ICD 172)

There are major racial differences, with much higher rates in whites than in blacks when living at the same latitude (*Lancet*, 1968). A familial tendency has been reported (Wallace, Exton and McLeod, 1971); in addition, a rare pigmented skin lesion that is genetically determined is a precursor for melanoma (Reimer *et al.*, 1978). There is also an increased risk of melanoma in subjects with xeroderma pigmentosa (Frichot *et al.*, 1977).

Collation studies indicate an association between latitude, or sunshine, and mortality rates for melanoma (Elwood *et al.*, 1974; Swerdlow, 1979). Migrants to Israel had increasing risk of melanoma the longer they stayed in the country (Movshovitz and Modan, 1973). Case-control studies indicate a relationship with light complexions and sensitivity to sunlight (Lancaster and Nelson, 1957; Klepp and Magnus, 1979). Less clearly defined are possible associations with: oestrogen consumption or parity (Sadoff, Winkley and Tyson, 1973; Rampen and Mulder, 1980), alcohol intake (Williams, 1976), and trauma (Lea, 1965). The latter is difficult to quantify, whilst the alcohol findings have been disputed (Lyon, Gardner and Klauber, 1976).

Two of the prospective studies of refinery workers (*see* 3.23 and *Table 3.5*) presented data for melanoma. There was a significantly increased number of deaths: O/E = 2.02, 95% CL = 1.3–3.0.

4.14 Skin: non-melanoma (ICD 173)

A racial difference exists, with whites having higher rates than blacks living at the same latitude (Schreek, 1944). There is an association with xeroderma and a number of other rare genetic skin disorders (Schimke, 1978).

The geographical variation accords with study of populations and patients indicating that increased ultraviolet radiation from sunlight is an aetiological factor (Jablon, 1975). Accepted but less frequent causes are: chronic bacterial infection (Davies, 1975); presence of scars (Templeton, 1975); irradiation (Ingram and Comaish, 1967); exposure to arsenic from medicinal use (Hutchinson, 1888); treatment with immunosuppressive drugs (Kinlen *et al.*, 1979).

The first occupational cancer to be recognized was scrotal cancer in chimney sweeps (Pott, 1775). There is still an increase in skin cancer in these workers (*see* 2.50.4). Related hazards have now been observed in workers in: petroleum refineries (3.23 and *Table 3.5*), and those exposed to mineral oils (2.50.7).

Another long-standing hazard has been from exposure to arsenic either in manufacture or use of various products (2.7).

Ultraviolet light is accepted as a causal agent of skin cancer, with increased risk in occupations involving prolonged exposure such as farming (3.14) and fishing (3.15). Some general issues are discussed in 2.57.

4.15 Breast (ICD 174)

There is a wealth of case reports indicating a familial association (e.g. Teasdale, Forbes and Baum, 1976); the genetic (rather than environmental) basis of this has been suggested by work showing very high risks in daughters where mothers and sisters have bilateral premenopausal cancer (Anderson, 1974). A Danish twin study estimated hereditability at about 0.3–0.40 (Holm, Hauge and Harvald, 1980). Parity and marital status had been associated with variation in risk (e.g. Fraumeni *et al.*, 1969); a 7 country study showed that the age at first pregnancy was the relevant factor, with risk rising with older childbearing (MacMahon *et al.*, 1970 a,b). Prospective studies have indicated that women with benign breast disease have an increased likelihood of subsequent cancer (Donnelly *et al.*, 1975; Hutchinson *et al.*, 1980); this has been disputed, partly on the basis of missed cancer in the original diagnosis and the validity of the calculated expected values (Levene, 1976). Artificial (early) menopause (Feinleib, 1968), thyroid disease (Mittra and Hayward, 1974), excess fat intake (Hill, Goddard and Williams, 1971; Miller *et al.*, 1978), use prior to first pregnancy of combination oral contraception in young women (WHO, 1978) and hormone replacement therapy (Hoover *et al.*, 1976) have all been suggested as risk factors.

Disputed evidence has been reported on the influence of: alcohol consumption (Lyon, Gardner and Klauber, 1976; Williams, 1976); treatment with rauwolfia (Boston Collaborative Drug Surveillance Program, 1974a; Christopher *et al.*, 1977); use of hair dyes (Kinlen *et al.*, 1977; Nasca *et al.*, 1980), or virus infection (Fraumeni and Miller, 1971; Henderson *et al.*, 1974). Irradiation from thorotrast, fluoroscopy, therapy for mastitis, and nuclear weapons increases the subsequent risk of breast cancer (Brody and Cullen, 1957; MacKenzie, 1965; Mettler *et al.*, 1969; Jablon and Kato, 1972; Boice and Monson, 1977).

4.16 Cervix (ICD 180)

Many epidemiological studies have been reported, which deal with 'risk factors' rather than explicit aetiological agents. There is a close inverse relationship of risk to age at first intercourse (Wynder *et al.*, 1954; Moghissi, Mack and Porzack, 1968); there is an inter-relationship of this to virginity (Gagnon, 1950), marital status (Leck, Sibary and Wakefield, 1978), parity (Boyd and Doll, 1964), number of marriages (Rotkin, 1967) and numbers of consorts (Stephenson and Grace, 1954).

Collation studies show a parallel trend in venereally transmitted infection (Beral, 1974); case-control studies have reported increased risk in prostitutes (Rojel, 1953) and persons having had a venereal infection such as syphillis, gonorrhoea, or trichomonas infection (Levin, Kress and Goldstein, 1942; Terris and Oalmann, 1960). A prospective study showed cervical cancer was more likely to develop in women with antibodies to herpes simplex type 2 (Choi *et al.*, 1977). This is more persuasive evidence than differences in prevalence of such

infections in cases compared with controls (Punnonen, Gronroos and Peltonen, 1974). Other lines of work have indicated the malignant potential of vulval warts (Zur Hausen, 1976) and the greatly increased frequency of cellular abnormalities associated with such lesions in cervical smears and mild dysplasia (Reid *et al.*, 1980).

Minor support for the role of infection is the suggestion that women are at lower risk of cervical cancer if their husbands use an obstructive method of contraception (Stern and Dixon, 1961; Aitken-Swan and Baird, 1965).

4.17 Uterus — body (ICD 182)

Case-control studies indicate higher risk in the nulliparous, those marrying late, first having intercourse at an 'older age', or having a 'late' menopause (Stewart *et al.*, 1966; Elwood *et al.*, 1977). The cancer is associated with obesity, diabetes, hypertension and arthritis (Elwood *et al.*, 1977); a syndrome exists with increased incidence of breast, ovary and uterine cancer in the same patients or in families (Thiessen, 1974).

All the above items relate to general indicators of risk. Quite different is an extensive series of studies that have explored the relationship to use of hormone replacement therapy. Nine studies noted a positive association, though there were queries about the selection of controls, the reason for therapy and the variation in case ascertainment. It was concluded that there was a genuine relationship because (*a*) the higher the dose of oestrogen, the higher the risk of endometrial cancer, (*b*) the risk increased with increasing duration of use, and (*c*) the risk decreased after hormone therapy ceased (*see Lancet*, 1979b).

A WHO study group concluded that there was some evidence of an increased risk of endometrial cancer among women using sequential oral contraceptives, which have now been withdrawn in a number of countries (WHO, 1978).

4.18 Ovary (ICD 183)

A minimal contribution is postulated for genetic factors, though family clusters have been reported (Lewis and Davidson, 1969; Li *et al.*, 1970) and a tenuous association of specific histological types with blood group A (Osborne and de George, 1963).

Case-control studies (Stewart *et al.*, 1966; Newhouse *et al.*, 1977; Casagrande *et al.*, 1979) have indicated an increased risk in women first having intercourse, pregnancy or marrying after the age of 20; having few children; having an early menopause; making limited use of oral contraceptives. These points can be aggregated into estimated 'total anovular time' which is indirectly related to risk of the cancer (Casagrande *et al.*, 1979). This agrees with collation data which indicated an indirect association between ovarian cancer mortality and average family size for 18 countries (Beral, Fraser and Chilvers, 1978). The increase in mortality this century in England and Wales could be 'accounted for' by the decrease in completed family size.

Two specific factors have been investigated. There is some suggestion of an increased risk in women who have been on hormone replacement therapy (Hoover, Gray and Fraumeni, 1977), though the analysis was disputed (Anneggers, O'Fallon and Kurland, 1977). In a limited study it was suggested that talc particles occurred more frequently in ovaries involved in cancer than normal ovaries (Henderson *et al.*, 1971). These tentative findings were criticized on publication (*Lancet*, 1977) and no definitive support for the hypothesis has since appeared (Roe, 1979).

There has been an indication of higher frequency of obesity and gallbladder disease in ovarian cancer patients (West, 1966; Casagrande *et al.*, 1979). Limited support for this comes from international collation studies which showed a high correlation between total fat intake and mortality from ovarian cancer (Armstrong and Doll, 1975).

In the section on asbestos exposure (*see* 2.31), there are 5 studies from England with follow-up of women exposed to asbestos in whom observed and expected deaths from ovarian cancer are given (*see Table 2.11*). Four of the 5 show increased risk, with the pooled data indicating a significant excess: O/E = 1.70, 95% CL = 1.2–2.4. Though there is the possibility of misclassification of peritoneal mesothelioma as ovarian cancer, this was not thought to account for these results.

4.19 Vagina (ICD 184)

A very rare, clear cell adenocarcinoma was reported in 7 adolescent girls (Herbst and Scully, 1970). The following year this was associated with prior consumption of diethylstilbestrol during pregnancy (Herbst, Ulfelder and Poskanzer, 1971). This therapy had been widely used in the US in 1948–70 for threatened miscarriage and an increasing number of affected patients has been reported (Herbst *et al.*, 1972). Less extensive use had been made of this in England and Wales (Kinlen *et al.*, 1974), but cases have now been identified (Monaghan and Sirisena, 1978; Shepherd, Dewhurst and Pryse-Davies, 1979).

4.20 Prostate (ICD 185)

Family clusters have been reported (Lynch *et al.*, 1966) and an increased risk in blood group A

subjects (Bourke and Griffin, 1962). However, the genetic influence is thought to be minor (Wynder, Mabuchi and Whitmore, 1971).

Case-control studies have reported differences in sexual habits (Wynder, Mabuchi and Whitmore, 1971; Rotkin, 1977; Schumann *et al.*, 1977); though the items examined have varied, there appears to be consistency in the reported excess risk with aspects of sexual drive: age at first intercourse, number of consorts, coital frequency, age at marriage, number of children, prior venereal disease. Two rather different hypotheses have been suggested; one associates dietary differences with altered hormone profile and thus sexual behaviour and risk of prostate cancer. Collation studies had indicated a broad association with fat intake (Blair and Fraumeni, 1978); though no detailed dietary studies have been reported, one case-control study did find an indication of high lipid/cholesterol intake (Rotkin, 1977). Another hypothesis suggests that the behaviour affects the risk of sexually transmitted infection (Zeigel *et al.*, 1977); there is some limited information on variation in prevalence of virus antibodies in cases and controls (Schumann *et al.*, 1977).

Conflicting findings from two prospective studies on patients with benign prostatic hypertrophy suggest no increased risk (Greenwald *et al.*, 1974) and about a four-fold increase (Armenian *et al.*, 1974). This discrepancy has not been resolved.

A number of studies have commented on the excess of patients who have been circumcised (Gibson, 1954). Prostate cancer is uncommon in Jews (Ravich and Ravich, 1951; Seidman, 1970); no report has been able to confirm whether the practice of circumcision or another aspect of behaviour is the key factor.

Following the initial suggestion of an increased risk of prostate cancer in cadmium workers, 5 studies have followed up exposed workers (2.13 and *Table 2.6*). The most recent study (which is also the largest) shows no increase, but the pooled results are at the borderline of significance: O/E = 1.29, 95% CL = 1.0–1.7.

Three of the 7 prospective studies of printing workers (2.50.12 and *Table 2.20*) report results on prostate cancer. The pooled data show an increase in deaths of borderline significance (O/E = 1.28, 95% CL = 1.0–1.6).

4.21 Testis (ICD 186)

There is extensive literature on the relationship of cryptorchism to risk of testicular cancer, with considerable inconsistency in the findings (Gilbert and Hamilton, 1940; Campbell, 1959; Morrison, 1976). This may be partly due to the difficulty in obtaining either a valid history from the cancer patients or of determining the prevalence in the general population. The weight of evidence supports an association between the 2 conditions.

Antecedent orchitis has also been suggested as an aetiological factor, but 2 major studies were negative (Gilbert, 1944; Ehrengut and Schwartau, 1977).

Other case-control studies have noted differences between cases and controls, but with no consistency to clearly identify risk factors or causal agents. There was an indication of association with trauma (Mustacchi and Millimore, 1976), though the latter is very difficult to document in an unbiased way.

4.22 Penis (ICD 187)

Studies in East Africa and India have both shown that the 'incidence' of the condition varies in relation to circumcision practice, being rare in those communities practicing this (Dodge and Linsell, 1963; Paymaster and Gangadharan, 1967).

A number of years ago, there was a suggestion of excess cervical cancers in wives of men with penile cancer (Martinez, 1969). Two prospective studies of wives of such men have confirmed this (Graham *et al.*, 1979; Smith *et al.*, 1980); this association only involved a very small proportion of cervical cancer patients. Neither study was appropriate to determine the mechanism, but it was thought to be compatible with a common virological aetiology for both cancers.

4.23 Bladder (ICD 188)

A number of studies have indicated a relative risk of 2.0–4.0 for smokers (*see* Morrison and Cole, 1976, for a review). Because of the prevalence of smoking, this makes an appreciable contribution to the overall toll from this site.

Coffee drinking has been suggested as increasing the risk of bladder cancer (Simon, Yen and Cole, 1975). Other studies have tentatively implicated alcohol, artificial sweeteners, Coca-Cola, and opium (Morgan and Jain, 1974; Miller, 1977; Sadeghi and Behmard, 1978). These suggestions have not been substantiated.

It was postulated that nitrosamines might be formed in an infected bladder and support came from studies on Egyptian and English patients (Hicks *et al.*, 1977). However, more recent studies of bladder cancer patients and controls showed no significant difference in levels of various nitrosamine compounds (IARC, 1978c).

Egypt has a considerably higher bladder cancer mortality than other countries. This is thought to be due to the endemic schistosomiasis. Patients with this infection have an appreciably raised risk of bladder cancer (Hashem, 1961; Dunham, Bailar and Lacquer, 1973).

The potential hazard of bladder cancer in certain dye workers was recognized at the end of the nineteenth century (Rehn, 1895).

Extensive studies have demonstrated the hazard from exposure to a variety of aromatic amines: 2-naphthylamine, magenta, benzidine, and auramine; it is not clear whether the increase in bladder cancer in those exposed to 1-naphthylamine was due to contamination with 2-naphthylamine (2.6). A related hazard stemmed from the use of an antioxidant in rubber manufacture containing the carcinogenic aromatic amines. A number of prospective studies confirmed the increase in bladder cancer in rubber workers (3.30 and *Table 3.6*). Pooled data from the 9 most recent studies in 4 countries show borderline increased risk of bladder cancer: O/E =1.11, 95% CL = 1.0–1.3.

Death from bladder cancer is also increased in the prospective studies of coke workers (2.50.5 and *Table 2.18*). Five studies combined showed: O/E = 1.5, 95% CL = 1.1–2.1. It has been suggested that this is because oven workers were exposed to 2-naphthylamine in the fumes from the plant. An increased risk has been identified in workers exposed to acrylonitrile (2.1 and *Table 2.1*) which was of borderline significance: O/E = 3.12, 95% CL = 1.0–7.3. Leather workers (3.20 and *Table 3.3*) have an increased occupational mortality from 3 counties, and raised risk for 5 case-control studies in 2 countries.

Early recognition of the bladder cancer risk in workers exposed to 4-aminobiphenyl (xenylamine) was sufficient to prevent widespread use of the chemical (2.3).

4.23.1 Case-control studies — 'fishing'

A number of general case-control studies have been reported in the past 20 years, which have included questions on occupation. Though some of these have concentrated on testing hypotheses already reported in the literature, others have been exploratory — searching for risk associated with many occupations, often only reported by very few of the subjects in the studies. *Table 4.1* is provided to show the main characteristics of 16 of these studies, whilst the results are set out in standard form in *Table 4.2*. It must be emphasized that the specific approaches in these studies have varied, which makes derivation of an overview difficult. In particular, the detail provided on occupation and the way of classifying this differs greatly between the studies. An attempt has been made to bring together results for occupational exposures, set out in alphabetical order; for any given occupation the results are ordered in size of relative risk.

Table 4.1 Main characteristics of 16 case-control studies of the aetiology of bladder cancer

Country	Authors	Data–years	No. pts	Source of controls	Matching factors
Canada: 1	Miller *et al.* (1978)	?	188	Urological patients	Sex, age, country of birth
Canada: 2	Howe *et al.* (1980)	1974–76	480	Population sample	Sex, age, address
Denmark	Mommsen, Asgaard and Sell (1982)	1972–79	165	Population sample	Sex, age, address
England and Wales: 1(*a*)	Anthony and Thomas (1970)	1959–67	340	Surgical patients	Sex, age, address, smoking
England and Wales: 1(*b*)	Anthony and Thomas (1970)	1959–67	312	Other cancer patients	Sex, age, address, smoking
England and Wales: 2	Cartwright (1982)	1978–80	991	Hospital patients	Sex, age, health district
England and Wales: 3	Coggon, Pannett and Acheson (1984)	1975–79	291	Deaths from any other cause	Sex, DoB, year of death, district of residence
Ireland	Tyrell, McCaughey and MacAirt (1971)	1967–68	200	Urological patients	Sex, age
Italy	Vineis *et al.* (1982)	1970s	225	Urological patients	Sex, age, hospital
US: 1	Wynder, Onderdonk and Mantel (1963)	1957–61	300	Hospital pts, excluding smoking-related diseases	Sex, age
US: 2	Dunham *et al.* (1968)	1958–64	265	Hospital patients	
US: 3	Cole, Hoover and Friedell (1972)	1967–68	461	Population sample	Sex, age
US: 4	Wynder and Goldsmith (1977)	1969–74	574	Hospital pts, excluding smoking-related diseases	Sex, age, race, hospital status
US: 5	Najem *et al.* (1978)	1978	75	Hospital patients excluding cancer	Sex, age, race, address, hospital
US: 6	Silverman *et al.* (1983)	1977–78	303	Population sample	Male, age
US: 7	Schoenberg *et al.* (1984)	1981–82	658	Population sample	Sex, age, county; whites only

DoB = date of birth.

A number of other case-control studies on bladder cancer are not included in *Tables 4.1* and *4.2*. Morgan and Jain (1974) studied 232 patients in Canada, but merely report that 'there was no association of disease with occupation'. Miller (1977), in another report from Canada, presented results on risk from occupation; however, these results were republished in a more extensive form by Howe *et al.* (1980). The latter are included in the table, but not the former. Also excluded are some other general case-control studies on bladder cancer, as the reports have not included any results of occupation; Lockwood (1961) — 396 patients in Denmark; Cartwright *et al.* (1981) — 841 patients in West Yorkshire; Kantor *et al.* (1984) — nearly 3000 patients in 10 localities in the US.

Davies, Sommerville and Wallace, (1976) analysed the occupational histories of 1000 patients with bladder tumours who had been referred to the Royal Marsden Hospital. It was thought that the following had been exposed to carcinogens: 44 in rubber manufacture, 21 in cable manufacture, 26 in gasworks, and 12 in miscellaneous activities. Because of the very special referral patterns and absence of control data, these results are impossible to interpret as far as estimating risk is concerned.

Study of bladder cancer patients who had been exposed to dye stuff intermediates showed that an excess had the low phenotype for *N*-acetyltransferase. It was suggested that acetylator status identified susceptible individuals, who might either be more likely to develop tumours when exposed to N-substituted aryl compounds or that this combination leads to invasive lesions (Cartwright *et al.*, 1982).

4.24 Kidney (ICD 189)

Collation studies have shown association with beer (Breslow and Enstrom, 1974), coffee drinking (Armstrong and Doll, 1975), and lead levels in water (Berg and Burbank, 1972).

Children developing Wilms' tumour are more likely to have a range of other congenital abnormalities, whilst adult renal tumours occur in excess in the rare congenital tuberous sclerosis (Mulvihill, 1975).

Table 4.2 Risk of bladder cancer from various occupations, reported in 16 case-control studies

Occupation	Exposure	RR	95% CL	Study
Agriculture	n.s.	1.2	(0.9–1.5)	US: 7
	n.s.	1.1	(0.8–1.5)	Canada: 2
	Crop spraying	7.0	(0.9–315.5)	Canada: 2
	Farming	1.1	(0.5–2.2)	E & W: 1(a)
		0.9	(0.4–1.9)	E & W: 1(b)
		0.8	(0.6–1.2)	US: 6
		0.7	(0.5–1.1)	US: 3
	Nurseryman	5.5	(1.2–51.1)	Canada: 2
Alcohol	n.s.	0.8	(0.3–2.7)	US: 1
Arsenic	n.s.	0.4	(0.1–1.2)	US: 2
Asbestos	n.s.	1.1	(0.5–2.5)	E & W: 3
Chemicals	n.s.	7.5	(1.7–67.6)	Canada: 2
	n.s.	2.0	(0.6–6.2)	E & W: 3
	n.s.	1.6	(1.0–2.5)	Denmark
	n.s.	1.6	(0.7–3.6)	US: 1
	n.s.	1.5	(1.0–2.3)	Canada: 1
	n.s.	1.2	(0.2–6.3)	US: 4
	n.s.	1.0	(0.7–1.5)	US: 9
	n.s.	0.1	(0.0–1.0)	US: 6
	Dry cleaner	1.3	(0.5–3.6)	US: 7
	Dye manufacture	3.5	(2.2–5.3)	E & W: 2
		3.0	(0.6–13.7)	Italy
	Dye worker	∞	(n.a.)	E & W: 1(a)
		∞	(n.a.)	E & W: 1(b)
		3.1	(1.2–8.1)	US: 5
		2.9	(1.6–5.3)	US: 1
		2.2	(0.7–7.6)	US: 3
		1.3	(0.8–2.4)	E & W: 2
		1.1	(0.0–169.4)	US: 2
		1.0	(0.3–2.9)	US: 4
		0.9	(0.4–2.2)	Ireland
	(2-naphthylamine)	0.5	(0.1–4.7)	US: 2
		0	(n.a.)	US: 6
	Insecticides	0.9	(0.4–1.7)	US: 2
	Pharmaceuticals	1.2	(0.3–4.5)	US: 5
	Solvents	0.8	(0.4–1.7)	US: 2
Clerks	n.s.	2.3	(0.9–6.6)	Canada: 2
	n.s.	2.1	(0.9–4.8)	E & W: 1(b)
	n.s.	1.5	(1.1–1.9)	E & W: 2
	n.s.	1.0	(0.7–1.6)	US: 6
	n.s.	0.8	(0.4–1.5)	E & W: 1(a)
	Other	1.2	(0.6–2.4)	US: 3
	Postal	1.5	(0.7–3.1)	US: 3
	Shipping	1.4	(0.8–2.4)	US: 3
		0.6	(0.4–1.1)	US: 6
Construction	n.s.	1.2	(0.9–1.7)	US: 3
	n.s.	1.2	(0.8–1.9)	US: 6
	n.s.	0.7	(0.3–1.5)	E & W: 1(a)
	n.s.	0.6	(0.2–1.3)	E & W: 1(b)
Cooking	n.s.	1.5	(0.9–2.7)	US: 3
	n.s.	1.1	(0.3–4.3)	US: 1
	Cook/counter work	2.5	(0.8–4.5)	US: 6
		1.8	(1.2–2.7)	US: 7
Dust	n.s.	1.0	(0.5–2.1)	US: 4
	Boiler worker	0.9	(0.6–1.6)	US: 7
Electrical	n.s.	2.5	(0.5–12.2)	E & W: 1(a)
	n.s.	2.0	(0.5–7.8)	E & W: 1(b)
	n.s.	0.8	(0.4–1.6)	US: 6

Table 4.2 Continued

Occupation	Exposure	RR	95% CL	Study
Fire	n.s.	1.8	(0.7–5.0)	US: 6
	n.s.	1.0	(0.4–2.4)	US: 1
Food processing	n.s.	1.8	(0.6–5.3)	E & W: 1(a)
	n.s.	1.6	(0.6–4.8)	Canada: 2
	n.s.	1.0	(n.a.)	E & W: 1(b)
Formaldehyde	n.s.	1.5	(0.9–2.5)	E & W: 3
Gas production	n.s.	∞	(n.a.)	E & W: 1(b)
	n.s.	2.0	(0.2–21.0)	E & W: 1(a)
	n.s.	0.5	(0.1–5.3)	Italy
Glass production	n.s.	6.0	(0.7–276.0)	Canada: 2
	n.s.	3.0	(0.3–25.8)	E & W: 1(b)
	n.s.	0.6	(0.1–2.5)	E & W: 1(a)
Hairdressing	Barbers	∞	(0.4–∞)	Canada: 2
		2.8	(0.4–17.0)	US: 2
		1.3	(0.6–2.7)	US: 6
		0.6	(0.2–1.8)	US: 3
	Hairdressers	∞	(n.a.)	E & W: 1(b)
		∞	(n.a.)	US: 1
		4.0	(0.5–30.3)	E & W: 1(a)
		1.5	(0.2–8.9)	US: 6
		0.9	(0.3–3.2)	E & W: 2
Leather	n.s.	∞	(n.a.)	US: 1
	n.s.	5.0	(0.7–34.5)	Italy
	n.s.	2.0	(1.4–2.9)	US: 3
	n.s.	1.8	(0.9–3.5)	US: 7
	n.s.	1.2	(0.5–3.1)	E & W: 2
	n.s.	0.0	(n.a.)	E & W: 1(a)
	n.s.	0.0	(n.a.)	E & W: 1(b)
	Shoe maker/repairer	2.7	(0.5–13.5)	US: 1
		1.0	(n.a.)	Italy
		0.7	(0.2–3.3)	US: 6
	Tanning	1.2	(0.3–6.3)	Canada: 2
Metals	n.s.	1.6	(0.8–3.0)	US: 1
	n.s.	1.1	(0.8–1.5)	US: 6
	n.s.	1.1	(0.8–1.5)	US: 4
	n.s.	0.8	(0.5–1.4)	US: 3
	n.s.	0.8	(0.5–1.3)	US: 4
	n.s.	0.7	(0.2–3.4)	Ireland
	Chromates	1.3	(0.5–3.6)	E & W: 3
	Engineers' fitters	4.7	(1.5–14.5)	E & W: 1(a)
		3.2	(1.1–9.4)	E & W: 1(b)
	Fabricators	∞	(0.8–∞)	Canada: 2
	Fitters	3.6	(1.2–10.7)	E & W: 3
	Forge, foundry, furnace	0.8	(0.3–2.1)	E & W: 1(a)
		0.6	(0.2–1.9)	E & W: 1(b)
		0.5	(0.2–1.4)	US: 6
	Machinists	2.7	(1.1–7.6)	Canada: 2
		4.1	(0.5–30.8)	US: 2
	Mechanics	1.6	(0.9–2.8)	Canada: 2
	Plumbers	3.2	(0.5–21.6)	US: 2
	Polisher	1.4	(0.9–2.3)	US: 6
	Structural steel workers	3.2	(0.0–145.3)	US: 2
	Tin/copper smiths	7.6	(0.7–85.7)	US: 2
		1.8	(0.6–5.4)	US: 6
	Welders	2.8	(1.1–8.8)	Canada: 2
		1.8	(0.9–3.6)	E & W: 3
		0.6	(0.3–1.0)	US: 6

Table 4.2 Continued

Occupation	Exposure	RR	95% CL	Study
Mining	Coal	7.1	(0.8–62.4)	US: 1
	Miners, quarrymen	1.3	(0.8–2.3)	E & W: 1(a)
		1.2	(0.7–2.0)	E & W: 1(b)
		1.0	(0.5–2.0)	US: 6
PAH	Coal/tar	4.6	(0.9–23.8)	US: 1
		0.7	(0.2–2.1)	Ireland
	Cutting oils	1.5	(0.8–2.8)	E & W: 3
	Engine fumes	2.8	(0.8–11.8)	Canada: 2
		2.1	(0.7–6.0)	Ireland
		1.7	(0.9–3.3)	E & W: 3
		1.4	(0.8–2.6)	US: 1
		1.0	(0.2–5.3)	US: 2
	Gasoline/oil	2.7	(1.2–6.1)	Denmark
		2.3	(1.5–3.8)	US: 7
		1.2	(0.6–2.4)	US: 6
	Grease/oil	1.4	(0.3–6.2)	US: 4
		1.3	(0.9–1.8)	US: 7
		0.9	(0.4–2.2)	Ireland
		0.8	(0.3–1.9)	US: 1
	Tar	0.9	(0.2–5.0)	US: 2
Paint	n.s.	1.5	(0.6–3.7)	US: 1
	n.s.	1.2	(0.7–1.9)	US: 3
	n.s.	1.0	(0.5–2.2)	US: 6
	n.s.	0.8	(0.2–2.6)	US: 4
	n.s.	0.7	(0.3–2.1)	E & W: 1(b)
	n.s.	0.6	(0.2–1.6)	E & W: 1(a)
	n.s.	0.5	(0.0–14.2)	Ireland
	Commercial painters	1.0	(0.6–2.3)	Canada: 2
	Painter/artist	1.5	(1.0–2.4)	US: 7
	Spray painters	1.8	(0.7–4.6)	Canada: 2
Petroleum	n.s.	5.3	(1.5–28.6)	Canada: 2
	n.s.	2.5	(1.2–5.4)	US: 5
	n.s.	1.0	(0.7–1.3)	US: 3
	Petroleum/asphalt	3.1	(0.9–10.7)	Denmark
	Refinery	1.3	(0.6–2.8)	US: 7
		0.5	(0.1–5.3)	Italy
Photography	n.s.	∞	(n.a.)	E & W: 1(a)
	n.s.	∞	(n.a.)	E & W: 1(b)
Printing	n.s.	3.1	(1.4–6.8)	E & W: 2
	n.s.	3.0	(0.6–14.8)	US: 6
	n.s.	2.7	(0.8–9.6)	US: 5
	n.s.	1.1	(0.6–2.0)	US: 3
	n.s.	0.3	(0.1–1.2)	E & W: 1(a)
	n.s.	0.2	(0.0–1.9)	E & W: 1(b)
	Ink	5.0	(1.0–25.8)	E & W: 3
Professional	n.s.	0.9	(0.3–2.5)	E & W: 1(a)
	n.s.	0.5	(0.2–1.4)	E & W: 1(b)
	Administration	2.0	(0.2–21.0)	E & W: 1(a)
		2.0	(0.2–21.0)	E & W: 1(b)
	Architect	0.7	(0.3–1.8)	US: 6
	Bank staff	0.7	(0.3–1.7)	US: 6
	Chemist	3.0	(0.3–25.8)	Italy
		1.4	(0.8–2.6)	US: 7
	Civil engineers	3.5	(0.4–32.4)	US: 2
	Engineer	1.5	(1.2–1.8)	E & W: 2
	Manager	1.1	(0.8–1.7)	US: 6

Table 4.2 Continued

Occupation	Exposure	RR	95% CL	Study
	Medical field	2.6	(0.9–9.3)	Canada: 2
		0.3	(0.1–1.2)	US: 6
	Medical lab. techn.	5.0	(0.7–34.5)	E & W: 1(a)
		2.0	(0.4–10.6)	E & W: 1(b)
Radiation	n.s.	∞	(n.a.)	US: 1
	n.s.	1.8	(0.7–4.2)	US: 2
	n.s.	1.6	(1.0–2.9)	Canada: 1
Retail trade	n.s.	6.0	(1.2–29.2)	E & W: 3
	n.s.	1.3	(0.8–2.2)	US: 6
	n.s.	1.0	(0.6–1.9)	E & W: 1(a)
	n.s.	0.9	(0.5–1.6)	E & W: 1(b)
Rubber	n.s.	∞	(n.a.)	E & W: 1(a)
	n.s.	∞	(n.a.)	E & W: 1(b)
	n.s.	∞	(n.a.)	US: 6
	n.s.	5.0	(0.6–236.5)	Canada: 2
	n.s.	3.0	(0.0–230.0)	US: 4
	n.s.	2.1	(0.9–4.8)	US: 7
	n.s.	1.9	(0.4–8.4)	US: 5
	n.s.	1.7	(0.8–3.4)	Italy
	n.s.	1.6	(1.0–2.4)	US: 3
	Cable workers	2.5	(0.9–6.8)	US: 5
		0.5	(0.0–9.6)	Canada: 2
	Rubber/cable/plastic	1.0	(n.a.)	Canada: 1
Security	Armed services	1.8	(1.2–2.7)	Canada: 2
		0.6	(0.3–1.3)	US: 6
	Guards	4.0	(1.3–16.4)	Canada: 2
		0.9	(0.4–1.9)	US: 6
	Janitor	1.2	(0.6–2.3)	US: 6
Service, sports etc.	n.s.	1.0	(0.9–1.1)	US: 3
	Recreation	1.4	(0.5–3.8)	US: 6
Stationary engine driver	n.s.	1.0	(n.a.)	E & W: 1(a)
	n.s.	0.9	(0.3–2.4)	E & W: 1(b)
Stone	n.s.	2.5	(0.7–8.3)	Ireland
	n.s.	2.3	(0.5–9.7)	US: 4
	n.s.	1.4	(0.5–4.3)	US: 1
Textiles	n.s.	2.7	(0.5–13.5)	US: 1
	n.s.	1.7	(0.4–6.9)	Italy
	n.s.	1.4	(0.5–4.2)	US: 4
	n.s.	0.9	(0.3–2.7)	US: 5
	n.s.	0.5	(0.1–2.7)	US: 6
	Dyers	∞	(n.a.)	E & W: 1(b)
		2.0	(0.1–118.0)	Canada: 2
		1.0	(n.a.)	E & W: 1(a)
	Fabricated textiles	1.7	(1.0–2.9)	US: 7
	Finishers	1.5	(0.2–8.9)	E & W: 1(a)
		1.5	(0.2–8.9)	E & W: 1(b)
	Mill workers	0.6	(0.3–1.2)	US: 7
	Tailors	∞	(n.a.)	E & W: 1(a)
		∞	(n.a.)	E & W: 1(b)
		1.5	(0.2–18.0)	Canada: 2
		1.1	(0.4–3.1)	US: 3
	Tailors cutters	0.5	(0.1–1.9)	E & W: 1(a)
		0.5	(0.1–2.6)	E & W: 1(b)
	Tailors pressers	6.0	(0.9–38.5)	E & W: 1(b)
		3.5	(0.8–15.3)	E & W: 1(a)

Table 4.2

Occupation	Exposure	RR	95% CL	Study
	Weavers	∞	(n.a.)	E & W: 1(*a*)
		5.0	(0.7–34.5)	E & W: 1(*b*)
Transport	n.s.	0.8	(0.5–1.3)	E & W: 1(*b*)
	n.s.	0.7	(0.4–1.1)	E & W: 1(*a*)
	Bus driver	1.5	(0.4–5.3)	US: 6
	Driver/delivery man	1.2	(0.9–1.5)	US: 7
	Railroad	9.0	(1.2–394.5)	Canada
	Sailors	8.2	(1.2–54.1)	US: 2
	Sailors and fishermen	0.8	(0.5–1.3)	US: 3
		0.4	(0.1–0.9)	US: 6
	Taxi driver	2.0	(0.7–5.4)	US: 6
	Truck driver	2.5	(1.4–4.4)	US: 6
UV light	n.s.	1.2	(0.5–2.9)	US: 1
Warehousemen	n.s.	1.0	(n.a.)	E & W: 1(*b*)
	n.s.	0.9	(0.4–2.2)	E & W: 1(*a*)
Woodwork	n.s.	3.4	(1.0–11.5)	Ireland
	n.s.	2.3	(0.6–8.6)	US: 2
	n.s.	1.1	(0.6–2.0)	US: 3
	n.s.	0.9	(0.3–2.4)	E & W: 1(*b*)
	n.s.	0.7	(0.3–1.8)	E & W: 1(*a*)
	n.s.	0.5	(0.2–1.2)	US: 1
	Carpenter	1.5	(0.7–3.2)	US: 6

n.s. = not specified.
n.a. = cannot be calculated.

Three quite different genito-urinary conditions are associated with increased frequency of renal tumours: Balkan nephropathy (Petrovic, Tomic and Mutavozic, 1966), phenacetin abuse (Johansson *et al.*, 1974), and renal stone (MacLean and Fowler, 1965). These are relatively rare or restricted conditions and together they can only account for a small proportion of all renal tumours. It is not clear whether the cause of each of the three conditions directly affects the risk of renal tumours, or indirectly via the long-standing changes that occur in the kidney.

Smoking has been suggested as relevant, but the large British prospective study showed no indication of this (Doll and Peto, 1976).

4.25 Central nervous system (ICD 190–191)

Collation studies show an association with fat intake, for which no adequate explanation exists (Armstrong and Doll, 1975).

Case reports have indicated the occasional family clusters of brain tumours; better data exist for a number of rare syndromes, such as tuberous sclerosis in which there is an increased risk of central nervous system tumours (Mulvihill, 1975). A study of children with brain tumours showed that their siblings and mothers were more likely to have suffered from seizures, epilepsy or stroke (Gold *et*

al., 1979). It is accepted that exposure to ionizing radiation can increase the risk of brain tumours (Jablon *et al.*, 1971; Preston-Martin *et al.*, 1980).

Trauma has been reported prior to development of brain tumours, but there is great difficulty in assessing the validity of such a history. A case-control study suggested a history was associated with double the risk of brain tumours (Preston-Martin *et al.*, 1980).

Follow-up of 3 groups of professional chemists in Sweden, the UK and US showed an increased mortality from brain tumours: O/E = 2.40, 95% CL = 1.8–3.1 (3.10 and *Table 3.1*). Follow-up of 11 groups of workers from petroleum refineries showed an increase of CNS neoplasms of borderline significance: O/E = 1.16, 95% CL = 1.0–1.3 (3.23 and *Table 3.5*). In neither of these occupational groups was there any indication of the aetiological factors involved. Some studies have suggested an increase of brain tumours in vinyl chloride workers (2.58); pooled data from 6 prospective studies in 4 countries showed a non-significant increase: O/E = 1.37, 95% CL = 0.9–2.0 (*see Table 2.22*).

4.26 Thyroid (ICD 192)

It is accepted that there is a rare familial medullary thyroid cancer (Hillyard, Evans and Hill, 1978). Also thyroid cancer can occur as one of the manifestations of the rare familial syndrome of multiple endocrine adenoma (Schimke, 1976).

There is evidence that some patients have an enhanced likelihood of tumours of the breast and thyroid (Schottenfeld, Berg and Vitsky, 1971), though the mechanism of this remains obscure. Somewhat more controversial is whether individuals who have suffered goitre are at increased risk of cancer of the thyroid. Some population statistics suggest an association (Wegelin, 1928), though this has been disputed (Saxen and Saxen, 1954). Histology reports of the prevalence of thyroid abnormalities in patients with cancer are compatible with a common aetiology (Wahner *et al.*, 1966), rather than a direct sequence of benign lesions later becoming malignant.

A well-defined aetiological agent is ionizing radiation; this has been shown in several countries for children given treatment for 'enlarged thymus' in infancy, scalp ringworm, or other disease of the head and neck (Duffy and Fitzgerald 1950; Hempelmann *et al.*, 1975; Modan, Ron and Werner, 1977). Therapeutic irradiation of adults has also been followed by cancer of the thyroid, but has not been numerically such a problem (Goolden, 1958). There is no evidence from large-scale prospective studies that ^{131}I has been associated with increased risk of cancer when used for diagnostic or therapeutic purposes (Pochin, 1960; Dobyns *et al.*, 1974).

4.27 Reticulo-endothelial system (ICD 200–208)

A number of occupational studies have grouped all malignant neoplasms of the RES together when presenting these results.

Workers exposed to acrylonitrile show a borderline increased risk: O/E = 2.29, 95% CL = 1.0–4.5 (2.1 and *Table 2.1*).

Follow-up of 4 groups of professional chemists in Sweden, UK, and US showed an increased mortality from RES neoplasms: O/E = 1.79, 95% CL = 1.6–2.0 (3.10 and *Table 3.1*). Follow-up of 11 groups of workers from petroleum refineries showed an excess of deaths from RES neoplasms of borderline significance: O/E = 1.10, 95% CL = 1.0–1.2 (3.23 and *Table 3.5*). The studies on farming (3.14) showed increased risk of RES neoplasms in 7 out of 10 that were reviewed. In none of these 3 occupational groups was there any clear indication of the aetiological factors involved.

Although it has been suggested that vinyl chloride exposure increases the risk of RES neoplasms, the pooled data from 6 studies in 3 countries only showed an increase of borderline significance: O/E = 1.11, 95% CL = 0.9–1.4 (2.15 and *Table 2.22*).

4.28 Hodgkin's disease (ICD 201)

There are studies indicating an excess of patients in families; this is more commonly around the same period rather than when members achieve the same age, suggesting an environmental factor (Razis, Diamond and Craver, 1959).

Circumstantial evidence suggested an infective origin to the disease; formal mathematical tests for clustering have been negative (Fraumeni and Li, 1969; Alderson and Nayak, 1971). An episode in New York suggested that the family and friends of an original group of patients had a raised incidence of the disease (Vianna, Greenwald and Davies, 1971); interpretation of such observational data is extremely difficult. A more rigorous examination of school pupils suggested an association between affected pupils or schools with cases and subsequent development of Hodgkin's disease (Vianna and Polan, 1973). An examination of the network of contacts in patients and controls in Oxford failed to identify any difference (Smith *et al.*, 1977). Very different to these studies is the follow-up of large numbers of patients with infectious mononucleosis; a small but significant excess of Hodgkin's disease has been observed (Rosdahl, Larsen and Clemmesen, 1974; Kvale, Hoiby and Pederson, 1979). A number of studies have suggested that children or young adults with Hodgkin's are more likely to have had tonsillectomy than their siblings (Vianna, Greenwald and Davies, 1971; Gutensohn *et al.*, 1975).

A case-control study suggested excess consumption of amphetamines (Newell *et al.*, 1973), but this was not confirmed in other work (Boston Collaborative Drug Surveillance Program, 1974b). Follow-up of college students indicated that those who were obese or drank and smoked more than others were at increased risk of developing Hodgkin's (Paffenbarger, Wing and Hyde, 1977); it is possible that this reflects confounding with affluence.

Nine studies of woodworkers reviewed in 3.38 included results on risk of Hodgkin's disease. These involved different methods and 3 countries. Eight of the studies showed an increased risk; the 95% CL was available for 6 of these and the risk was significantly raised in 4. The consistency of these results suggests they are unlikely to be due to chance, though there is no indication of the specific factor involved.

4.29 Lymphoma (ICD 200,202)

Limited evidence indicates a possible familial association (Freedlander, Kissen and McVie, 1978). The disease also occurs in excess in patients with coeliac disease — in itself a familial condition (Gough, Read and Nash, 1962; Whorwell *et al.*, 1976).

Follow-up of patients treated with immunosuppressive drugs shows a significant excess of lymphoma (Kinlen *et al.*, 1979; 1980), some occurring a relatively short while after initial treatment associated with renal transplant. Increase in lymphoma has been reported in patients with rheumatoid arthritis (Isomaki, Hakulinen and Joutsenlahti, 1979); this observation has not been confirmed, nor has it been indicated whether this is thought to be a reflection of the cause of the arthritis, the presence of the arthritis, or the treatment given.

Very different is the lymphoma in children described by Burkitt (1958–59). This occurs in restricted localities in Africa, shows space–time clustering (Williams *et al.*, 1978) and marked seasonal variation (Williams, Day and Geser, 1974). A prospective study of a large number of children in Uganda, who had sera collected on entry to the study, showed higher titres of viral capsid antigen than matched controls (de Thé *et al.*, 1978). The disease only occurs in areas where malaria is endemic (apart from very rare cases of rather different nature in developed countries). It has been suggested that neonatal infection with Epstein–Barr virus may initiate the malignancy, which is then promoted by major immunological stress such as from malaria (de Thé, 1977).

4.30 Leukaemia (ICD 204–207)

If one child develops leukaemia, the likelihood of a second child so doing in the sibship is twice that of the population risk (Draper, Heaf and Kinnier Wilson, 1977). Patients with Down's syndrome have a chromosomal abnormality and are at greatly increased risk of leukaemia (Stewart, Webb and Hewitt, 1958). No adequate sized twin study is available to permit familial and genetic factors to be distinguished (Cederlof, Friberg and Lundman, 1977).

Ionizing radiation from various sources has been shown to be leukaemogenic. Diagnostic investigation in early pregnancy (Stewart, Webb and Hewitt, 1958; MacMahon, 1962), therapeutic irradiation for malignant (Li, Cassady and Jaffe, 1975) or benign disease (Brinkley and Haybittle, 1969; Smith and Doll, 1976) are all confirmed hazards. Diagnostic X-ray other than of the fetus (Gibson *et al.*, 1972) or use of ^{131}I (Pochin, 1967) has not been shown to constitute a hazard in controlled use. There is no evidence that background irradiation ever reaches an adequate level for a measurable leukaemogenic risk (Court Brown *et al.*, 1960).

Leukaemia is associated with certain immunological deficiencies (Kersey, Spector and Good, 1973) and other rare syndromes (Mulvihill, 1975). Excess mortality has been recorded in subjects with rheumatoid arthritis (Lea, 1964) and pernicious anaemia (Blackburn *et al.*, 1968), but this is as yet unexplained.

Medical treatment with immunosuppressive drugs (Sieber and Adamson, 1976; Stutman, 1976), cytotoxic drugs for chronic disease (Sieber and Adamson, 1976), or chemotherapy for other malignant disease (Canellos *et al.*, 1975) have been shown to increase the risk of leukaemia. A similar hazard has been suggested from butazolidine and chloramphenicol (Fraumeni, 1967), but this is not confirmed.

The most confusing area has been the search for an infective agent. There is some indication that virus infections in pregnancy increase the risk of the child developing leukaemia (Stewart, Webb and Hewitt, 1958; Fedrick and Alberman, 1972; Hakulinen *et al.*, 1973); other studies have produced negative results (Leck and Steward, 1972; McCrea Curnen *et al.*, 1974). Patients have reported excess contact with hospitals (Timonen and Ilvonen, 1978), farm animals (Fasal, Jackson and Klauber, 1968; Milham, 1971), and sick pets (Bross, Berteu and Gibson, 1972) compared with controls; there is little consistency in these studies (Schneider and Riggs, 1973; Linos *et al.*, 1980). Many studies of mathematical clustering in space and time of incident cases in populations have failed to confirm the original suggestive findings from the north-east of England (Knox, 1964; Gunz and Spears, 1968; Glass and Mantel, 1969). This may be due partly to the inappropriateness of the mathematical approach; alternative examination of networks of case and control contacts has also been substantially negative (Schimpff *et al.*, 1976; Zack *et al.*, 1977). Laboratory studies have produced results that as yet fail to demonstrate an infective aetiology (Karpas, Wreghitt and Nagington, 1978).

There has been circumstantial evidence that exposure to benzene led to increased risk of leukaemia for over 50 years. It is accepted that levels of more than 100 ppm were associated with risk of acute myelogenous leukaemia; more recent reports have suggested the hazard may extend down to lower levels and involve other cytological types (2.8 and *Table 2.4*).

Irradiation is an accepted cause of leukaemia and 2.39.1 reviewed data on increased risk in health professionals exposed to ionizing radiation.

Three other occupational groups appear to have consistent reports of increased risk of leukaemia, based on studies using a variety of methods: electrical workers (3.12); printing workers (2.50.12 and *Table 2.20*); the rubber industry (3.30 and *Table 3.6*). There is no indication of the agent that might be involved in these reports.

Recommended reading

ALDERSON, M.R. (1982) In *Prevention of Cancer*. Ed. M.R. Alderson. pp. 20–71. London: Arnold

BOURKE, G.J. (1983) *The Epidemiology of Cancer*. London: Croom Helm

DOLL, R. and PETO, R. (1981) *The Causes of Cancer*. Oxford: Oxford University Press

SCHOTTENFELD, D. and FRAUMENI, J.F. (1982) *Cancer Epidemiology and Prevention*. Philadelphia: Saunders

5

Towards control of occupational cancer

This chapter discusses the role of research on occupational cancer control, the three main approaches to cancer prevention, the place of legislation, the contribution from various national and international bodies, and practical steps that have been taken to control specific occupational hazards.

5.1 The role of research

This section covers aspects of the organization of research, the funding of research, the information required on a suspect hazard, and risk assessment.

5.1.1 The organization of research

Alderson (1978) emphasized the need to have central coordination of an agreed research strategy. It was necessary to include the following:

(a) Quantification of the extent of the problem.
(b) Identification of topics suitable to study.
(c) Selection of good research projects and proposals.
(d) Provision of research facilities.
(e) Monitoring of control of cancer.

The application of these activities will not be linear, but is an iterative process; a constant check is needed to see, for example, if facilities provided are used, and that results are reviewed to determine their effect upon cancer control. Thus an active strategy is required; a passive organization which merely vets projects in isolation when they are submitted is of limited value. A prime concern must be the periodic assessment of the topic of occupational cancer, viewed as a subset of (a) cancer in

general, and (b) the broad issues of health and welfare of all employed persons.

5.1.2 Funding of research

The research strategy will be influenced by a variety of people and bodies whose interests range from general concern for health and welfare to a specific concern with the identification, removal, or alleviation of a particular hazard. Funding in England and Wales may be through the following:

Government funds: Health and Safety Executive, Department of Health and Social Security; Medical Research Council; Department of Environment; University Grants Committee (via university support).
Voluntary sources: Cancer Research Campaign; Imperial Cancer Research Fund; other funds.
Industry: Through internal or external projects.

Some of this research is coordinated by the Cancer Coordinating Committee, but the role of this Committee is very wide and specific attention to occupational cancer is unlikely to loom large in its deliberations. A recent report from the House of Lords (Gregson, 1984) emphasized that the research effort in this field was ill-coordinated in Britain. Reference was made to the approach in the US and it was suggested that there should be planning of priorities of research in occupational disease.

In considering the funding of research, it is essential that the study must be acceptable to the financial sponsors, but at the same time scientifically sound. The funding body must not impose constraints which would result in a study whose design would not provide valid results.

Another issue is that of agreement on publication of the final results, which must be clarified in the commissioning phase. Management and union representatives must be shown a draft report, but the final decision on wording of the research report would be in the hands of the scientists heading the research team and they alone would have the final responsibility for publication. If there is any suggestion of a specific hazard and how this might be overcome, the management and the unions are the people who will have to translate the research findings into action. Unilateral publication by the scientist, in an atmosphere of friction, is unlikely to result in dispassionate consideration of the research findings, let alone translation into practical steps of prevention.

5.1.3 Local facilities required

The organization for coordinating research should have the responsibility for ensuring that the staff and research facilities are mobilized for the particular piece of work. However, there then remains the crucial issue of the opportunities that are required at local level in order to carry out a satisfactory study. This will partly depend on the nature of the specific study design. Some may only require access to stored records, such as historical prospective studies (*see* 1.1.7); even for these, there will usually be the important task of ensuring that the method of recording potential exposure in the works records is clearly understood by the research team. In many studies still being carried out there are no documented results from environmental measurements, and few studies are prospective in nature with the planned collection of requisite measurements.

Once the study has been accepted as warranting exploration, it must be given full support from the company's management and the representatives of the staff and unions. The specific points requiring clearance will depend upon the design of the study: 2 main epidemiological approaches entail either access to retrievable records or the investigation of individuals. The former will require (*a*) access to personal records, (*b*) the availability of environmental data, and the facility to follow-up those workers who have left the industry. The access to personal records is one of the issues which requires the approval of both management and union. Approval is required also for permission to release information to trace individuals who have left the industry; the tracing of leavers raises the issues of confidentiality and personal records. The Medical Research Council (1973) has clearly identified guidelines for carrying out research that comes into this field.

There must be continuing dialogue throughout the study from the preparation of the initial research proposal, through commissioning the study and the field work, until data analysis and interpretation are complete. This often requires considerable goodwill, patience, and ability to understand the pressures and concerns of the very different groups involved.

The US Department of Health and Human Services (1983) produced a comprehensive plan for promoting health and preventing disease. This included implementation of plans for (*a*) toxic agents and radiation control, and (*b*) occupational safety and health. Each of these plans had a short statement of the problem, a list of priority objectives and, for each objective, various implementation steps showing the responsible DHHS agencies and the year of initiation of the plan. One given high priority was the need for a broad-scale surveillance and monitoring system to discern known environmental hazards.

Davies (1982) has drawn attention to the pace of detection of carcinogenic hazards in the workplace and the change in attitude that has occurred to occupational cancers over the past 50 years.

5.1.4 Information required on suspect hazards

Before clearcut plans can be laid to prevent a given hazard, research should have identified a causal agent and quantified the relative influence of the agent itself and other intervening and confounding factors. It is important to quantify:

(*a*) The dose–response relationship.
(*b*) Individual variation in susceptibility.
(*c*) The pathways of exposure from the process to the individual.
(*d*) Facets of worker behaviour that can influence risk.
(*e*) The mechanisms of carcinogenesis.

The more information that is available on these points, the more likely it is that a sound programme for preventive action can be introduced.

The *Lancet* (1984b) discussed the interaction that could occur between the smoking of an individual and occupational exposures to hazardous substances such as asbestos. It is suggested that there was no shortage of research into the question of which workers were particularly at risk from occupational exposures (asbestos and smoking, atopic status and response to allergens, pregnancy and exposure to teratogens etc). Strategies for reducing ill-health should therefore consider exclusion (or specific protection) of workers susceptible to particular exposures. Elmes (1981) assessed the importance of cigarette smoking in occupational lung disease. He suggested that in British coal mining, and the iron and steel industry, dust exposure contributes little to risk of disease compared with the workers' smoking habits, whilst in the slate industry smoking and dust were perhaps of equal importance.

5.1.5 Risk assessment

There is a growing body of literature on risk assessment. The issues that require consideration extend way beyond the scientific determination of the potential hazard from a carcinogenic hazard to which workers may be exposed. There is need to consider:

(a) The numbers exposed.
(b) The degree of individual risk.
(c) The dose–response relationship.
(d) Viability of an alternative substance.
(e) Possibility of achieving safe levels with the substance.
(f) The financial liability of the hazard.
(g) Public opinion.
(h) Pressure groups.
(i) Social responsibility.

A US Government Agencies' report (Rodricks *et al.*, 1979) has discussed the scientific bases for identifying potential carcinogens and estimating risks. This emphasized the philosophy of using approaches that, if they erred, aimed to overemphasize the potential hazard to man. However, the hazard from falsely exaggerating risks was not discussed. The great difficulty in risk assessment has been emphasized by Paddle (1980), who drew attention to a number of examples where extrapolation from animals to man could be cross-checked by actual human data. On one particular hazard, the Panel on Nitrates (1978) produced estimates of risk that differed by two orders of magnitude.

Attention has already been drawn to the difficulty in assessing environmental levels of many potential carcinogens. For any given environmental level, there may be many other factors that contribute to variation in actual exposure (or ingestion, respiration, or absorption) of the compound. Recent work on carcinogen metabolism by human tissue specimens (IARC, 1978c) shows a 60-fold variation between individuals. This confirms that individual responses to the same level of an environmental carcinogen may differ widely.

The gross divergence between laboratory studies and human data for nitrosamines and arsenic indicates that extrapolation from animals to man, or even the assessment of human data can be difficult, if not impossible. Pochin (1975) has emphasized that the risk of a particular circumstance may add a trivial increment to the risk of death from natural causes, but such a risk operating upon a large group of individuals might lead to an appreciable number of deaths. This is a powerful argument for quantifying the absolute levels of risk. He presented data for

fatality rates in various occupations from accidents and occupational diseases; non-fatal accident and disease rates in various occupations and a range of non-occupational risks (from accidents, sports, medication, alcohol, drugs, smoking, pregnancy, and acts of God). Attention is drawn to the paucity of the data, although further statistics have been published by Pochin (1978).

The acceptance of risk seems to be determined by personal preference rather than evaluation of risk. Pochin (1978) pointed out that it was important to consider the anxiety of the worker and his family as well as hard data on morbidity or mortality when assessing estimates of 'harm'. Starr (1969) has described an approach to comparing benefit to society with risks from technological change. He suggested that the public would accept self-imposed risks (from sport, hobbies, or ways of life) that generated risks 1000 times greater than risks introduced by government or industry. He also pointed out that social acceptance of a risk appeared to be directly influenced by public awareness of potential for benefit.

The role of the epidemiologist should be that of an impartial scientist endeavouring to assess, in quantified terms, the risk of cancer from any particular chemical or physical agent. He should contribute to reviews of the overall perspective of health and welfare and place the additional hazard (should one be demonstrated) in the context of this perspective. Whatever subsequent preventive action is taken, it is essential that some evaluation be instituted to quantify the benefits and costs to individuals. These issues have been discussed by Alderson (1980b).

Jones and Grendon (1975) suggested that a cancer might develop after an interval that varied as the cube-root of the dose. If this was so, low dose exposure might be without risk, if the calculated latent interval was greater than the expectation of life.

Lerch (1980) emphasized that perception of risk often had greater impact on actions than objective analysis of probabilities. A similar point was made by Lee (1980), who suggested that a hazard could not be evaluated except in terms of human values and emotions.

The report of the study group of the Royal Society (1983) considered that risk assessment involved:

(a) Risk estimation — the identification of the outcomes; estimation of the magnitude of the associated consequences of these outcomes; estimation of the probabilities of these outcomes.
(b) Risk evaluation — the complex process of determining the significance or value of the identified hazards and estimated risks to those concerned or affected by the decision.

The Faculty of Occupational Medicine (1983) advocated that a Hazard Evaluation and Risk Assessment Unit should be established in the Health and Safety Commission, which should be independent and advise the Commission of the scientific conclusions of the risk and acceptable risk of work. The Commission would then discuss the issues in the forum of representatives of management, trade unions, and local authorities; decisions would then be taken, after considering the wider political and societal aspects of the issue.

5.2 Prevention

Control of many diseases may be achieved by:

(*a*) Primary prevention, which aims to remove the causative agent.

(*b*) Secondary prevention, which has the general aim of improving the results from therapy, partly by early detection.

(*c*) Tertiary prevention, which covers the alleviation of the problems associated with the disease.

These general aspects need to be considered in more detail, with the specific topic of occupational cancer in mind.

5.2.1 Primary prevention

Primary prevention aims at removing the agent or reducing exposure. Removal of the agent may involve closure of specific plants or the replacement of the hazardous substance by an innocuous or less dangerous one. If either of these two approaches is not feasible, then ways of reducing the workers' exposure to the agent should be considered. This might mean modification of the plant, modification of the environment, or direct protection of the worker.

Each of these aspects requires different decisions to be taken by different categories of people. Closure of the plant may have to be decided by top management, weighing the financial implications of closing the plant against the hazard of continuing production. Replacement of the hazardous agent may be carried out without involving the individual workers, if a safe substitute can be found. In general, where the plant is closed or the agent replaced, the chance of successful prevention is much higher than where steps have been taken merely to reduce exposure. Unless reduction of exposure can be carried out entirely by modification of the plant, it will usually mean that the individual worker has to change his way of working. Modification of the environment and protection of the worker may result in various disadvantages to the individual; he may have to wear a mask or thick heavy clothing, he may require positive pressure ventilation, or he may have to alter his pace of working and thus his productivity. Many of these issues have ramifications that go far beyond the impact on the individual of the risk of his developing cancer.

The DHSS (1977) stressed that the effectiveness of a preventive strategy depended to a large extent on peoples attitudes and behaviour.

5.2.2 Secondary prevention

This term is used to approaches that do not require any information about the cause of a specific cancer nor removal of the carcinogenic agent, but aim to identify disease at a stage at which treatment can be applied and will be successful. The evidence as to whether early diagnosis can reduce morbidity and mortality has been questioned; some people maintain that early diagnosis merely lengthens the time over which a person knows he suffers from the disease, but does nothing to alter the natural history of the condition, or the ultimate fatality. This is discussed in some detail by Chamberlain (1982).

Secondary prevention must always be considered whenever a long-standing hazard has been identified. Even if the suspect plant is immediately closed, there will be a number of workers who have been exposed to the agent in the past. Alterations to the plant may come too late for most of these workers and, with a lengthy latent interval, many of the exposed individuals may have retired for a number of years.

There are 2 aspects of secondary prevention: the first is to screen the workers to identify disease that they may not have recognized themselves. This screening can be carried out by physical examination, by investigation that requires minimal collaboration with the individuals (e.g. urine cytology or chest X-ray), or by investigations that place the individual at discomfort (e.g. periodic cystoscopy). The higher the relative risk of the disease the more effort should be made to ensure that the workers attend for screening at sufficiently frequent intervals. Of course, it is no use suggesting screening unless there is (*a*) an appropriate test with adequate sensitivity and specificity that is acceptable and cost-effective, and (*b*) treatment which can alter the natural history of the disease.

The second course of action is to introduce an educational programme to reduce the delay in diagnosis in patients developing symptoms of disease. This will require a planned campaign which draws attention of individuals to the risk of disease and to the early warning signs. It must be accompanied by provision of appropriate facilities for diagnosis and treatment, otherwise there is no point in encouraging workers to come forward with symptoms. As with other aspects of cancer control, secondary prevention requires collaboration between management, individuals, and the health care system.

5.2.3 Tertiary prevention

Although this is beyond the scope of the present work, this third phase of prevention is mentioned for completeness. It has been discussed briefly by Alderson (1982) and more fully by Saunders (1978).

A recent development of prevention has been the line of work that tests chemoprevention of cancer. The US NCI has now instituted a comprehensive programme, which emphasizes the potential of vitamin supplements. In addition to testing this for primary prevention, studies are being carried out on: (*a*) 2500 men with asbestosis, to determine the influence on risk of subsequent cancer; (*b*) groups with basal cell cancer of the skin, to see if there is reduction in subsequent development of further skin primaries (Greenwald, 1984).

5.2.4 Threshold limit values

Waldron (1979) described how the physical monitoring of work hazards is based on keeping environmental levels below some predetermined level, which in the UK are the threshold limit values (TLV). These have been adapted from a list originally prepared by the American Conference of Governmental Industrial Hygienists (the ACGIH standards). The TLV is a time-weighted average concentration which may safely be inhaled over an 8-hour working day. An excursion factor is given which limits 'above swing' permissible and is related to the actual TLV (the higher the TLV, the smaller the excursion factor).

There are 2 approaches to setting such levels:

(*a*) Start with a high level and work down to a 'no effect' level.
(*b*) Start with a very low level and work up to some effect.

The former is the US approach, whilst the latter has been the approach in Russia. A WHO/ILO committee found only 24 substances with adequate agreement within a factor of 2 (Waldron, 1979).

The ACGIII had begun to produce an annual revision of their standards when the British Occupational Hygiene Society formed a Hygiene Standards Committee in 1965 to advise on standards. In general, this Committee recommended the use of the ACGIH list of standards and supplements, with particular comments where the standards were thought to be unsatisfactory for British workers (Roach, 1970). The main committee formed various subcommittees with responsibility for particular hazards and associated standards.

Davies (1982) pointed out the difficulty that could occur if one country officially declares a substance a potential occupational carcinogen; there then may be some groups in other countries which find it hard to believe that it can be safely used even with appropriate precautions.

Robinson *et al.* (1976) pointed out the need to clarify the units involved in any threshold value, rather than use undefined ppm. They suggest that for air pollution, the values should be $\mu g/l$ (or mg/m^3); for concentrations of one chemical in another this should be quoted as $\mu g/g$ or mg/kg.

5.2.5 Implementation of prevention

The implementation of prevention of occupational cancer requires the participation of a wide number of different agencies and the development of good practice, preferably in advance of changes in legislation. Subsequent sections cover the role of (*a*) the legislation, and (*b*) various national and international organizations.

Davies (1982) has indicated the powerful influence of the attitudes of various groups in the situation; a particular point that warrants careful consideration is the genuine independence of the opinions of the research workers, who must be unaligned with any of the groups involved.

5.3 Legislation

This section begins with consideration of UK legislation, and then turns to consideration of the EEC, US, and other national legislation.

5.3.1 UK legislation

There are 3 different aspects to legislation or the application of the law in the prevention of cancer:

(*a*) Primary legislation.
(*b*) Regulations introduced under various statutes.
(*c*) Recourse to common law.

The main acts are set out in *Table 5.1*, which cover the span from the first that had a particular bearing upon cancer prevention to more general ones of recent origin. The Factories Act (1961) obliged the doctors treating lead, phosphorus, arsenical, or mercurial poisoning, or anthrax contracted in a factory to report this to the Chief Inspector of Factories. Provision was made for regulations to extend the list of diseases. Formal inspection could be initiated into causes and

Table 5.1 Acts and regulations particularly relevant to occupational cancers in England and Wales

1931	Asbestos Regulations
1936	Factory and Workshop (Notification of Disease) Order
1938	Factories (Notification of Disease) Regulations
1946	National Insurance (Industrial Injuries) Act
1946	Patent Fuel Manufacture (Health and Welfare) Special Regulations
1948	The Radioactive Substances Act
1953	Mule Spinning (Health) Special Regulations
1965	Nuclear Installations Act
1965	Nuclear Installations (Dangerous Occurrences) Regulations
1967	Carcinogenic Substances Regulations
1969	Asbestos Regulations
1969	Ionising Radiations (Sealed Sources) Regulations
1973	Notice of Industrial Diseases Order
1974	The Health and Safety at Work Act
1974	The Radioactive Substances (Modification) Regulations
1977	The Safety Representatives and Safety Committees Regulations
1978	The Packaging and Labelling of Dangerous Substances Regulations
1981	1983 Amendments to above Act
1982	Notification of New Substances Regulations
1982	Notification of Toxic Substances Regulations
1982	The Notification of Installations Handling Hazardous Substances Regulations

circumstances of each case reported. There was also a general duty placed upon the appointed factory doctor to report death or injury caused by exposure to fumes or other noxious substance. In addition to formal notification, informal arrangements have developed to establish registers of angiosarcoma of the liver and mesothelioma of the liver.

An EEC recommendation (Annex 1 to EC Regulation 23/7/62 — revision) provided a list of occupational diseases, which member states were urged 'to insert into their legislation...'. A further recommendation (20/7/66) proposed that restrictive conditions should generally be removed from the terms in which diseases were prescribed.

The Robens report (1972) stressed that real progress towards safety and health at work is impossible without full cooperation and commitment of all employees. They discussed the role of safety representatives, joint safety committees, and periodic meetings for all employees to discuss safety. It was recommended that there should be a general statutory obligation on employers to consult with their workforce on measures for promoting safety and health. Regulations introduced under the Health and Safety Act (1974) set out the function of the Safety Representatives and Safety Committees in 1979.

A particular note should be made of the Carcinogenic Substances Regulations (1967), which

included the requirement to keep a register of those individuals exposed to certain controlled substances, and the requirement to offer 6-monthly cytology to those exposed to carcinogenic aromatic amines. These regulations were emphasizing the base for research, some aspects of primary prevention, and also secondary prevention.

In an attempt to identify hazards before the workers are exposed, there has been the recent Notification of New Substances Regulations (1982), which has been accompanied by the provision of Approved Codes of Practice, issued by HSE (*see* 5.4.2).

The latest regulations just published have introduced a warning labels scheme, with the aim of reducing the number of accidents that occur, and also improving the protection of workers dealing with hazardous substances. These are due to come into force on 1/1/86.

It is possible to bring legal action for negligence against the manufacturer of, or employer using, a carcinogen. Examples of such action have been (*a*) a case against ICI and Dunlop Ltd for the use of a rubber antioxidant containing 2-naphthylamine until 1949; (*b*) an engineering firm was found negligent for failing to institute 6-monthly medicals before a worker exposed to mineral oils died of scrotal cancer. In discussing these, Davies (1982) emphasized how court cases may attract publicity and draw attention to the problem of industrial cancer.

5.3.2 EEC

The Commission of the European Community set up an Advisory Committee on Safety, Hygiene, and Health Protection at Work. The aim has been to produce 'Directives', which are statutory instruments, binding upon the member states, which (*a*) set down the principles that have to be observed, but (*b*) leave the implementation to the discretion of the national bodies.

Examples have been the 1979 Directive requiring member states to establish notification schemes for new substances, whilst more recently there have been directives on labelling, packaging, and safety symbols on chemical containers.

Hunter (1978, 1982) described the EEC programme, whilst the Confederation of British Industry (1980) has produced an employers' guide to safety and health regulations from the EEC.

5.3.3 US legislation

The move towards cancer control began with the formation of the American Society for the Control of Cancer in 1913 (this later became the American Cancer Society). In 1937 the National Cancer Institute Act was passed, giving this body the responsibility for the application of research to the development of widespread use of the most effective methods for the prevention, diagnosis, and treatment of cancer (Breslow and Breslow, 1982).

The main advance in the field of occupational health was the 1970 Occupational Safety Act, which led to the formation of the Occupational Safety and Health Administration (OSHA), which had the power to prescribe mandatory occupational safety and health standards. These can apply if OSHA determines that a material or process in use imperils health. This is typically to set a maximum level of employee exposure to a chemical, and prescribe changes in work procedure or equipment to achieve this. The standard may also require the provision and use of equipment. The 1970 Act also led to the formation of the National Institute of Occupational Safety and Health (NIOSH), which had the responsibility for conducting research designed to produce recommendations for safety standards. On the basis of such and other research, OSHA sets, promulgates, and enforces the standards.

Bates and Merrill (1982) emphasized an important point in that the Food, Drug and Cosmetic Act requires the demonstration of safety before a chemical may be used, but the OSHA standards can only operate successfully after a substance has been in use and then been shown to be hazardous. They can only then prescribe that levels are reduced.

In 1977, OSHA published 'Draft rules for the identification, classification, and regulation of toxic substances posing an occupational carcinogenic risk' (*see* Bates and Merrill, 1982). By this time the NIOSH had identified about 1500–2000 suspect carcinogens, but in the period since 1971, only 17 had been covered by OSHA regulatory action. It was pointed out that it would thus take 100 years to regulate all known occupational carcinogens at this rate (McElheny, 1981). It was therefore suggested that substances would be categorized such that:

Category I — Potentially occupational carcinogens for which an emergency temporary standard would be introduced, followed by mandatory permanent standards. Where substitution was possible a substance might be banned. The emergency standard would be released prior to any public hearing and was likely to be less stringent than the final level of control.

Category II — With incomplete evidence of carcinogenicity, standards would be set to avoid known acute or chronic effects.

This classification was finally published in 1980 (OSHA, 1980); this was followed by bitter criticism from industry. It seems more likely (as a result of a Supreme Court decision on benzene and a recent Presidential directive) that OSHA will have to balance the risk of carcinogens at varying levels against the cost of the control measures and the associated health benefits (Bates and Merrill, 1982).

5.3.4 Legislation in other countries

Montesano and Tomatis (1977) surveyed legislation in 24 countries with an appreciable degree of industrialization that: (*a*) related to chemical carcinogens in the workplace, or (*b*) dealt with compensation from occupational cancers in individuals. They pointed out that prohibition of manufacture of known carcinogens was limited, some major hazards were not covered, legislation based on experimental data was overexclusive, and some permissible levels seemed very high.

5.4 National and International bodies

5.4.1 DHSS

Unlike many other countries, in the UK there is a split between responsibility for prevention of occupational hazards and the compensation of those inflicted with work-generated disease and injury. The DHSS is responsible for the scheme of compensation. The first Workmens' Compensation Act of 1897 made no provision for industrial disease as such. In 1905, a House of Lords decision confirmed that in certain circumstances contracting a disease could constitute 'personal injury by accident'. The following year the Workmens' Compensation Act set out 6 industrial diseases for which compensation could be paid, but none directly involved the hazard of cancer.

The prescribed disease schedule has been periodically under review since that time, with additional diseases appearing on the list, and also changes being made in the occupational coverage. The Social Security (Industrial Injuries) (Prescribed Diseases) Regulations (1980) have been modified since then. A major review of the scheme (Industrial Injuries Advisory Council, 1981) recommended restructuring the schedule, with the adoption of a revised classification. They also discussed the need to speed prescription of newly recognized hazards, but accepted the great difficulty where a disease is common in the general population, but may sometimes carry an occupational component in the history of some of the subjects. The report also pointed out that the identification and measurement of the occupational component in both rare and common diseases depends on costly, exacting, and time-consuming epidemiological investigation — including follow-up of groups of workers over long periods. This could lead to delay between suspecting and concluding that there was an occupational risk. The report did not favour individuals bringing claims for a condition not covered by the schedule and endeavouring to establish the proof of industrial causation.

DHSS accepted the recommendations of the restructured schedule of prescribed diseases. This was accompanied by the issue of a revised booklet *Notes on the Diagnosis of Occupational Diseases* (DHSS, 1983).

Where an occupation caused or materially accelerated death a benefit was payable to the dependent, either under the Industrial Injuries Provision of the Social Security Act (1975) or the earlier Pneumoconiosis, Byssinosis, and Miscellaneous Diseases Benefit Scheme (which covers cancer from exposure to tar, pitch, other specific substances, irradiation, nickel cancer, papilloma of the bladder, mesothelioma, or carcinoma of the nose where the causative employment took place before 1948). Also disablement benefit is payable after 90 days incapacity from the prescribed disease.

Somerville *et al.* (1980) have described the difficulties of claiming for benefit for bladder cancer following exposure to aromatic amines. It is not clear if the particularly long latent interval, other aspects for claiming for this condition, or under-claiming in general accounted for their findings.

Since the report was published in 1983, there have been further changes in the regulations. Carcinoma *in situ* and invasive bladder cancer is now covered including all forms of transitional cell carcinoma. The notes on the chemicals covered were also modified, with inclusion of manufacture of magenta and suramine, but not of handling these chemicals.

5.4.2 The Health and Safety Commission and the Health and Safety Executive

Following the Health and Safety at Work Act (1974), the Health and Safety Commission and Executive were established. The HSE is responsible for enforcement of the regulations made under the 1974 Act. This is through the activities of 6 inspectorates: Agriculture, Alkalis and Clean Air, Factories, Mines, Quarries, and Nuclear Installations. Where work conditions do not conform to specific regulations or codes of practice the inspector may:

(*a*) Serve an Improvement Notice, requiring remedy within a specified period.
(*b*) Serve a Prohibition Order, if serious risk to health exists, which takes immediate effect.
(*c*) Prosecute in the Magistrates Court for breach of regulations.

The HSE (1984a) has an Epidemiological and Medical Statistics unit, which is responsible for:

Setting up, processing, analysing, and reporting on in-house epidemiological studies.
Collection, maintenance, and collation of routine statistics on occupational ill-health.
Running the Mesothelioma, Asbestosis, and Angiosarcoma Registers.
Providing advice to other parts of HSE on epidemiology and an assessment of published work relevant to HSE policy.

A Data Appraisal Unit has recently been set up to serve as scientific back-up to handle the action required under the Notification of New Substances Regulations (1982).

The HSE has published an extensive series of pamphlets and reports that are relevant to the prevention of occupational disease. Those specifically linked to malignant disease that appeared in the December 1983 list of the HSE library and information service are:

Best practical means leaflets
BPM 10 Amine Works.
Codes of practice
COP 3 Work with Asbestos Insulation and Asbestos Coating, 1983.
Guidance notes
EH 1 Cadmium (Health and Safety Precautions).
EH 2 Chromium (Health and Safety Precautions).
EH 10 Asbestos — Control Limits and Measurements of Airborne Dust Concentrations.
EH 27 Acrylonitrile: Personal Protective Equipment.
EH 34 Benzidine-based Dyes: Health and Safety Precautions.
MH 13 Asbestos.
Guidance booklets
HS(G) 18 Portable Grinding Machines: Control of Dust.
Regulations booklets
HS(B) 1 Packaging and Labelling of Dangerous Substances.
HS(R) 14 A Guide to the Notification of New Substances Regulations, 1982.
Health and Safety at Work booklets
44 Asbestos: Health Precautions in Industry.
Safety Health and Welfare leaflets
SHW 397 Effects of Mineral Oils on the Skin.
Toxicity reviews
TR 1 Styrene, 1981.
TR 2 Formaldehyde, 1981.
TR 4 Benzene, 1982.
TR 6 Trichloroethylene, 1982.
TR 7 Cadmium and its Compounds, 1983.

Approved Codes of Practice
Methods of Determining Ecotoxicity: Notification of New Substances Regulations, 1982.
Methods for the Determination of Toxicity: Notification of New Substances Regulations, 1982.

The first Technical Report (HSE, 1982d) considered the control of the hazards from the use of carcinogens; this presently depends upon the Carcinogenic Substances Regulations (1967). The various ways of controlling hazards are discussed, and then the rather new approach in the report on asbestos was considered (HSC, 1979). This emphasized that specific control limits should be set down, but then considered that there should be confirmation in the legislation that there was an over-riding requirement to reduce the exposure to the minimum that is reasonably practicable in conjunction with the need to meet the control limits.

HSE (1984c) published a document on *Control of Substances Hazardous to Health.* This included draft regulations and codes of practice to cover hazardous substances including those which were carcinogenic, teratogenic, or mutagenic. As part of the control mechanisms the document advocated health surveillance of workers including the collection, storage, and use of data to detect hazards to health.

5.4.3 National Radiological Protection Board (NRPB)

The NRPB was established in 1970, under the authority of the Radiological Protection Act, as a successor to the Radioactive Substances Advisory Committee, but with a wider role. The NRPB was responsible for the acquisition of knowledge on the protection of mankind from radiation hazards; this was subsequently extended to cover non-ionizing electromagnetic radiation. The Board has a duty to advise on the acceptability to the UK of standards recommended by international bodies and the principles involved in such standards.

An important aspect has been through Advice on Standards for Protection (ASPs), particularly in response to recommendations of the International Commission of Radiological Protection. Much of the work is reflected in scientific publications, including those produced by the NRPB. These included scientific and technical reports, research and development reports, and a radiological protection bulletin.

5.4.4 International Labour Organization/Office

The International Labour Organization (ILO) was established in 1919, following the Peace Conference. This organization has a long history of contribution to the study and control of occupational hazards. This is through the publication of scientific documents on the hazards from various substances, and via conventions, which national governments are expected to adopt.

Workmens' compensation was initially set out for 3 diseases in 1925. The ILO Convention No. 42 (ILO, 1934) carried an obligation to recognize 10 scheduled occupational diseases; this was ratified by the UK in 1936 and is therefore legally binding on the government. (The 10 diseases have since appeared in the UK schedule of Prescribed Industrial Disease.) This convention was subsequently amended in 1964, with addition of 4 further diseases.

In 1949, a Model Code of Safety Regulations for industrial establishments was issued for the guidance of governments and industry. This was followed in the 1950s by a range of codes of practice and guides for practice. In the 1960s specific provisions were set out for particular risks; those for radiation were published jointly with IAEA. More recently the work has been combined with that of WHO (*see below*) in setting out criteria documents on specific hazards. A specific contribution to cancer prevention was ILO Recommendation No. 147 (1947), which contained provision on: the main preventive measures of occupational cancer; the need to medically supervise workers; the role of information for and education of workers.

In fulfilling its educational and informative role, ILO has produced an *Encyclopedia of Occupational Health and Safety.* The first edition appeared in 1930–34, with the aim of providing a comprehensive guide and survey of workers' health and safety. It is now thought that there are about 10 000 publications each year over the entire field of workers' health appearing from about 1000 different institutions in the world. The third edition of the encyclopedia (Parmeggiani, 1983) is an impressive collaborative venture, which involved more than 1000 authors who participated in drafting material covering 6000 references on occupational disease published in the past 5 years; 15 international organizations also participated in preparation of material.

ILO (1982) published the report of a symposium on prevention of occupational cancer. Much of this (*pp. 17–515*) was devoted to papers on occupational carcinogenesis. The remainder of the report discussed general methods for monitoring the extent of the problem and identifying associations between occupation and cancer, national policies and international cooperation. Very little space was devoted to specific steps to be taken to control identified hazards.

5.4.5 United Nations Scientific Committee on the Effects of Atomic Radiation

The UN Scientific Committee on the Effects of Atomic Radiation (UNSCEAR) was established by the General Assembly of the UN in 1955. With the help of a small staff and advice from consultants and other agencies, UNSCEAR carries out a periodic review of the sources of radiation, the population exposures from these sources, and the effects of radiation. This work has been published in a series of official reports, with extensive annexes on the scientific analyses upon which the Committee's conclusions rest. An appendix lists the reports received from Governments. The recent reports have been: UNSCEAR, 1972, 1977, 1982.

The 1982 report has an annex on occupational exposures, which provides information on sources and doses to workers. This deals particularly with nuclear power, medical, industrial, and research use of radiation. No discussion on safe levels appears.

5.4.6 US Committee on the Biological Effects of Ionizing Radiations (BEIR)

The US National Research Council, established in 1916, is the principle operating agency of the National Academy of Sciences, of Engineering, and the Academy of Medicine. As a result of Government requests, a subcommittee (the BEIR committee) has evaluated information on the effects of human exposure to low levels of ionizing radiation. Three reports have been published:

> 1972—The effects on populations of exposure to low levels of ionizing radiation (BEIR I).
> 1977—Consideration of health benefit–cost analysis of activities involving ionizing radiation exposure and alternatives (BEIR II).
> 1980—The effects on populations of exposure to low levels of ionizing radiation (BEIR III).

5.4.7 World Health Organisation

The WHO has made a major contribution to study of health in industry through its series of technical reports published on various topics. A more specific role was confirmed in 1979, when the Thirtieth Assembly passed a resolution on chemical safety that led to the setting up of the International Program on Chemical Safety (IPCS).

The IPCS is a joint endeavour of the UN Environmental Program, the ILO, and WHO. The principle objectives of the programme are:

(*a*) Carry out and disseminate evaluations of the risk to human health from exposure to chemicals, based on existing data.
(*b*) Encourage the use and improvement and, in some cases, the validation of methods for the laboratory testing and epidemiological studies

that are suitable for health risk evaluations; propose appropriate methods for assessing health risks, hazards, benefits, and exposures.
(*c*) Promote effective international cooperation with respect to emergencies and accidents involving chemicals.
(*d*) Promote training of the manpower needed for testing and evaluating health effects of chemicals and for regulatory and other control of chemical hazards.

A major contribution from this programme has been the preparation of Environmental Health Criteria. About 50 of these are in the process of drafting and revision, with a very careful cycle of revision. The first draft is prepared by an author, and this is then reviewed by a small group of experts, and after emendation is sent to the national focal points for comment. All comments are then reviewed by a further group of experts before publication. Twenty-eight criteria documents have now been published, the last in the series dealing with acrylonitrile. The intention is to cover those substances that may influence the environment and human health.

In response to a 1977 Executive Board resolution, WHO implemented a programme on internationally recommended health-based limits for occupational exposure to toxic substances. The appropriate methods were set out in a report from an expert group (WHO, 1977 — TRS 601). By convening study groups, this had led to consensus reports providing recommendations. To date, these have been:

> TRS 647 (1980) — Heavy metals (cadmium, inorganic lead, manganese, inorganic mercury).
> TRS 664 (1981) — Organic solvents (toluene, xylene, carbon disulphide, trichloroethylene)
> TRS 667 (1982) — Pesticides (malathion, carboryl, lindane, dinitro-*o*-cresol).

5.5 Control of specific occupational carcinogens

The emphasis of this volume is on the developing epidemiological literature on the contribution of occupation to risk of cancer. Though it was thought essential to include a chapter of the issues of prevention (for that is the rationale for carrying out epidemiological studies), it is not possible to provide much detail on the possible steps that should be taken in the prevention of hazards from every specific agent, in the space available. Some general points have already been covered in this chapter, and a few selected examples are now discussed.

These have been chosen because the agent involved is thought to be important either (*a*) as a large number of workers are exposed, or (*b*) the role of the agent in causing cancer is well defined, and the risk of a specific cancer hazard is high and well quantified and recognized by all as valid.

A further reason for not attempting a systematic detailed and comprehensive coverage of all possible agents is that many excellent reports and books already cover this subject. Some have already been indicated, but a list of recommended reading on this topic is given at the end of the chapter.

An important point to remember is that many of the substances are toxic and thus provision for control of the work environment may have already been proposed to prevent either acute or long-term chronic disease, quite apart from any evidence of a cancer hazard. Sometimes an occupation may have a clearly recognized excess of cancer without the specific factor being identified. In this situation, general engineering control may be instituted to improve the work environment.

5.5.1 Acrylonitrile

This is the latest substance to be covered by a criteria document from the IPCS (*see* WHO in previous section). The *Lancet* (1984c) pointed out that until recently the occupational exposure limits had been 45 mg/m^3 in most countries, but that the UK had proposed lowering this to 4 and the US to 4.5 mg/m^3. In addition to providing information about the ways of biological monitoring for exposure, the need for further laboratory and epidemiological studies is indicated in the IPCS document.

5.5.2 Asbestos

The link between exposure to asbestos and the development of respiratory disease became clear in the first 2 decades of the century. This was followed by legislation in the UK on the compensation for affected workers and the need to provide initial and periodic examinations of exposed workers. The Asbestos Industry Regulations (1931) came into force in 1933 and only applied to the manufacture of asbestos. Laggers and other insulation workers were not covered by the provisions. There have been many modifications of the compensation and hygiene standards since the 1930s.

Initially there was optimism that the 1931 regulations had satisfactorily dealt with the lung cancer hazard (Doll, 1955). However, a number of factors may have contributed to the continuing problems: (*a*) the long latent interval, (*b*) the reduction of deaths from tuberculosis or asbestosis increased the number at risk of lung cancer, (*c*) the multiplicative effect of smoking with asbestos exposure, (*d*) the many different jobs that were not initially covered by the 1931 regulations.

A further standard for chrysotile dust was put forward by the British Occupational Hygiene Society (1968), which was followed by the new regulations in 1969, which gave more strict control over crocidolite (which was then unprofitable in many uses). The 1969 regulations also covered the removal of waste from factories and disposal in a dust-free manner.

The *British Medical Journal* (1976) drew attention to the hazard from steam pipes and boilers where insulation was flaking off and also the problem of alteration and demolition of buildings insulated with crocidolite-containing material. The *Lancet* (1976), in discussing the enquiry of the Parliamentary Commissioner for Administration into an asbestos factory at Hebden Bridge, emphasized that the 1931 regulations were from the outset 'no more than a pious hope'.

Peto (1978) reviewed the 1969 standard and suggested that the work that led to this may have underestimated the risk of morbidity and mortality following exposure to low levels of asbestos dust. He suggested that accurate dose–response data below 2 fibres/cm^3 were unlikely to be available for the foreseeable future; the biologically plausible assumption that excess cancer mortality is approximately proportional to dust levels should be provisionally accepted. However, he considered that a safe threshold may reasonably be postulated.

Acheson and Gardner (1983) point out that a wide range of factors need to be considered when setting control limits. These relate to policy, cost etc. in addition to the scientific data. They also point out that because of the wide range in slope of the dose relationship between asbestos and lung cancer, a single control limit may not be appropriate throughout the industry. They felt that chrysotile may be more dangerous than had been previously recognized and that stricter control might be more appropriate than in the remainder of the industry. However, there were many uncertainties in the validity of the historical dust measurements and the external mortality used in many studies. Also textile production only accounts for about 4% of the British asbestos industry. Studies from other parts of the industry do not suggest the need for a reduction in the control limit set in 1979; however, further reductions might be made when advances in engineering make this reasonably practicable.

They emphasized that public policy should take into account the fact that all types of asbestos are extremely durable and that products containing them may require further processing, servicing, and demolition in circumstances where dust control may be difficult.

Following study by an advisory committee (Health and Safety Commission, 1979), and a further report on control limits (Acheson and Gardner, 1983), the Commission made a number of recommendations: the control limit in the workplace should be reduced to 0.2 fibres/ml of air for brown (amosite), 0.5 for white (chrysotile), and remain at 0.2 for blue asbestos (crocidolite). The marketing and use of brown and blue asbestos and their products should be prohibited after 1/6/84. Asbestos removal by contractors will require a licence and workers will have a medical every 2 years. These regulations were also in line with 2 directives by the European Commission in 1983 on the marketing and use of asbestos, and control of the workplace.

The above recommendations of the Commission were included in control limits from 1/8/84 (Health and Safety Executive, 1984b). Guidance was also provided on control measures to achieve such levels, and details on the techniques to be used for dust sampling and testing.

Various issues of prevention were discussed at a conference on dust and diseases by the US Society for Occupational and Evnironmental Health (Lemen and Dement, 1979). Selikoff and Hammond (1979) emphasized that examination of scientific information provides guidance for public health control of asbestos on topics such as: dose–response, family contact, the use of mesothelioma registers, surveillance of exposed workers, environmental contamination, and waste disposal. This was in a short forward to a report on the conference 'Health Hazards of Asbestos Exposure'; a number of papers in the full report cover detailed aspects of control of the hazard.

Kobusch *et al.* (1984) reported on the sputum cytology results for asbestos miners in Quebec, but they failed to indicate whether this was a suitable screening technique for such workers. Chamberlain (1982) has reviewed the general use of methods for the detection of lung cancer; asbestos-exposed workers are one group in which a satisfactory technique would be of value.

5.5.3 Aromatic amines

There was evidence from the early part of the century of a hazard of increased bladder cancer to workers exposed to various aromatic amines. Ferguson (1934) described the US industry acceptance that there was a cancer hazard from dye works and (*a*) the search for a specific agent, and (*b*) the intention to remove such an agent from the industrial process. In 1947, the Association of British Chemical Manufacturers set up and financed a major project on this subject. The results from the epidemiological studies of the industry (*see* 2.6) were passed to the Ministry of Pensions and National Insurance and led to the prescription of papilloma of the bladder as an industrial disease if it followed contact with 2-naphthylamine, 1-naphthylamine, and benzidine, or the manufacture of auramine or magenta.

The ABCM produced a draft code of industrial practice in 1953, which was then revised (Scott and Williams, 1957). After discussing the background on the hazard, the recommendations were divided into 2 sections: Part I was medical, and covered the need for good records, selection of new entrants, education and training of workers, protective measures including clothing and hygiene, hours of work, and limitation of the number of workers exposed. Part II covered plant and operating precautions — including plant and building, environment, work practice, transport, and waste disposal. Specific comments were provided about particular chemicals.

In 1967, the importation was prohibited of 2-naphthylamine, benzidine, 4-aminodiphenyl, 4-nitrodiphenyl, and their salts and substances containing them, unless these chemicals were present at concentrations of 1%. At the same time the system of warning all workers and offering 6-monthly cytology was instituted.

In the light of knowledge of the potential hazard of certain of these chemicals, new enclosed plants were built for handling benzidine and 1-naphthylamine; however, the design was not adequate to control the bladder cancer risk of the workers and the new plants had to be closed (*Lancet*, 1965).

5.5.4 Benzene

The US ACGIH recommended a TLV of 100 ppm in 1946, which was quickly reduced to 50 ppm in 1947, and then to 35 ppm in 1948. This standard then remained until 1963, when it was reduced to 25 ppm, and then in 1974 to 10 ppm. These standards were adopted in the UK; they were based on evidence of the haematological effect of exposure to benzene, but not on consideration of the specific risks of leukaemia.

In 1977 the OSHA in the US moved to control benzene as an occupational carcinogen with lowering of the TLV to 1 ppm, which is around the limit of detection. This standard was challenged by the oil, rubber and other industries in the US which produce benzene, or use it for solvents, pesticides, detergents, and other products.

The International Academy of Environmental Safety with the help of the International Association of Occupational Health and other bodies held a workshop on the hazards from benzene in 1976 (Truhaut and Murray, 1978). This recommended that the standard should be an 8-h TWA occupational exposure limit of 10 ppm, with a ceiling limit of 25 ppm measured using a 10–15-minute sampling period. It was suggested that the use of benzene should be limited to those applications where it is clearly essential for technical reasons. Other uses should be avoided and, in those essential applications, benzene should be used in such a way that human exposure is kept to the lowest practical level and certainly within the proposed working guidelines.

The Chemical Industries Association (1980) and the Institute of Petroleum published guidelines for benzene exposure in the petroleum refining and chemical industries, including bulk distribution. This included suggestions on the control of exposure, and the monitoring of the health of workers exposed to benzene.

OSHA attempted to move the temporary standard of 1 ppm to a permanent standard of 1 ppm, but was challenged in the US courts. The action moved to the Supreme Court, which ruled in 1980 (European Chemical News, 7/7/80 and 14/7/80) that OSHA could not introduce the 1 ppm standard. One important point that emerged from this was that OSHA might have to consider the cost–benefit of any new standard before it could be introduced.

The International Academy of Environmental Safety and Permanent Commission of the International Association of Occupational Health held further workshops in 1980 and 1983 and made no further suggestions of any need for change in the 10 ppm TWA standard.

5.5.5 Formaldehyde

In 1980 the US Chemical Industry Institute of Toxicology held a conference on the hazard from exposure to formaldehyde; the evidence was reviewed, but no carcinogenic hazard to man was confirmed that would suggest the TLV of 2 ppm was inadequate as a level for protection. This present level was determined by the need to avoid acute and chronic toxicity.

5.5.6 Irradiation

The sources of irradiation should all be identified and precautions taken to ensure that workers who are potentially exposed are appropriately shielded. The permissible levels are laid down by ICRP and national regulations. Specific proposals were set out by HSC (1978).

A crucial step in prevention of hazard is that all workers potentially exposed to ionizing irradiation should wear badges to permit regular measurement of dose received. This permits detailed investigations to occur whenever the level of exposure of an individual is above that set down in safety regulations. The NRPB use a technique of chromosome aberration analysis to investigate all reported accidental excess exposures. Out of 55 suspected overdoses in 1977 (Lloyd *et al.*, 1978), the largest group of 36 (55%) came from industrial use of radiation sources, particularly for non-destructive

testing of welds and joints. Six (11%) incidents were from the nuclear industry, and 13 (24%) from research and health institutions.

The UK Health and Safety Commission (1978), following on the Euratom Treaty of 1976, proposed that all workers who receive more than 10% of the maximum permissible dose would have to be supervised by appropriately qualified staff, whilst those exposed to more than 30% would be subject to medical surveillance and close monitoring of dose of radiation incurred. A UK registry has been set up for all 'radiation' workers; the intention is that this will cover individuals employed by the Atomic Energy Authority, British Nuclear Fuels, the Ministry of Defence, electricity generating boards, and in mines with dust-bearing radon decay products (NRPB, 1978).

5.5.7 Leather and wood

IARC (1981) discussed the mucociliary clearance of dusts from the respiratory passages, and the extent to which inhaled dusts will be distributed to the nose, tracheobronchial or alveolar regions. It was emphasized that there had been very little research on the effect of inspired leather and wood dusts. No comment was made on the value of protective masks to reduce the hazard from nasal cancer.

Acheson (1983) stated that he knew of no quantitative evidence to suggest that concentrations of dust inhaled by British furniture workers had diminished since the disease was prescribed in 1968.

Examples of TLVs for wood dust were set out for different countries (IARC, 1981). It was pointed out that TLVs and other comparable regulations apply to pure wood and leather dust only (for example, those of the ACGIH). However, if the dust contains substances which are more toxic than the dust itself, the TLVs of these other substances should be applied. The ILO (1977) has provided TLVs for some of the chemicals used in leather, wood, and associated industries.

5.5.8 Petroleum industry

The following notes cover a small selection of the papers that have dealt with the control of potential hazards in this industry. Page (1955) reviewed the growth of the industry from the drilling of the first well in 1859. He emphasized that there was a wide range of jobs involved in production, refining, transport, and marketing. General points on maintaining health were set out.

Meyer and Church (1961) emphasized that maintenance staff and craftsmen may have relatively greater exposure to various chemicals than process operators in refineries. Listings were provided of potential hazards and means of avoiding risks. A more specific contribution on cancer prevention was set out by Eckardt (1967), whilst Sherwood (1971) described the essential features of safe practice in specific plants. He covered: design for containment, safe working procedures, education and training of workers, monitoring of environment and workers, and investigation of atypical results.

Reports from 2 annual conferences of the Institute of Petroleum (1977, 1983) have covered a number of general issues of health and safety in the industry.

5.5.9 Polycyclic aromatic hydrocarbons

The hazard from exposure to mineral oils was recognized early in this century and in 1914 mineral oil was added to the list of carcinogenic agents in the Workmens' Compensation Act. In 1920, it became compulsory to notify occupational skin cancer due to paraffin or mineral oil or their compounds, residues, or products. In 1924, a Lancashire County Court judge decided that the disease which arose out of employment in cotton spinning was attributable to the mineral oil. This was subsequently the view of a departmental committee, after discussion of the relative part played by mechanical friction, temperature, humidity, cleanliness, use of coloured overalls, and the material they were made from, and contamination of the oil by metallic and carbon particles.

The industry introduced a number of protective measures, which were subsequently followed by the 1953 legislation; this enforced the use of refined oil for lubricating spindles and 6-monthly examination of cotton spinners.

Apart from the introduction of less carcinogenic oils, the problem of skin and scrotal cancer from occupation has been tackled by a variety of steps. Cookson (1971) concluded that a solvent-refined oil was acceptable, but that soluble oils were also an important step. Cookson (1971) also discussed the changes in working conditions that were required. Cruikshank and Squire (1950), Fife (1962) and Kipling (1968) discussed the part played by protective clothing, the use of barrier creams, and washing and changing facilities. A more controversial issue is the need for periodic medicals. This has been enforced for mule spinners, and Fife (1962) advocated this for others exposed to mineral oils, including those who had retired. However, Kipling (1968) emphasized that no cases had occurred in the majority of firms and that it was unlikely that general introduction of examination was justified. Kipling also discussed the need for an educational programme, so that individuals know the risk from mineral oil, the need for preventive steps, and also the early signs of skin cancers.

Sexton (1960) described a control programme for skin cancer in workers involved in coal hydrogenation. Lippman and Goldstein (1970) carried out a survey of ink mist in pressrooms in New York, and tested the effect of electrostatic mist suppressors at the ink rollers and local exhaust ventilation. The general precautions for those exposed to oil mists were described by Waldron (1977).

In a study of workers in coke ovens exposed to coal tar pitch volatiles, Mazumdar *et al.* (1975) suggested that a TLV of 0.2 mg/m^3 was adequate; at this working level for 30 years, there should not be an increase in risk of dying of lung cancer.

5.5.10 Nickel

Though there was no evidence of a hazard from nasal cancer until the 1930s, Morgan (1958) has described the measures taken in the 1920s which altered the work environment of men employed in the South Wales nickel smelter.

In a series of studies of the workers initiated after 1945 (*see* 2.44) there was evidence of markedly increased risk of nasal cancer in those men who had worked before 1924 and a moderate risk from lung cancer. The *Lancet* (1971) discussed the findings available at the time and described this as 'a cancer prevented', suggesting that this was an example where the risk had been lowered before the cause was fully understood and in the absence of documented evidence of the risks involved. It was emphasized that the elimination of dust and fumes which cause dirty and unpleasant working conditions may also prove lifesaving.

A subsequent report (Doll, Matthews and Morgan, 1977) indicated that the risk may have persisted until about 1930, which accorded better with historical information of the environmental changes in the plant.

5.5.11 Skin cancer

Sanderson (1984) pointed out that industrial ocupational causes of skin cancer from fossil fuels and their derivatives are now well recognized and, in general, the premalignant changes of the skin due to mineral oils and tar derivatives are rarely seen. He emphasized that this was certainly true of the larger factories, although isolated cases are still observed in older workers who have been employed in small 'backyard' factories with no medical advisers.

5.5.12 Vinyl chloride

Though chronic effects from exposure to vinyl chloride (acro-osteolysis) were identified in 1966, it was not until 1974 that an association with angiosarcoma of the liver was recorded (*see* 2.58). A TLV of 50 ppm was imposed, which was reduced to 10 ppm in 1975, with a ceiling of 30 ppm. In March 1977, angiosarcoma of the liver in workers exposed to VCM polymerization plants was prescribed as an industrial disease.

The *British Medical Journal* (1976) suggested there had not been a better example of swift cooperative reaction to evidence that a hitherto unsuspected process carried a carcinogenic risk.

The initial reports stimulated great activity in examining the long-term risk of cancer in exposed workers. Various aspects of the control of the hazard were discussed by:

Corn (1975) — general and local considerations.
Rowe (1975) — reducing industrial exposure.
Perkel, Mazzocchi and Beliczky (1975) — surveillance of exposed workers.

Recommended reading

ALDERSON, M.R. (1982) *The Prevention of Cancer*. London: Arnold (*see* especially chapters by Chamberlain, and Davies)

ASSOCIATION OF SCIENTIFIC, TECHNICAL AND MANAGERIAL STAFFS (1980) *The Prevention of Occupational Cancer*. London: ASTMS

EDDY, D.M. (1980) *Screening for Cancer. Theory, Analysis, and Design*. New Jersey: Prentice Hall

INTERNATIONAL AGENCY FOR RESEARCH IN CANCER (1979) *Carcinogenic Risks: Strategies for Intervention*. Scientific publ. 25. Lyon: IARC

INTERNATIONAL LABOUR OFFICE (1974) *Control and Prevention of Occupational Hazards caused by Carcinogenic Substances and Agents*. Geneva: ILO

MILLER, A.B. (1978) *Screening in Cancer*. Technical Report 40. Geneva: UICC

SCHOTTENFELD, D. and FRAUMENI, J.F. (1982) *Cancer Epidemiology and Prevention*. Philadelphia: Saunders (*see* especially chapters by Bates and Merrill, and Miller)

References

ABRAHAMSON, J.H., PRIDAN, H., SACKS, M.I., AVITZOUR, M. and PERITZ, E. (1978) *Journal of the National Cancer Institute,* **61**, 307–314

ACHESON, E.D. (1967) *Lancet,* **ii**, 988–989

ACHESON, E.D. (1983) *Job-exposure Matrices.* Southampton: MRC Environmental Epidemiology Unit

ACHESON, E.D., BARNES, H.R., GARDNER, M.J., OSMOND, C., PANNETT, B. and TAYLOR, C.P. (1984b) *Lancet,* **i**, 611–616

ACHESON, E.D., BARNES, H.R., GARDNER, M.J., OSMOND, C., PANNETT, B. and TAYLOR, C.P. (1984c) *Lancet,* **i**, 1066–1067

ACHESON, E.D., BARNES, H.R., GARDNER, M.J., OSMOND, C., PANNETT, B. and TAYLOR, C.P. (1984d) *Lancet,* **ii**, 403

ACHESON, E.D., BENNETT, C., GARDNER, M.J. and WINTER, P.D. (1981) *Lancet,* **ii**, 1403–1405

ACHESON, E.D., COWDELL, R.H., HADFIELD, E. and MACBETH, R.G. (1968) *British Medical Journal,* **ii**, 587–596

ACHESON, E.D., COWDELL, R.H. and JOLLES, B. (1970) *British Medical Journal,* **i**, 385–393

ACHESON, E.D., COWDELL, R.H. and RANG, E. (1972) *British Journal of Industrial Medicine,* **29**, 21–30

ACHESON, E.D., COWDELL, R.H. and RANG, E. (1981) *British Journal of Industrial Medicine,* **38**, 218–224

ACHESON, E.D. and GARDNER, M.J. (1979) *Archives of Environmental Health,* **34**, 240–242

ACHESON, E.D. and GARDNER, M.J. (1980) *Lancet,* **i**, 706

ACHESON, E.D. and GARDNER, M.J. (1983) *Asbestos: The Control Limits for Asbestos.* London: HMSO

ACHESON, E.D., GARDNER, M.J., PIPPARD, E.C. and GRIME, L.P. (1982) *British Journal of Industrial Medicine,* **39**, 344–348

ACHESON, E.D., GARDNER, M.J., WINTER, P.D. and BENNETT, C. (1984a) *International Journal of Epidemiology,* **13**, 3–10

ACHESON, E.D., HADFIELD, E.H. and MACBETH, R.G. (1967) *Lancet,* **i**, 311–312

ACHESON, E.D., PANNETT, B. and PIPPARD, E.C. (1984) *Lancet,* **i**, 1126

ACHESON, E.D. and PIPPARD, E.C. (1984) *Lancet,* **i**, 563

ACHESON, E.D., PIPPARD, E.C. and WINTER, P.D. (1982) *British Journal of Cancer,* **46**, 940–946

ACQUAVELLA, J.F., TIETJEN, G.L., WILKINSON, G.S., KEY, C.R. and VOELZ, G.L. (1982) *Lancet,* **i**, 883–884

ADAMS, E.E. and BRUES, A.M. (1980) *Journal of Occupational Medicine,* **22**, 583–587

ADVISORY COMMITTEE ON PESTICIDES (1983) *The Safety of Phenoxy Herbicides: Report to the Minister.* London: Ministry of Agriculture, Fisheries and Food

AIRD, I., BENTALL, H.H., MEHIGAN, J.A. and ROBERTS, J.A.F. (1954) *British Medical Journal,* **ii**, 315–321

AITKEN-SWAN, J. and BAIRD, D. (1965) *British Journal of Cancer,* **19**, 217–227

AKSOY, M. (1978) *Lancet,* **i**, 441

AKSOY, M., ERDEM, S. and DINCOL, G. (1974) *Blood,* **44**, 837–841

ALBERT, R.E., PASTERNAK, B.S. and SHORE, R.E. (1975) *Environmental Health Perspectives,* **11**, 209–215

ALBERT, R.E., PASTERNAK, B.S., SHORE, R.E. and NELSON, N. (1979) *Journal of the National Cancer Institute,* **63**, 1289–1290

ALDERSON, M.R. (1965) *The Accuracy of the Certification of Death.* MD thesis, London University

ALDERSON, M.R. (1972) *British Journal of Industrial Medicine,* **29**, 245–254

ALDERSON, M.R. (1978) *Annals of Occupational Hygiene,* **21**, 285–291

ALDERSON, M.R. (1979) In *Perspectives and Progress in Occupational Health.* Ed. W. Gardner. pp. 151–186. Bristol: Wright

ALDERSON, M.R. (1980a) *Journal of Epidemiology and Community Health,* **34**, 182–185

ALDERSON, M.R. (1980b) In *Health and Environmental Toxicity.* Ed. L. Wood. pp. 107–125. London: Academic Press

ALDERSON, M.R. (1981a) *International Mortality Statistics.* Macmillan: London

ALDERSON, M.R. (1981b) In *Quantification of Occupational Cancers.* Ed. R. Peto and M. Schneiderman. pp. 590–610. New York: Cold Spring Harbour Laboratory

ALDERSON, M.R. (1982) *The Prevention of Cancer.* London: Arnold

ALDERSON, M.R. (1983) *An Introduction to Epidemiology,* 2nd ed. London: Macmillan

ALDERSON, M.R. and MEADE, T.W. (1967) *British Journal of Preventive and Social Medicine,* **21**, 22–29

ALDERSON, M.R. and NAYAK, R. (1971) *British Journal of Preventive and Social Medicine,* **25**, 168–173

ALDERSON, M.R. and RATTAN, N. (1980) *British Journal of Industrial Medicine,* **37**, 85–89

ALDERSON, M.R., RATTAN, N. and BIDSTRUP, L. (1981) *British Journal of Industrial Medicine*, **38**, 117–124

AMERICAN OCCUPATIONAL MEDICAL ASSOCIATION (1977) Report July/August 1977. NIOSH advises handling acrylonitrile as though a human carcinogen. Washington: American Occupational Medical Association

AMES, R.G., AMANDUS, H., ATTFIELD, M., GREEN, F.Y. and VALLYATHAN, V. (1983) *Archives of Environmental Health*, **38**, 331–333

AMOR, A.J. (1939) *Beright uber den VIII internationalen Kongress fur Unfallmedizin und Berufskrankheiten*. Leipzig: Thieme

ANDERSEN, H.C. (1975) *Ugeskrift fur Laeger*, **137**, 2567–2571

ANDERSEN, H.C., ANDERSEN, I. and SOLGAARD, J. (1977) *British Journal of Industrial Medicine*, **34**, 201–207

ANDERSEN, H.C., SOLGAARD, J. and ANDERSEN, I. (1976) *Acta Otolaryngolica*, **82**, 263–265

ANDERSON, A., DAHLBERG, B.E., MAGNUS, K. and WANNAG, A. (1982) *International Journal of Cancer*, **29**, 295–298

ANDERSON, D.E. (1974) *Cancer*, **34**, 1090–1097

ANDERSON, H.A., LILIS, R., DAUM, S.M., FISHBEIN, A.S. and SELIKOFF, I.J. (1976) *Annals of the New York Academy of Science*, **271**, 311–323

ANDERSON, H.A., LILIS, R., DAUM, S.M. and SELIKOFF, I.J. (1979) *Annals of the New York Academy of Science*, **330**, 387–399

ANDERSON, T.W. (1978) *Health Physics*, **35**, 743–750

ANDJELKOVIC, D., TAULBEE, J. and BLUM, S. (1978) *Journal of Occupational Medicine*, **20**, 409–413

ANDJELKOVIC, D., TAULBEE, J. and SYMONS, M. (1976) *Journal of Occupational Medicine*, **18**, 387–394

ANDJELKOVIC, D., TAULBEE, J., SYMONS, M. and WILLIAMS, T. (1977) *Journal of Occupational Medicine*, **19**, 397–405

ANDREWS, P. (1983) *Journal of Otolaryngology*, **12**, 255–256

ANDREWS, P.A.J. and MICHAELS, L. (1968) *Lancet*, **ii**, 85–87

ANNEGERS, J.F., O'FALLON, W. and KURLAND, L.T. (1977) *Lancet*, **ii**, 869–870

ANTHOINE, D., BRAUN, P., CERVONI, P., SCHWATZ, P. and LAMY, P. (1979) *Revue Francaise Maladie Respiratoire*, **7**, 63–65

ANTHONY, H.M. and THOMAS, G.M. (1970) *Journal of the National Cancer Institute*, **45**, 879–895

ANTHONY, P.P., VOGEL, C.L., SADIKALI, F., BARKER, L.F. and PETERSON, M.R. (1972) *British Medical Journal*, **i**, 403–406

AOKI, K. (1978) *World Health Statistics Quarterly*, **31**, 28–50

ARCHER, V.E. (1977) *Cancer*, **39**, 1802–1806

ARCHER, V.E., GILLAM, J.D. and WAGONER, J.K. (1976) *Annals of the New York Academy of Science*, **271**, 280–293

ARIES, V., CROWTHER, J.S., DRASAR, B.S., HILL, M.J. and WILLIAMS, R.E.O. (1969) *Gut*, **10**, 334–335

ARMENIAN, H.K., LILIENFELD, A.M., DIAMOND, E.L. and BROSS, I.D.J. (1974) *Lancet*, **ii**, 115–117

ARMIJO, R., ORELLANA, M., MEDINA, E., COULSON, A.H., SAYRE, J.W. and DETELS, R. (1981) *International Journal of Epidemiology*, **10**, 53–56

ARMSTRONG, B. and DOLL, R. (1975) *International Journal of Cancer*, **15**, 617–631

ARMSTRONG, B.G. and KAZANTZIS, G. (1983) *Lancet*, **i**, 1425–1427

ARMSTRONG, B.K., McNULTY, J.C., LEVITT, L.J., WILLIAMS, K.A. and HOBBS, M.S.T. (1979) *British Journal of Industrial Medicine*, **36**, 199–205

ARP, E.W., WOLF, P.H. and CHECKOWAY, H. (1983) *Journal of Occupational Medicine*, **25**, 598–602

ASHLEY, D.J.B. (1969) *British Journal of Preventive and Social Medicine*, **23**, 187–189

ASKROG, V. and HARVALD, B. (1970) *Nordisk Medicin*, **83**, 498–500

ASK-UPMARK, E. (1955) *Diseases of the Chest*, **27**, 427–435

ASSOCIATION OF DUTCH CHEMICAL INDUSTRY (1980) *Mortality in Acrylonitrile Workers*. The Hague: Association of Dutch Chemical Industry

AUB, J.C., EVANS, R.D., HEMPLEMANN, L.H. and MARTLAND, H.S. (1952) *Medicine*, **31**, 221–329

AUSTIN, D.F., REYNOLDS, P.J., SNYDER, M.A., BIGGS, M.W. and STUBBS, H.A. (1981) *Lancet*, **ii**, 712–716

AUSTIN, S.G. and SCHATTER, A.R. (1983) *Journal of Occupational Medicine*, **25**, 304–312

AVELLAN, L., BRIENE, U., JACOBSSON, B. and JOHANSON, B. (1967) *Scandinavian Journal of Plastic and Reconstructive Surgery*, **1**, 135–140

AXELSON, O. (1981) In *Quantification of Occupational Cancer*. Eds R. Peto and M. Schneidermann. p. 693. New York: Cold Spring Harbour Laboratory

AXELSON, O., ANDERSSON, K., HOGSTEDT, C., HOLMBERG, B., MOLINA, G. and DE VERDIER, A. (1978b) *Journal of Occupational Medicine*, **20**, 194–196

AXELSON, O., DAHLGREN, E., JANSSON, C-D. and REHNLUND, S.O. (1978a) *British Journal of Industrial Medicine*, **35**, 8–15

AXELSON, O., JOSEFSON, H., REHN, M. and SUNDELL, L. (1971) *Lakartidningen*, **68**, 5687–5693

AXELSON, O. and REHN, M. (1971) *Lancet*, **ii**, 706–707

AXELSON, O. and SUNDELL, L. (1974) *Work and Environmental Health*, **11**, 21–28

AXELSON, O. and SUNDELL, L. (1978) *Scandinavian Journal of Work and Environmental Health*, **4**, 46–52

AXELSON, O., SUNDELL, L., ANDERSON, K., EDLING, C., HOGSTEDT, C. and KLING, H. (1980) *Scandinavian Journal of Work and Environmental Health*, **6**, 73–79

AXELSSON, G., JEANSSON, S., RYLANDER, R. and UNANDER, M. (1980) *American Journal of Industrial Medicine*, **1**, 129–137

AXELSSON, G., LUTZ, C. and RYLANDER, R. (1984) *British Journal of Industrial Medicine*, **41**, 305–312

AXELSSON, G. and RYLANDER, R. (1984) *International Journal of Epidemiology*, **13**, 94–98

AXELSSON, G., RYLANDER, R. and SCHMIDT, A. (1980) *British Journal of Industrial Medicine*, **37**, 121–127

BAETJER, A.M. (1950a) *Archives of Industrial Hygiene*, **2**, 487–504

BAETJER, A.M. (1950b) *Archives of Industrial Hygiene*, **2**, 505–516

BAETJER, A., LEVIN, M. and LILIENFELD, A.M. (1975) *Federal Register*, **40**, 3392–3403

BAHN, A.K. (1974) *New England Journal of Medicine*, **291**, 207

BAHN, A.K., GROVER, P., ROSENWAIKE, I., O'LEARY, K. and STELLMAN, J. (1977) *New England Journal of Medicine*, **296**, 108

BAHN, A.K., ROSENWAIKE, I., HERRMANN, N., GROVER, P., STELLMAN, J. and O'LEARY, K. (1976) *New England Journal of Medicine*, **295**, 450

BAILAR, J.C. and EDERER, F. (1964) *Biometrics*, **20**, 630–643

BAIRD, J.C. (1967) *Journal of Occupational Medicine*, **9**, 415–420

BAKER, E.L., GOYER, R.A., FOWLER, B.A., KHETTRY, U., BERNARD, D.B., ADLER, S. *et al.* (1980) *American Journal of Industrial Medicine*, **1**, 139–148

BAKO, G., SMITH, E.S.O., HANSON, J. and DEWAR, R. (1982) *Canadian Journal of Public Health*, **73**, 92–94

BALARAJAN, R. (1983) *Journal of Epidemiology and Community Health*, **37**, 279–230

BALARAJAN, R. and ACHESON, E.D. (1984) *Journal of Epidemiology and Community Health*, **38**, 113–116

BALARAJAN, R. and McDOWALL, M. (1983) *Journal of Epidemiology and Community Health*, **37**, 316

BALL, M.J. (1967) *Lancet*, **ii**, 1089–1090

BALL, M.J. (1968) *British Medical Journal*, **ii**, 253

BAND, P., FELDSTEIN, M., SACCOMANNO, G., WATSON, L. and KING, G. (1980) *Cancer*, **45**, 1273–1277

BARTHEL, E. (1976) *Zeitschrift für Erkrankungen der Atmungsorgane mit Folia Bronchologia*, **146**, 266–274

BARTHOLOMEW, L.G., GROSS, J.B. and COMFORT, M.W. (1958) *Gastroenterology*, **35**, 473–477

BATES, R.R. and MERRILL, R.A. (1982) In *Cancer Epidemiology and Prevention*. Eds D. Schottenfeld and J.F. Fraumeni. pp. 1123–1137. Philadelphia: Saunders

BATTISTA, G., CAVALLOCCI, F., COMBA, P., QUERCIA, A., VINDIGNI, C. and SARTORELLI, E. (1983) *Scandinavian Journal of Work and Environmental Health*, **9**, 25–29

BAUM, J.K., HOLTZ, F., BOOKSTEIN, J.J. and KLEIN, E.W. (1973) *Lancet*, **ii**, 926–929

BAVERSTOCK, K.F., PAPWORTH, D. and VENNART, J. (1981) *Lancet*, **i**, 430–433

BAXTER, P.J., ANTHONY, P.P., MacSWEEN, R.N.M. and SCHEUER, P.J. (1977) *British Medical Journal*, **ii**, 919–921

BAXTER, P.J., ANTHONY, P.P., MacSWEEN, R.N.M. and SCHEUER, P.J. (1980) *British Journal of Industrial Medicine*, **37**, 213–221

BAXTER, P.J. and FOX, A.J. (1975) *Lancet*, **ii**, 27–28

BAXTER, P.J. and FOX, A.J. (1976) *Lancet*, **i**, 245–246

BAXTER, P.J. and WERNER, J.B. (1980) *Mortality in the Rubber Industry 1967–76*. London: HMSO

BAXTER, R.A. and HENSHAW, J.L. (1982) *Annals of Occupational Hygiene*, **25**, 95–100

BAYLISS, E.L., DEMENT, J.M., WAGONER, J.K. and BLEEJER, H.P. (1976) *Annals of the New York Academy of Science*, **271**, 324–335

BAYLISS, D.L. and LAINHART, W.S. (1972) *Mortality Patterns in Beryllium Production Workers*. OSHA exhibit no. 66, H-005, at American Industrial Hygiene Conference, 18/5/72

BAYLOR, C.H. and WEAVER, N.K. (1968) *Archives of Environmental Health*, **17**, 210–214

BEAUMONT, J.J. and WEISS, N.S. (1980) *American Journal of Epidemiology*, **112**, 775–786

BECK, G.J., SCHACHTER, E.N. and MAUNDER, L.R. (1981) *Chest*, **79**, 268–305

BECKMAN, G., BECKMAN, L. and NORDSON, I. (1977) *Environmental Health Perspectives*, **19**, 145–146

BECKMAN, L. and NORDSTROM, S. (1982) *Hereditas*, **97**, 1–7

BEEBE, G.W. (1960) *Journal of the National Cancer Institute*, **25**, 1231–1252

BEEBE, G.W. (1981) In *Quantification of Occupational Cancer*. Eds R. Peto and M. Schneiderman. pp. 661–673. New York: Cold Spring Harbour Laboratory

BELL, J. (1876) *Edinburgh Medical Journal*, **22**, 135–137

BENN, R.T., MANGOOD, A. and SMITH, A. (1979) *British Medical Journal*, **ii**, 1143

BERAL, V. (1974) *Lancet*, **i**, 1037–1040

BERAL, V., EVANS, S., SHAW, H. and MILTON, G. (1982) *Lancet*, **ii**, 290–293

BERAL, V., FRASER, P. and CHILVERS, C. (1978) *Lancet*, **i**, 1083–1087

BERAL, V. and ROBINSON, N. (1981) *British Journal of Cancer*, **44**, 886–891

BERG, J.W. and BURBANK, F. (1972) *Annals of the New York Academy of Science*, **199**, 249–262

BERRY, G. (1980) *Journal of Epidemiology and Community Health*, **34**, 217–222

BERRY, G. and MOLYNEUX, M.K.B. (1981) *Chest*, **79**, 11S–15S

BERRY, G. and NEWHOUSE, M.L. (1983) *British Journal of Industrial Medicine*, **40**, 1–7

BERRY, G., NEWHOUSE, M.L. and TUROK, M. (1972) *Lancet*, **ii**, 476–479

BERRY, G. and ROSSITER, C.E. (1976) *Lancet*, **ii**, 416

BERTAZZI, P.A. and ZOCCHETTI, C. (1980) *American Journal of Industrial Medicine*, **1**, 85–97

BERTAZZI, P.A., ZOCHETTI, C., GUERCILENA, S., FOGLIA, M.D., PESATORI, A. and RIBOLDI, L. (1982) In *Prevention of Occupational Cancer; International Sympsoium*. pp. 242–248. Geneva: ILO

BHAMARAPRAVATI, N. and VIRANUVATTI, V. (1966) *American Journal of Gastroenterology*, **45**, 267–275

BIAVA, C.G., SMUCKLER, E.A. and WHORTON, D. (1978) *Experimental and Molecular Pathology*, **29**, 448–458

BIDSTRUP, P.L. (1951) *British Journal of Industrial Medicine*, **8**, 302–305

BIDSTRUP, P.L. and CASE, R.A.M. (1956) *British Journal of Industrial Medicine*, **13**, 260–264

BINGHAM, S., WILLIAMS, D.R.R., COLE, T.J. and JAMES, W.P.T. (1979) *British Journal of Cancer*, **40**, 456–463

BINNIE, W.H., CAUSON, R.A., HILL, G.B. and SOAPER, A.E. (1972) *Oral Cancer in England and Wales*. London: HMSO

BISHOP, C.M. and JONES, A.H. (1981) *Lancet*, **ii**, 369

BJELKE, E. (1971) In *Oncology 1970: Proceedings of the 10th International Cancer Congress*. Eds R.L. Clarke, R.C. Cumley, J.E. McCoy and M.M. Copeland. pp. 320–334. Chicago: Chicago Year Book Medical

BJELKE, E. (1974) *Scandinavian Journal of Gastroenterology*, **9**, Supplement 31, 1–235

BJELKE, E. (1975) *International Journal of Cancer*, **15**, 561–565

BLACKBURN, E.K., CALLENDER, S.T., DACIE, J.V., DOLL, R., GIRDWOOD, R.H., MOLLIN, D.L. *et al.* (1968) *International Journal of Cancer*, **3**, 163–170

BLAIR, A. (1980) *Journal of Occupational Medicine*, **22**, 158–162

BLAIR, A., BERNEY, B.W., HEID, M.F. and WHITE, D.W. (1983b) *Archives of Environmental Health*, **38**, 223–228

BLAIR, A., DECOUFLE, P. and GRAUMAN, D. (1979) *American Journal of Public Health*, **69**, 508–511

BLAIR, A. and FRAUMENI, J.F. (1978) *Journal of the National Cancer Institute*, **61**, 1379–1384

BLAIR, A., GRAUMAN, D.J., LUBIN, J.H. and FRAUMENI, J.F. (1983a) *Journal of the National Cancer Institute*, **71**, 31–37

BLAIR, A. and HAYES, H.M. (1980) *International Journal of Cancer*, **25**, 118–125

BLAIR, A. and HAYES, H.M. (1982) *International Journal of Epidemiology*, **11**, 391–397

BLAIR, A. and MASON, T.J. (1980) *Archives of Environmental Health*, **35**, 92–94

BLAIR, A. and THOMAS, T.L. (1979) *American Journal of Epidemiology*, **110**, 264–273

BLAIR, A. and WHITE, D.W. (1981) *Journal of the National Cancer Institute*, **66**, 1027–1030

BLANK, C.E., COOKE, P. and POTTER, A.M. (1983) *British Journal of Industrial Medicine*, **40**, 87–91

BLATTNER, W.A., BLAIR, A. and MASON, T.J. (1981) *Cancer*, **48**, 2547–2554

BLEJER, H.P. and WAGNER, W. (1976) *Annals of the New York Academy of Science,* **271**, 179–186

BLOCK, J.B. (1977) In *Proceedings of NIOSH Styrene Butadiene Briefing.* Ed. L. Ede. pp. 28–29. Cincinnati; US Department of Health, Education and Welfare

BLOT, W.J., BRINTON, L.A., FRAUMENI, J.F. and STONE, B.J. (1977) *Science,* **198**, 51–53

BLOT, W.J., BROWN, L.M., POTTERN, L.M., STONE, B.J. and FRAUMENI, J.F. (1983) *American Journal of Epidemiology,* **117**, 706–716

BLOT, W.J., DAVIES, J.E., BROWN, L.M., NORDWALL, C.W., BUATTI, E., NG, A. et al. (1982) *Cancer,* **50**, 364–371

BLOT, W.J. and FRAUMENI, J.F. (1975) *Lancet,* **ii**, 142–144

BLOT, W.J. and FRAUMENI, J.F. (1976) *American Journal of Epidemiology,* **103**, 539–550

BLOT, W.J. and FRAUMENI, J.F. (1977) *Journal of Chronic Disease,* **30**, 745–757

BLOT, W.J., FRAUMENI, J.F. and STONE, B.J. (1978) *Cancer,* **42**, 373–380

BLOT, W.J., HARRINGTON, J.M., TOLEDO, A., HOOVER, R., HEATH, C.W. and FRAUMENI, J.F. (1978) *New England Journal of Medicine,* **299**, 620–624

BLOT, W.J., MORRIS, L.E., STROUBER, R., TAGNON, I. and FRAUMENI, J.F. (1980) *Journal of the National Cancer Institute,* **65**, 571–575

BLUM, S., ARP, E.W., SMITH, A.H. and TYROLER, H.A. (1979) In *Dusts and Diseases.* Eds R. Lemen and J.M. Dement. pp. 325–334. Illinois: Pathotox

BOHLIG, H., DABBERT, A.F., DALQUEN, P., HAIN, E. and HINZ, I. (1970) *Environmental Research,* **3**, 365–372

BOICE, J.D. and MONSON, R.A. (1977) *Journal of the National Cancer Institute,* **59**, 823–832

BOND, G.G., COOK, R.R., WIGHT, P.C. and FLORES, G.H. (1983) *Journal of Occupational Medicine,* **25**, 372–386

BONE, E., DRASAR, B.S. and HILL, M.J. (1975) *Lancet,* **i**, 1117–1120

BONNELL, J.A. (1982) *Journal of the Royal Society of Medicine,* **75**, 933–941

BONNELL, J.A. and HARTE, G. (1978) *Lancet,* **i**, 1032–1034

BOS, R.P., LEENAARS, A.O., THEUWS, J.L.G. and HENDERSON, P.TH. (1982) *International Archives of Occupational and Environmental Health,* **50**, 359–369

BOSTON COLLABORATIVE DRUG SURVEILLANCE PROGRAM (1974a) *Lancet,* **ii**, 669–671

BOSTON COLLABORATIVE DRUG SURVEILLANCE PROGRAM (1974b) *Journal of the American Medical Association,* **229**, 1462–1463

BOURKE, J.B. and GRIFFIN, J.P. (1962) *Lancet,* **ii**, 1279–1280

BOVET, P. and LOB, M. (1980) *Schweizerische Medizinische Wochenschrift,* **110**, 1277–1287

BOYD, J.T. and DOLL, R. (1954) *British Journal of Cancer,* **8**, 231–273

BOYD, J.T. and DOLL, R. (1964) *British Journal of Cancer,* **18**, 419–434

BOYD, J.T., DOLL, R., FAULDS, J.S. and LEIPER, J. (1970) *British Journal of Industrial Medicine,* **27**, 97–106

BRADY, J., LIBERATORE, F., HARPER, P., GREENWALD, P., BURNETT, W., DAVIES, J.N.P., BISHOP, M. et al. (1977) *Journal of the National Cancer Institute,* **59**, 1383–1385

BRANDT, L., NILSSON, P.G. and MITELMAN, F. (1978) *British Medical Journal,* **i**, 553

BRAUN, W. (1958) *German Medical Monthly,* **3**, 321–324

BRESLIN, P. (1979) In *Dusts and Diseases.* Eds R. Lemen and J.M. Dement. pp. 439–447. Illinois: Pathotox

BRESLOW, L. and BRESLOW, D.M. (1982) In *Cancer Epidemiology and Prevention.* Eds D. Schottenfeld and J.F. Fraumeni. pp. 1039–1048. Philadelphia: Saunders

BRESLOW, N.E. and ENSTROM, J.E. (1974) *Journal of the National Cancer Institute,* **53**, 631–639

BRIDGE, J.C. (1933) *Annual Report of the Chief Inspector of Factories and Workshops for 1932.* pp. 103–104. London: HMSO

BRIDGE, J.C. (1934) *Annual Report of the Chief Inspector of Factories and Workshops for 1933.* p. 57. London: HMSO

BRINKLEY, D. and HAYBITTLE, J.L. (1969) *British Journal of Radiology,* **42**, 519–521

BRINTON, L.A., BLOT, W.J., BECKER, J.A., WINN, D.M., BROWDER, J.P., FARMER, J.C. et al. (1984) *American Journal of Epidemiology,* **119**, 896–906

BRINTON, L.A., BLOT, W.J., STONE, B.J. and FRAUMENI, J.F. (1977) *Cancer Research,* **37**, 3473–3474

BRINTON, H.P., FRASIER, E.S. and KOVEN, A.L. (1952) *Public Health Reports,* **67**, 835–847

BRINTON, L.A., STONE, B.J., BLOT, W.J. and FRAUMENI, J.F. (1976) *Lancet,* **ii**, 628

BRITISH MEDICAL JOURNAL (1974) **ii**, 486–487

BRITISH MEDICAL JOURNAL (1975) **iii**, 396

BRITISH MEDICAL JOURNAL (1976) **i**, 1361–1362

BRITISH MEDICAL JOURNAL (1978) **i**, 1164–1165

BRITISH MEDICAL JOURNAL (1981) **282**, 504–505

BRITISH OCCUPATIONAL HYGIENE SOCIETY (1968) *Hygiene Standards for Chrysotile Asbestos Dust.* Oxford: British Occupational Hygiene Society

BRITTEN, R.H. (1934) *Public Health Reports,* **49**, 1101–1111

BRODY, H. and CULLEN, M. (1957) *Surgery,* **42**, 600–606

BROGAN, W.F., BROGAN, C.E. and DADD, J.T. (1980) *Lancet,* **ii**, 595

BROSS, I.D.J., BERTEU, R. and GIBSON, R. (1972) *American Journal of Public Health,* **62**, 1520–1531

BROSS, I.D.J., VIADANA, E. and HOUTEN, L. (1978) *Archives of Environmental Health,* **33**, 300–307

BROWN, A.J., WALDRON, H.A. and WATERHOUSE, J.A.H. (1975) *Study of Occupational Skin Cancer with Special Reference to Scrotal Cancer.* London: Institute of Petroleum

BROWN, D.P., DEMENT, J.M. and WAGONER, J.K. (1979) In *Dusts and Diseases.* Eds R. Lemen and J.M. Dement. pp. 317–324. Illinois: Pathotox

BROWN, D.P. and JONES, M. (1981) *Archives of Environmental Health,* **36**, 120–129

BROWN, L.M. and POTTERN, L.M. (1984) *Lancet,* **i**, 1356

BROWN, R.L., SUH, J.M. and SCARBOROUGH, J.E. (1965) *Cancer,* **18**, 2–13

BRUCE, D., EIDEM, K.A., LINDE, H.W. and ECKENHOFF, J.E. (1968) *Anesthesiology,* **29**, 565–569

BRUES, A.M. and KIRSH, I.E. (1977) *Transactions of the American Clinical Climatological Association,* **88**, 211–218

BRUUSGAARD, A. (1959) *Tiddskrift for den Norske Laegeforening,* **79**, 755–756

BUATTI, E., BACCETTI, S., CACCHI, F., TOMASSINI, A. and DOLARA, P. (1979) *Medicina Lavora,* **i**, 21–23

BUELL, P., DUNN, J.E. and BRESLOW, L. (1960) *Journal of Chronic Disease,* **12**, 600–621

BUESCHING, D.P. and WOLLSTADT, L. (1984) *Journal of the National Cancer Institute,* **72**, 503

BUFFLER, P.S., WOOD, S., EIFLER, C., SUAREZ, L. and KILIAN, D.J. (1979) *Journal of Occupational Medicine,* **21**, 195–203

BURCH, G.E. and ANSARI, A. (1968) *Archives of Internal Medicine*, **122**, 273–275

BURCH, J.D., HOWE, G.R., MILLERM, A.B. and SEMINCIW, R. (1981) *Journal of the National Cancer Institute*, **67**, 1219–1224

BURCH, P.R.J. (1980) *Journal of Chronic Disease*, **33**, 221–238

BURGES, D.C.L. (1980) In *Nickel Toxicology*. Eds S.S. Brown and S.W. Sunderman. pp. 15–18. New York: Academic Press

BURKITT, D. (1958/59) *British Journal of Surgery*, **46**, 218–223

BURMEISTER, L.F. (1981) *Journal of the National Cancer Institute*, **66**, 461–464

BURMEISTER, L.F., EVERETT, G.D., VAN LIER, S.F. and ISACSON, P. (1983) *American Journal of Epidemiology*, **118**, 72–77

BURMEISTER, L.F. and MORGAN, D.P. (1982) *Journal of Occupational Medicine*, **24**, 898–900

BURMEISTER, L.F., VAN LIER, S.F. and ISACSON, P. (1982) *American Journal of Epidemiology*, **115**, 720–728

BURRELL, R. (1974) *Environmental Health Perspectives*, **9**, 297–298

BURROWS, G.E. (1980) *Journal of the Society of Occupational Medicine*, **30**, 164–168

BUSSEY, H.J.R. (1975) *Familial polyposis coli.*, Baltimore: Johns Hopkins University

BUSUTTIL, A., KEMP, I.W. and HEASMAN, M.A. (1981) *Health Bulletin*, **39**, 146–152

BYREN, D., ENGHOLM, G., ENGLUND, A. and WESTERHOLM, P. (1976) *Environmental Health Perspectives*, **17**, 167–170

BYREN, D. and HOLMBERG, B. (1975) *Annals of the New York Academy of Science*, **246**, 249–250

CALDWELL, G.G. (1983) In *The Epidemiology of Cancer*. Ed. G.J. Bourke. pp. 292–326. London: Croom Helm

CALDWELL, G.G., BAMGARTENER, L., CARTER, C., COTTER, S., CURRIER, R., ESSEX, M. et al. (1976) *Bibliotheca Haematologica*, **43**, 238–241

CALDWELL, G.G., CANNON, S.B., PRATT, C.B. and ARTHUR, R.D. (1981) *Cancer*, **48**, 774–778

CAMERON, H.M. and MCGOOGAN, E. (1981) *Journal of Pathology*, **133**, 273–300

CAMPBELL, H.E. (1959) *Journal of Urology*, **81**, 663–668

CANELLOS, G.P., DEVITA, V.T., ARSENAAN, J.C., WHANG-PENG, J. and JOHNSON, R.E.C. (1975) *Lancet*, i, 947–949

CANTOR, K.P. (1982) *International Journal of Cancer*, **29**, 239–247

CAPURRO, P.U. and ELDRIDGE, J.E. (1978) *Lancet*, i, 942

CARLTON-FOSS, J.A. (1982) *Lancet*, ii, 818–819

CARTER, J.T. (1976) *British Journal of Industrial Medicine*, **33**, 9–12

CARTWRIGHT, R. (1982) *Scandinavian Journal of Work and Environmental Health*, **8**, Supplement 1, 79–82

CARTWRIGHT, R.A., ADIB, R., APPLEYARD, I., GLASHAN, R.W., GRAY, B., HAMILTON-STEWART, P.A. et al. (1983) *Journal of Epidemiology and Community Health*, **37**, 256–263

CARTWRIGHT, R.A., ADIB, R., GLASHAN, R. and GRAY, B.K. (1981) *Carcinogenesis*, **2**, 343–347

CARTWRIGHT, R.A. and BOYKO, R.W. (1984) *Lancet*, i, 850–851

CARTWRIGHT, R.A., GLASHAN, R.W., ROGERS, H.J., AHMAD, R.A., BARHAM-HALL, D., HIGGINS, E. et al. (1982) *Lancet*, ii, 842–845

CASAGRANDE, J.T., PIKE, M.C., ROSS, R.K., LOUIE, E.W., ROY, S. and HENDERSON, B.E. (1979) *Lancet*, ii, 170–173

CASARETT, L.J., FRYER, G.C., YAUGER, W.L. and KLEMMER, H. (1968) *Archives of Environmental Health*, **17**, 306–311

CASE, R.A.M. and HOSKER, M.E. (1954) *British Journal of Preventive and Social Medicine*, **8**, 39–50

CASE, R.A.M., HOSKER, M.E., McDONALD, D.B. and PEARSON, J.T. (1954) *British Journal of Preventive and Social Medicine*, **11**, 75–104

CASE, R.A.M. and LEA, A.J. (1955) *British Journal of Preventive and Social Medicine*, **9**, 62–72

CASE, R.A.M. and PEARSON, J.T. (1954)*British Journal of Preventive and Social Medicine*, **11**, 213–216

CECCHI, F., BUATTI, E., KRIEBEL, D., NASTAS, L. and SANTUCCI, M. (1980) *British Journal of Industrial Medicine*, **37**, 222–225

CEDERLOF, R., FRIBERG, L. and LUNDMAN, T. (1977) *Acta Medica Scandinavica, Supplement* **612**

CHADWICK, E. (1842) *Report on the Sanitary Condition of the Labouring Population of Great Britain*. London: Clowes

CHAMBERLAIN, J. (1982) In *Prevention of Cancer*. Ed. M.R. Alderson. pp. 227–258. London: Arnold

CHAN-YEUNG, M., WONG, R., MacLEAN, L., TAN, F., SCHULTZER, M., ENARSON, D. et al. (1983) *American Review of Respiratory Diseases*, **127**, 465–469

CHECKOWAY, H. SMITH, A.H., McMICHAEL, A.J., JONES, F.S., MONSON, R.R. and TYROLER, H.A. (1981) *British Journal of Industrial Medicine*, **38**, 240–246

CHEMICAL INDUSTRIES ASSOCIATION (1980) *Health Precaution Guidelines for Benzene Exposure in the Petroleum Refining and Chemical Industries*. London: Chemical Industries Association

CHEN, M-C., HU, J-C., CHANG, S-H., CHUANG, G-Y., TS'AO, P.F., CHANG, P'Y. et al. (1965) *Chinese Medical Journal*, **84**, 513–525

CHIAZZE, L., FERENCE, L.D. and WOLF, P.H. (1980) *Journal of Occupational Medicine*, **22**, 520–526

CHIAZZE, L., FERENCE, L.D. and WOLF, P.H. (1984) *Journal of Occupational Medicine*, **26**, 215–221

CHIAZZE, L., NICHOLS, W.E. and WONG, D. (1977) *Journal of Occupational Medicine*, **19**, 623–628

CHOI, N.W., SCHUMAN, L.M. and GULLEN, W.H. (1970) *American Journal of Epidemiology*, **91**, 238–259

CHOI, N.W., SHETTIGARA, P.T., ABU-ZEID, H.A.H. and NELSON, N.A. (1977) *International Journal of Cancer*, **19**, 167–171

CHOVIL, A. (1981) *Journal of Occupational Medicine*, **23**, 417–421

CHRISTOPHER, L.J., CROOKS, J., DAVIDSON, J.F., ERSKINE, Z.G., GALLON, S.C., MOIR, D.C. et al. (1977) *European Journal of Clinical Pharmacology*, **11**, 409–417

CLARK, C.G. and MITCHELL, P.E.G. (1961) *British Medical Journal*, ii, 1259–1262

CLARKE, C. and WHITFIELD, A.G.W. (1978) *British Medical Journal*, ii, 1063–1065

CLEMMESEN, J. (1977a) *Danish working party report on hair dyes*, pp. 93–95. Copenhagen: Ministry of Health

CLEMMESEN, J. (1977b) *Statistical studies in malignant disease*, V. Copenhagen: Munksgaard

CLEMMESEN, J. and HJALGRIM-JENSEN, S. (1981) *Ecotoxicology and Environmental Safety*, **5**, 15–23

CLEMMESEN, J. and HJALGRIM-JENSEN, S. (1983) *Journal of Ecotoxicology and Environmental Safety*, **5**, 15–23

CLOUGH, E.A. (1983) *Journal of the Society of Radiological Protection*, **3**, 24–27

COCHRANE, A.L. and MOORE, F. (1980) *British Journal of Industrial Medicine*, **37**, 226–233

COGGON, D. and ACHESON, E.D. (1982) *Lancet,* i, 1057–1059

COGGON, D., PANNETT, B. and ACHESON, E.D. (1984) *Journal of the National Cancer Institute,* **72,** 61–65

COHEN, E.N., BROWN, B.W., BRUSE, D.L., CASCORBI, H.F., CORBETT, T.H., JONES, T.W. *et al.* (1974) *Anesthesiology,* **41,** 321–340

COHEN, J. and HEIMANN, R.K. (1962) *Industrial Medicine and Surgery,* **31,** 115–120

COLE, P., HOOVER, R. and FRIEDELL, G.H. (1972) *Cancer,* **29,** 1250–1260

COLEMAN, M., BELL, J. and SKEET, R. (1983) *Lancet,* i, 982–983

CONFEDERATION OF BRITISH INDUSTRY (1980) *Safety and Health Legislation in the European Communities—an Employers' Guide.* London: Confederation of British Industry

CONTROLLER GENERAL (1981) *Problems in assessing the Cancer Risk of Low-level Ionizing Radiation Exposure.* , Washington: GAO–US

COOK, R. (1981) *Lancet,* i, 618–619

COOK, R., TOWNSEND, J.C., OTT, G. and SILVERSTEIN, L.G. (1980) *Journal of Occupational Medicine,* **22,** 530–532

COOK, R.R. (1979) *Journal of Occupational Medicine,* **21,** 784

COOK, R.R. (1980) *Journal of Occupational Medicine,* **22,** 369–370

COOK-MOZAFFARI, P.J., AZORDEGAN, F., DAY, N.E., RESSI-CAUD, A., SABAI, C. and ARAMESH, B. (1979) *British Journal of Cancer,* **39,** 293–309

COOKSON, J.O. (1971) *Annals of Occupational Hygiene,* **14,** 181–190

COOPER, W.C. (1976) *Annals of the New York Academy of Science,* **271,** 250–259

COOPER, W.C. and GAFFEY, W.R. (1975) *Journal of Occupational Medicine,* **17,** 100–107

CORBETT, T.H., CORNELL, R.G., ENDRES, J.L. and LIEDING, K. (1974) *Anesthesiology,* **41,** 341–344

CORBETT, T.H., CORNELL, R.G., LIEDLING, K. and ENDRES, J.L. (1973) *Anesthesiology,* **38,** 260–263

CORN, M. (1975) *Annals of the New York Academy of Science,* **246,** 303–305

COSTELLO, J., ORTMEYER, C.E. and MORGAN, W.K.C. (1974) *American Journal of Public Health,* **64,** 222–224

COUNCIL OF EUROPEAN COMMUNITIES (1979) *Official Journal,* **22,** C89/6–9

COURT BROWN, W.M. and DOLL, R. (1958) *British Medical Journal,* ii, 181–187

COURT BROWN, W.M., DOLL, R., SPIERS, F.W. and DUFFY, R.J. (1960) *British Medical Journal,* i, 1753–1759

COX, G.V. (1983) *An Industry-wide Mortality Study of Chemical Workers Exposed to Benzene.* Chemical Manufacturers Association report to US regulatory authorities, 16/12/83

COX, J.E., DOLL, R., SCOTT, W.A. and SMITH, S. (1981) *British Journal of Industrial Medicine,* **38,** 235–239

CREAGAN, E.T., HOOVER, R.N. and FRAUMENI, J.F. (1974) *Archives of Environmental Health,* **28,** 28–30

CREECH, J.L. and JOHNSON, M.N. (1974) *Journal of Occupational Medicine,* **16,** 150–151

CROFTON, E.C. (1969) *British Journal of Preventive and Social Medicine,* **23,** 141–144

CRUIKSHANK, C.N.D. and GOUREVITCH, A. (1952) *British Journal of Industrial Medicine,* **9,** 74–79

CRUIKSHANK, C.N.D. and SQUIRE, J.R. (1950) *British Journal of Industrial Medicine,* **7,** 1–11

CURTES, J.P., TROTEL, E. and BOURDINIERE, J. (1977) *Archives des Maladies Professionelles,* **38,** 773–786

DALAGER, N.A., MASON, T.J., FRAUMENI, J.F., HOOVER, R. and PAYNE, W.W. (1980) *Journal of Occupational Medicine,* **22,** 25–29

DALDERUP, L.L. and ZELLENRATH, D. (1983) *Lancet,* ii, 1134–1135

DALES, L.G., URY, H.K., FRIEDMAN, G.D. and EADS, W. (1979) *American Journal of Epidemiology,* **106,** 362–369

DAMBER, L. and LARSSON, L.G. (1982) *Acta Radiologica Oncologica,* **21,** 305–313

DANMARKS STATISTIKS (1979) *Occupational Mortality 1970–75.* Copenhagen: Danmarks Statistiks

DARBY, S.C. and REISSLAND, J.A. (1981) *Journal of the Royal Statistical Society,* part A, 144, 298–331

DAVIES, G.M. (1977) *British Journal of Industrial Medicine,* **34,** 291–297

DAVIES, J.M. (1965) *Lancet,* ii, 143–146

DAVIES, J.M. (1978) *Lancet,* i, 384

DAVIES, J.M. (1982) In *Prevention of Cancer.* Ed. M.R. Alderson. pp. 184–206. London: Arnold

DAVIES, J.M. (1984a) *British Journal of Industrial Medicine,* **41,** 158–169

DAVIES, J.M. (1984b) *British Journal of Industrial Medicine,* **41,** 170–178

DAVIES, J.M., SOMERVILLE, S.M. and WALLACE, D.M. (1976) *British Journal of Urology,* **48,** 561–566

DAVIES, J.M., THOMAS, H.F. and MASON, D. (1982) *British Medical Journal,* **285,** 927–931

DAVIES, J.P.N. (1975) In *Persons at High Risk of Cancer.* Ed. J.F. Fraumeni. pp. 373–381. New York: Academic Press

DAVIS, L.K., WEGMAN, D.H., MONSON, R.R. and FROINES, J. (1983) *American Journal of Industrial Medicine,* **4,** 705–723

DAVTYAN, R.M., FOMENKO, V.N. and ANDREYEVE, G.P. (1973) *Toksikologiia Novykh Promyshlennykh Khimicheskikh Veshchestv,* **13,** 58–62

DE FONSO, L.R. and KELTON, S.C. (1979) *Archives of Environmental Health,* **31,** 125–130

DE JONG, U.W., BRESLOW, N., GOH, E.H., SRIDHARAN, M. and SHANMUGARATHNAM, K. (1974) *International Journal of Cancer,* **13,** 291–303

DE LAJARTRE, M. and DE LAJARTRE, A.Y. (1979) *Annals of the New York Academy of Science,* **330,** 323–332

DE THÉ, G. (1977) *Lancet,* i, 335–338

DE THÉ, G., GESER, A., DAY, N.E., TUKEI, P.M., MANUBE, G., WILLIAMS, E.H. *et al.* (1978) *Nature,* **274,** 756–761

DEAN, G., MacLENNAN, R., McLOUGHLIN, H. and SHELLEY, E. (1979) *British Journal of Cancer,* **40,** 581–589

DEBOIS, J.M. (1969) *Tydschrift voor Geneeskunde,* **25,** 92–93

DECOUFLE, P. (1976) *Annals of the New York Academy of Science,* **271,** 94–101

DECOUFLE, P. (1978) *Journal of the National Cancer Institute,* **61,** 1025–1030

DECOUFLE, P. (1979) *Archives of Environmental Health,* **34,** 33–37

DECOUFLE, P. (1980) *Lancet,* i, 259

DECOUFLE, P., BLATTNER, W.A. and BLAIR, A. (1983) *Environmental Research,* **30,** 16–25

DECOUFLE, P., STANISLAWEZYK, K., HOUTEN, L., BROSS, I.D.J. and VIADANA, E. (1977) *A Retrospective Survey of Cancer in Relation to Occupation.* Washington: Government Printing Office

DECOUFLE, P. and WOOD, D.J. (1979) *American Journal of Epidemiology*, **109**, 667–675

DELEMARRE, J.F.M. and THEMANS, H.H. (1971) *Nederlands Tijdschrift voor Geneeskunde*, **115**, 688–689

DELORE, P. and BORGAMANO, C. (1928) *Journal Medicin de Lyon*, **9**, 227–235

DELORME, F. and THERIAULT, G. (1978) *Journal of Occupational Medicine*, **20**, 338–340

DELZELL, E., ANDJELKOVIC, D. and TYROLER, H.A. (1982) *American Journal of Industrial Medicine*, **3**, 393–404

DELZELL, E. and GRUFFERMAN, S. (1983) *Journal of the National Cancer Institute*, **71**, 735–740

DELZELL, E., LOUIK, C., LEWIS, J. and MONSON, R.R. (1981) *American Journal of Industrial Medicine*, **2**, 209–219

DELZELL, E. and MONSON, R.R. (1982a) *Journal of Occupational Medicine*, **24**, 767–769

DELZELL, E. and MONSON, R.R. (1982b) *Journal of Occupational Medicine*, **24**, 539–545

DEMENT, J.M., HARRIS, R.L., SYMONS, M.J. and SHY, C. (1982) *Annals of Occupational Hygiene*, **26**, 869–887

DEMENT, J.M., HARRIS, R.L., SYMONS, M.I. and SHY, C.M. (1983) *American Journal of Industrial Medicine*, **4**, 421–423

DEPARTMENT OF HEALTH AND HUMAN SERVICES (1983) Promoting health and preventing disease. *Public Health Reports Supplement*, September/October

DEPARTMENT OF HEALTH AND SOCIAL SECURITY (1977) *Prevention and Health*, Cmnd 7047. London: HMSO

DEPARTMENT OF HEALTH AND SOCIAL SECURITY (1983) *Notes on the Diagnosis of Occupational Diseases*. London: HMSO

DEPUE, R.H. and MENCK, H.R. (1980) *Journal of the National Cancer Institute*, **65**, 495–496

DESNOS, J. and MARTIN, A. (1973) *Correspondence Otorinolaryngologie*, **8**, 367–374

DESPLANQUES, G. (1976) *La mortalité des adultes suivant le milieu social, 1955–1971*. Paris: Institut National de la Statistique et des Etudes Economiques

DINGWALL-FORDYCE, I. and LANE, R.E. (1963) *British Journal of Industrial Medicine*, **20**, 313–315

DITRALGIA, D., BROWN, D.P., NAMEKATA, T. and IVERSON, N. (1981) *Scandinavian Journal of Work and Environmental Health*, **7**, 140–146

DOBYNS, B.M., SHELINE, G.E., WORKMAN, J.B., TOMKINS, E.A., McCONAHEY, W.M. and BECKER, D.V. (1974) *Journal of Clinical Endocrinology and Metabolism*, **38**, 976–998

DODGE, O.G. and LINSELL, C.A. (1963) *Cancer*, **16**, 1255–1263

DOERKEN, H. and REHPENNING, W. (1982) *Lancet*, **i**, 561

DOLL, R. (1952) *British Journal of Industrial Medicine*, **9**, 180–185

DOLL, R. (1955) *British Journal of Industrial Medicine*, **12**, 81–86

DOLL, R. (1958) *British Journal of Industrial Medicine*, **15**, 217–223

DOLL, R. and COOK, P. (1967) *International Journal of Cancer*, **2**, 269–279

DOLL, R., DRANE, H. and NEWELL, A.C. (1961) *Gut*, **2**, 352–359

DOLL, R., FISHER, R.E.W., GAMMON, E.J., GUNN, W., HUGHES, G.O., TYRER, F.H. *et al.* (1965) *British Journal of Industrial Medicine*, **22**, 1–12

DOLL, R., GRAY, R., HAFNER, B. and PETO, R. (1980) *British Medical Journal*, **280**, 967–971

DOLL, R. and HILL, A.B. (1950) *British Medical Journal*, **ii**, 739–748

DOLL, R., MATHEWS, J.D. and MORGAN, L.G. (1977) *British Journal of Industrial Medicine*, **34**, 102–105

DOLL, R., MORGAN, L.G. and SPEIZER, F. (1970) *British Journal of Cancer*, **24**, 623–632

DOLL, R. and PETO, R. (1976) *British Medical Journal*, **i**, 1525–1536

DOLL, R. and PETO, R. (1977) *British Medical Journal*, **i**, 1433–1436

DOLL, R., VESSEY, M.P., BEASLEY, R.W.R., BUCKLEY, A.R., FEARS, E.C., FISHER, R.E.W. *et al.* (1972) *British Journal of Industrial Medicine*, **29**, 394–406

DOLPHIN, G.W. (1976) *A Comparison of the Observed and Expected Cancers of the Haemopoietic and Lymphatic Systems among Workers at Windscale: a First Report.* London: HMSO

DONHAM, K.J., VAN DER MAATEN, M.J., MILLER, J.M., KRUSE, B.C. and RUBINO, M.J. (1977) *Journal of the National Cancer Institute*, **59**, 851–853

DONHAM, K.J., BERG, J.W. and SAWIN, R.S. (1980) *American Journal of Epidemiology*, **112**, 80–92

DONNELLY, P.K., BAKER, K.W., CARNEY, J.A. and O'FALLON, W.M. (1975) *Mayo Clinic Proceedings*, **50**, 650–656

DORKEN, H. and VOLLMER, J. (1968) *Archiv Geschwulstforschung*, **31**, 18–38

DORN, H.F. and BAUM, W.S. (1955) *Industrial Medicine and Surgery*, **24**, 239–241

DRAPER, G.J., HEAF, M.M. and KINNIER WILSON, L.M. (1977) *Journal of Medical Genetics*, **14**, 81–90

DRUCKREY, H., PREUSSMANN, R., NASHED, N. and IVANKOVIC, S. (1966) *Zeitschrift fur Krebsforschung*, **68**, 103–111

DUBROW, R. and WEGMAN, D.H. (1983) *Journal of the National Cancer Institute*, **71**, 1123–1142

DUCK, B.W., CARTER, J.T. and COOMBES, E.J. (1975) *Lancet*, **ii**, 1197–1199

DUFFY, B.J. and FITZGERALD, P.J. (1950) *Journal of Clinical Endocrinology*, **10**, 1296–1308

DUNCAN, K.P. and HOWELL, R.W. (1970) *Health Physics*, **19**, 285–291

DUNHAM, L.J., RABSON, A.S., STEWART, H.L., FRANK, A.S. and YOUNG, J.L. (1968) *Journal of the National Cancer Institute*, **41**, 683–709

DUNHAM, L., BAILAR, J.C. and LACQUER, G.L. (1973) *Journal of the National Cancer Institute*, **50**, 1119–1128

ECKARDT, R.E. (1967) *International Journal of Cancer*, **2**, 656–661

ECHARDT, R.E. (1974) *Journal of Occupational Medicine*, **16**, 472–477

EDGE, J.R. (1979) *Annals of the New York Academy of Science*, **330**, 289–294

EDLING, C. (1982) *American Journal of Industrial Medicine*, **3**, 191–199

EDLING, C. and AXELSON, O. (1983) *British Journal of Industrial Medicine*, **40**, 182–187

EDLING, C. and GRANSTAM, S. (1980) *Journal of Occupational Medicine*, **22**, 403–406

EGAN, B., WAXWEILER, R.J., BLADE, L., WOLFE, J. and WAGONER, J.K. (1979a) *Journal of Environmental Pathology and Toxicology*, **2**, 259–272

EGAN, B., WAXWEILER, R.J., BLADE, L., WOLFE, J. and WAGONER, J.K. (1979b) In *Dusts and Diseases*. Eds R. Lemen and J.M. Dement. pp. 417–428. Park Forest, Illinois: Pathotox

EGAN-BAUM, E., MILLER, B.A. and WAXWEILER, R.J. (1981) *Scandinavian Journal of Work and Environmental Health*, **7**, Suppl 4, 147–155

EHRENGUT, W. and SCHWARTAU, M. (1977) *British Medical Journal*, **ii**, 191

EISENBUD, M., GOLDWATER, L.J., HIGGINS, I., McMAHON, B., ROGERS, A.E., ROTH, H.O. *et al.* (1978) *Journal of Occupational Medicine*, **20**, 434–435

ELLIS, F.P. (1969) *British Journal of Industrial Medicine*, **26**, 190–201

ELMES, P.C. (1981) *British Journal of Industrial Medicine*, **38**, 1–13

ELMES, P.C. and SIMPSON, M.J.C. (1971) *British Journal of Industrial Medicine*, **28**, 226–236

ELMES, P.C. and SIMPSON, M.J.C. (1977) *British Journal of Industrial Medicine*, **34**, 174–180

ELWOOD, J.M. (1981) *Canadian Medical Association Journal*, **124**, 1573–1577

ELWOOD, P.D., COCHRANE, A.L., BENJAMIN, I.T. and SEYS-PROSSER, D. (1964) *British Journal of Industrial Medicine*, **21**, 304–307

ELWOOD, J.M., COLE, P., ROTHMAN, K.J. and KAPLAN, S.D. (1977) *Journal of the National Cancer Institute*, **59**, 1055–1060

ELWOOD, J.M., LEE, J.A.H., WALTER, S.D., MO, T. and GREEN, A.E.S. (1974) *International Journal of Epidemiology*, **3**, 325–332

ELY, T.S., PEDLEY, S.F., HEARNE, F.T. and STILLE, W.T. (1970) *Journal of Occupational Medicine*, **12**, 253–261

EMERY, A.E.H., ANAND, R., DANFORD, N., DUNCAN, W. and PATON, L. (1978) *Lancet*, **i**, 470–472

ENGELS, F. (1845) *The Condition of the Working Class in England*. Leipzig: Druck and Wigand

ENGLUND, A. (1980) *Journal of Toxicology and Environmental Health*, **6**, 1267–1273

ENGLUND, A., EKMAN, G. and ZABRIELSKI, L. (1982) *Annals of the New York Academy of Science*, **381**, 188–196

ENGZELL, U., ENGLUND, A. and WESTERHOLM, P. (1978) *Otolaryngology*, **86**, 437–442

ENSTROM, J.E. (1977) *British Journal of Cancer*, **35**, 674–683

ENSTROM, J.E. (1978) *Cancer*, **42**, 1943–1951

ENSTROM, J.E. (1983) *American Journal of Public Health*, **73**, 83–92

ENTERLINE, P.E. (1964) *American Journal of Public Health*, **54**, 758–768

ENTERLINE, P.E. (1965) *Annals of the New York Academy of Science*, **132**, 156–165

ENTERLINE, P.E. (1970) *Journal of Occupational Medicine*, **12**, 34–37

ENTERLINE, P.E. (1972) *Annals of the New York Academy of Science*, **200**, 260–272

ENTERLINE, P.E. (1974) *Journal of Occupational Medicine*, **16**, 523–526

ENTERLINE, P.E. (1975) *Journal of Occupational Medicine*, **17**, 127–128

ENTERLINE, P.E. (1976a) *American Review of Respiratory Disease*, **113**, 175–181

ENTERLINE, P.E. (1976b) *Journal of Occupational Medicine*, **18**, 150–156

ENTERLINE, P.E. (1982) *Annals of the New York Academy of Science*, **381**, 344–349

ENTERLINE, P.E., DECOUFLE, P. and HENDERSON, V. (1972) *Journal of Occupational Medicine*, **14**, 897–903

ENTERLINE, P.E., DECOUFLE, P. and HENDERSON, V. (1973) *British Journal of Industrial Medicine*, **30**, 162–160

ENTERLINE, P. and HENDERSON, V. (1973) *Archives of Environmental Health*, **27**, 213–217

ENTERLINE, P.E. and KENDRICK, M.A. (1967) *Archives of Environmental Health*, **15**, 181–186

ENTERLINE, P.E. and MARSH, G.M. (1980a) *American Journal of Industrial Medicine*, **1**, 251–259

ENTERLINE, P.E. and MARSH, G.M. (1980b) In *Biological Effects of Mineral Fibres*. Ed. J.C. Wagner. Vol. 2, pp. 965–972. Lyon: IARC

ENTERLINE, P.E. and MARSH, G.M. (1982a) *American Journal of Epidemiology*, **116**, 895–911

ENTERLINE, P.E. and MARSH, G.M. (1982b) *Journal of the National Cancer Institute*, **68**, 925–933

ENTERLINE, P.E., MARSH, G.M. and ESMEN, N.A. (1983) *American Review of Respiratory Disease*, **128**, 1–7

ENTERLINE, P.E. and WEILL, H. (1973) In *Biological Effects of Asbestos*. Eds P. Bogovski, J.C. Gilson, V. Timbrell, J.C. Wagner and W. Davis. pp. 179–183. Lyon: IARC

ENTICKNAP, J.B. and SMITHER, J.W. (1964) *British Journal of Industrial Medicine*, **21**, 20–31

ENZENWA, A.O. (1982) *Canadian Journal of Public Health*, **73**, 310–312

EPIDEMIOLOGICAL PROJECT STUDY GROUP (1979) *Report on the Collection and Handling of Occupational Information*. The Hague: Medical Division, Shell International

ERIKSSON, M., HARDELL, L., BERG, N.O., MOLLER, T. and AXELSON, O. (1981) *British Journal of Industrial Medicine*, **38**, 27–33

ERNSTER, V.L., SELVIN, S., BROWN, S.M., SACKS, S.T., WINKELSTEIN, W. and AUSTIN, D.F. (1979) *Journal of Occupational Medicine*, **21**, 175–183

ESPING, B. and AXELSON, O. (1980) Cited by IARC (1980b)

EVANS, C.C., LEWINSOHN, H.C. and EVANS, J.M. (1977) *British Medical Journal*, **i**, 603–605

EVANS, H.J., BUCKTON, K.E., HAMILTON, G.E. and CAROTHERS, A. (1979) *Nature*, **277**, 531–534

FABIA, J. and THUY, T.D. (1974) *British Journal of Preventive and Social Medicine*, **28**, 98–100

FACULTY OF OCCUPATIONAL MEDICINE (1982) *Guidance on Ethics for Occupational Physicians*. London: Royal College of Physicians

FACULTY OF OCCUPATIONAL MEDICINE (1983) *Evidence to the House of Lords Select Committee*. London: Faculty of Occupational Medicine

FALK, H. and BAXTER, P.J. (1981) In *Quantification of Occupational Cancer*. Eds R. Peto and M. Schneiderman. pp. 543–551. New York: Cold Spring Harbour Laboratory

FALK, H., CREECH, J.L., HEATH, C.W., JOHNSON, M.N. and KEY, M.M. (1974) *Journal of the American Medical Association*, **230**, 59–63

FALK, H., THOMAS, L.B., POPPER, H. and ISHAK, K.G. (1979) *Lancet*, **ii**, 1120–1124

FARR, W. (1875) *35th Annual Report of the Registrar General*. London: HMSO

FASAL, E., JACKSON, E.W. and KLAUBER, M.R. (1966) *Journal of Chronic Disease*, **19**, 293–306

FASAL, E., JACKSON, E.W. and KLAUBER, M.R. (1968) *American Journal of Epidemiology*, **87**, 267–274

FAULDS, J.S. and STEWART, M.J. (1956) *Journal of Pathology and Bacteriology*, **72**, 353–366

FEDRICK, J. and ALBERMAN, E. (1972) *British Medical Journal*, **ii**, 485–488

FEINLEIB, M. (1968) *Journal of the National Cancer Institute*, **41**, 315–329

FERGUSON, R.S. (1934) *Journal of Urology*, **31**, 121–126

FERRIS, B.G., PULEO, S. and CHEN, H.Y. (1979) *British Journal of Industrial Medicine*, **36**, 127–134

FIELD, B. and KERR, C. (1979) *Lancet*, **i**, 1341–1342

FIFE, J.G. (1962) *British Journal of Industrial Medicine*, **19**, 123–125

FIGUEROA, W.G., RASZKOWSKI, R. and WEISS, W. (1973) *New England Journal of Medicine*, **288**, 1096–1097

FINEGOLD, S.M., ATTEBERY, H.R. and SUTTER, V.L. (1974) *American Journal of Clinical Nutrition*, **27**, 1456–1469

FINKE, W. (1956) *International Record of Medicine*, **169**, 61–72

FINKELSTEIN, M.M. (1983) *British Journal of Industrial Medicine*, **40**, 138–144

FINKELSTEIN, M., KUSIAK, R. and SURANYI, G. (1982) *Journal of Occupational Medicine*, **24**, 663–667

FISHBECK, W.A., TOWNSEND, J.C. and SWANK, M.G. (1978) *Journal of Occupational Medicine*, **20**, 539–542

FLANDERS, W.D., CANN, C.I., ROTHMAN, K.J. and FRIED, M.P. (1984) *American Journal of Epidemiology*, **119**, 23–32

FLANDERS, W.D. and ROTHMAN, K.J. (1982) *American Journal of Public Health*, **72**, 369–372

FLEIG, I. and THIESS, A.M. (1978a) *Journal of Occupational Medicine*, **20**, 745–746

FLEIG, I. and THIESS, A.M. (1978b) *Scandinavian Journal of Work and Environmental Health*, **4**, Suppl. 2, 254–258

FLETCHER, D.E. (1972) *British Journal of Industrial Medicine*, **29**, 142–145

FLETCHER, A.C. and ADES, A. (1984) *Scandinavian Journal of Work and Environmental Health*, **10**, 7–16

FLODIN, U., ANDERSON, L., ANJOU, C-G., PALM, U.B., VIKROT, O. and AXELSON, O. (1981) *Scandinavian Journal of Work and Environmental Health*, **7**, 169–178

FOMBEUR, J-P. (1972) *Archives Maladie Professionelle*, **33**, 453–455

FONTE, R., GRIGIS, L., GRIGIS, P. and FRANCO, G. (1982) *Lancet*, **ii**, 50

FOX, A.J. (1976) *Lancet*, **ii**, 416–417

FOX, A.J. and ADELSTEIN, A.M. (1978) *Journal of Epidemiology and Community Health*, **32**, 73–78

FOX, A.J. and COLLIER, P.F. (1976a) *British Journal of Industrial Medicine*, **33**, 249–264

FOX, A.J. and COLLIER, P.F. (1976b) *British Journal of Preventive and Social Medicine*, **30**, 225–230

FOX, A.J. and COLLIER, P.F. (1977) *British Journal of Industrial Medicine*, **34**, 1–10

FOX, A.J. and GOLDBLATT, P.O. (1982) *Longitudinal Study: Sociodemographic Mortality Differentials*. London: HMSO

FOX, A.J., GOLDBLATT, P.O. and KINLEN, L.J. (1981) *British Journal of Industrial Medicine*, **38**, 378–380

FOX, A.J. and LEON, D.A. (1982) *Routine Statistical Sources for the Detection of Occupational Cancer Hazards in the UK and Scandinavia*. IARC Meeting on the Use of Statistical Sources for the Detection of Occupational Cancers, London, 12/12/82

FOX, A.J., LINDARS, D.C. and OWEN, R. (1974) *British Journal of Industrial Medicine*, **31**, 140–151

FOX, A.J., LYNGE, E. and MALKER, H. (1982) *Lancet*, **i**, 165–166

FOX, A.J. and WHITE, G.C. (1976) *Lancet*, **i**, 1009–1011

FRASER, P., CHILVERS, C. and GOLDBLATT, P. (1982) *British Journal of Industrial Medicine*, **39**, 323–329

FRAUMENI, J.F. (1967) *Journal of the American Medical Association*, **201**, 828–834

FRAUMENI, J.F. and LI, F.P. (1969) *Journal of the National Cancer Institute*, **42**, 681–691

FRAUMENI, J.F., LLOYD, J.W., SMITH, E.M. and WAGNER, M.S. (1969) *Journal of the National Cancer Institute*, **42**, 455–468

FRAUMENI, J.F. and MILLER, R.W. (1971) *Lancet*, **ii**, 1196–1197

FRAZIER, T.M., SESISTO, J.P., MULLAN, R.J. and WHORTON, M.D. (1984) *American Journal of Public Health*, **74**, 622

FREEDLANDER, E., KISSEN, L.H. and McVIE, J.G. (1978) *British Medical Journal*, **i**, 80–81

FRENTZEL-BEYME, R. (1983) *Journal of Cancer Research and Clinical Oncology*, **105**, 183–188

FRENTZEL-BEYME, R. and CLAUD, J. (1980) *American Journal of Epidemiology*, **112**, 423

FRENTZEL-BEYME, R., THIESS, A.M. and WIELLAND, R. (1978) *Scandinavian Journal of Work and Environmental Health*, **4**, Suppl. 2, 231–239

FRICHOT, B.C., LYNCH, H.T., GUIRGIS, H.A., HARRIS, R.E. and LYNCH, J.F. (1977) *Lancet*, **i**, 864–865

FRIEDLANDER, B.R., HEARNE, F.T. and NEWMAN, B.J. (1982) *Journal of Occupational Medicine*, **24**, 605–613

FROST, J. (1972) *Cancerriskoen Blandt Stoberierbejdere 1968–72*. Copenhagen: Danish Labour Ministry

FULTON, J.P., COBB, S., PREBLE, L., LEONE, L. and FORMAN, E. (1980) *American Journal of Epidemiology*, **111**, 292–296

FUNES-CRAVIOTO, F., ZAPATA-GAYON, C., KOLMODIN-HEDMAN, B., LAMBERT, B., LINDSTEN, J., NORBERG, E. *et al.* (1977) *Lancet*, **ii**, 322–325

GADIAN, T. (1975) *Chemistry and Industry*, 4/10/75, 821–831

GAFAFER, W.M. (1953) *Health of Workers in Chromate Producing Industry*. Washington, DC: US Public Health Service

GAFAFER, W.M. and SITGREAVES, R. (1940) *Public Health Reports*, **55**, 1517–1526

GAFFEY, W.R. (1975) *Journal of Occupational Medicine*, **17**, 128

GAGNON, F. (1950) *American Journal of Obstetrics and Gynaecology*, **60**, 516–522

GALLAGHER, R. and THRELFALL, W. (1983) *Canadian Medical Association Journal*, **129**, 1191–1194

GALLAGHER, R. and THRELFALL, W. (1984) *Lancet*, **i**, 48

GALLAGHER, R.P., SPINELLI, J.J., ELWOOD, J.M. and SKIPPEN, D.H. (1983) *British Journal of Cancer*, **48**, 853–857

GALLAGHER, R.P., THRELFALL, W.J., JEFFERIES, E., BAND, P.R., SPINELLI, J. and COLDMAN, A.J. (1984) *Journal of the National Cancer Institute*, **72**, 1311–1315

GALY, P., TOURAINE, R., BRUNE, J., ROUDIER, P. and GALLOIS, P. (1963) *Medicaux de Clinique et Therapeutique*, **17**, 303–311

GAMBILL, E.E. (1971) *Mayo Clinic Proceedings*, **46**, 174–177

GARDINER, J.S., WALKER, S.A. and MacLEAN, A.J. (1982) *British Journal of Industrial Medicine*, **39**, 355–360

GARDNER, M.J., ACHESON, E.D. and WINTER, P.D. (1982) *British Journal of Cancer*, **46**, 81–88

GARDNER, M.J., CRAWFORD, M.D. and MORRIS, J.N. (1969) *British Journal of Preventive and Social Medicine*, **23**, 133–140

GARDNER, M.J., WINTER, P.D. and ACHESON, E.D. (1982) *British Medical Journal*, **284**, 784

GARFINKEL, J., SELVIN, S. and BROWN, S.M. (1977) *Journal of the National Cancer Institute*, **58**, 141–143

GAU, D.W. and DIEHL, A.K. (1981) *British Medical Journal*, **284**, 239–241

GENERAL REGISTER OFFICE (1968) *Census, 1961—Great Britain, General Report*. London: HMSO

GENIN, V.A. (1974) *Gigiena Truda i Professoonalnye Zabolevaniia*, **6**, 18–22

GERARDE, H.W. and GERARDE, D.F. (1974) *Journal of Occupational Medicine*, **16**, 322–344

GHANDUR-MNAYMNEH, L. and GONZALEZ, M.S. (1981) *Cancer*, **47**, 1318–1324

GHEZZI, I., ARESINI, G. and VIGLIANI, E.C. (1972) *Medicina del lavoro*, **5–6**, 33–56

GIBBS, G.W. and HOROWITZ, I. (1979) *Journal of Occupational Medicine*, **21**, 347–353

GIBSON, E.C. (1954) *British Journal of Urology*, **26**, 227–229

GIBSON, E.S., LOCKINGTON, J.N. and MARTIN, R.H. (1979) In *Dusts and Diseases*. Eds R. Lemen and J.M. Dement. pp. 429–438. Illinois: Pathotox

GIBSON, E.S., MARTIN, R.H. and LOCKINGTON, J.N. (1977) *Journal of Occupational Medicine*, **19**, 807–812

GIBSON, E.S., McCALLA, D.R., KAISER-FARRELL, C., KERR, A.A., LOCKINGTON, J.N., HERTZMAN, C. *et al.* (1983) *Journal of Occupational Medicine*, **25**, 573–578

GIBSON, R., GRAHAM, S., LILIENFELD, A., SCHUMAN, L., DOWD, J.E. and LEVIN, M.L. (1972) *Journal of the National Cancer Institute*, **48**, 301–311

GIGNOUX, M. and BERNARD, P. (1969) *Journal de Medicine Lyon*, **50**, 731–736

GILBERT, J.B. (1944) *Journal of Urology*, **51**, 296–300

GILBERT, J.B. and HAMILTON, J.B. (1940) *Surgery, Gynaecology and Obstetrics*, **71**, 731–743

GILLIS, C.R., BOYLE, P. and MacINTYRE, I. (1982) In *Prevention of Occupational Cancer*. pp. 338–390. Geneva: ILO

GILSON, J.C. (1966) *Transactions of the Society of Occupational Medicine*, **16**, 62–74

GIRARD, R., TOLOT, F., MARTIN, P. and BOURRET, J. (1969) *Journal de Medicine Lyon*, **50**, 771–773

GLASS, A.G. and MANTEL, N. (1969) *Cancer Research*, **29**, 1995–2001

GLASS, R.I., LYNESS, R.N., MENGLE, D.C., POWELL, K.E. and KAHN, E. (1979) *American Journal of Epidemiology*, **109**, 346–351

GLATZEL, H. (1943) *Deutsches Archiv fur Klinische Medicin*, **190**, 418–428

GLOAG, D. (1981a) *British Medical Journal*, **282**, 551–553

GLOAG, D. (1981b) *British Medical Journal*, **282**, 623–626

GLOAG, D. (1981c) *British Medical Journal*, **282**, 970–972

GLOVER, J.R., BEVAN, C., COTES, J.E., ELWOOD, P.C., HODGES, N.G., KELL, R.L. *et al.* (1980) *British Journal of Industrial Medicine*, **37**, 152–162

GLOYNE, S.R. (1933) *Tubercle*, **14**, 550–558

GOFMAN, J.W. (1979) *Health Physics*, **37**, 617–639

GOGUEL, A., CAVIGNEAUX, A. and BERNARD, J. (1967) *Nouvelle Revue Francais Hematologie*, **7**, 465–480

GOLD, C. and CUTHBERT, J. (1966) *Public Health*, **80**, 261–270

GOLD, E., GORDIS, L., TONACSIA, J. and SZKLO, M. (1979) *American Journal of Epidemiology*, **109**, 309–319

GOLDBLATT, M.W. (1949) *British Journal of Industrial Medicine*, **6**, 65–81

GOLDMAN, K.P. (1965) *British Journal of Industrial Medicine*, **22**, 72–77

GOLDMAN, P., FLACH, H., HEY, W., HOCHADEL, H., PETRI, N. and STRASSBURGER, K.U. (1982) *Zentral fur Arbeitsmedizin Arbeitschutz Prophylaxe und Ergonomie*, **32**, 250–252 and 254–258

GOLDSMITH, D.F., GUIDOTTI, T.L. and JOHNSON, D.R. (1982) *American Journal of Industrial Medicine*, **3**, 423–440

GOLDSMITH, D.F., SMITH, A.H. and McMICHAEL, A.J. (1980) *Journal of Occupational Medicine*, **22**, 533–541

GOLDSMITH, J.R. (1975) *Journal of Occupational Medicine*, **17**, 126–127

GOLDSMITH, J.R. (1982) *American Journal of Industrial Medicine*, **3**, 341–348

GOLDSMITH, J.R. and GUIDOTTI, T.L. (1977) *Pathology Annual*, **12**, 411–425

GOLDSTEIN, D.H., BENOIT, J.N. and TYROLER, H.A. (1970) *Archives of Environmental Health*, **21**, 600–603

GOOLDEN, A.W.G. (1958) *British Medical Journal*, **ii**, 954–955

GOTTLIEB, M.S. (1980) *Journal of Occupational Medicine*, **22**, 384–388

GOTTLIEB, L.S. and HUSEN, L.A. (1981) *Chest*, **81**, 449–452

GOTTLIEB, M.S., PICKLE, L.W., BLOT, W.J. and FRAUMENI, J.F. (1979) *Journal of the National Cancer Institute*, **63**, 1131–1137

GOUGH, K.R., READ, A.E. and NASH, J.M. (1962) *Gut*, **3**, 232–239

GRACE, M., LARSON, M. and HANSON, J. (1980) *Health Physics*, **38**, 657–661

GRAHAM, S., DAYAL, H., ROHRER, T., SWANSON, M., SULTZ, H., SHEDD, D. *et al.* (1977) *Journal of the National Cancer Institute*, **59**, 1611–1618

GRAHAM, S. and LILIENFELD, A.M. (1958) *Cancer*, **11**, 945–958

GRAHAM, S., PRIORE, R., GRAHAM, M., BROWNE, R., BURNETT, W. and WEST, D. (1979) *Cancer*, **44**, 1870–1884

GREENBERG, M. (1972) *British Journal of Industrial Medicine*, **29**, 15–20

GREENBERG, M. and LLOYD DAVIES, T.A. (1974) *British Journal of Industrial Medicine*, **31**, 91–104

GREENE, M.H., BRINTON, L.A., FRAUMENI, J.F. and D'AMICO, R. (1978) *Lancet*, **ii**, 626–627

GREENE, M.H., HOOVER, R.N., ECK, R.L. and FRAUMENI, J.F. (1979) *Environmental Research*, **20**, 66–73

GREENWALD, P. (1984) *Public Health Reports*, **99**, 259–264

GREENWALD, P., KIRMSS, V., POLAN, A.K. and DICK, V.S. (1974) *Journal of the National Cancer Institute*, **53**, 335–340

GREGOR, O., TOMAN, R. and PRUSOVA, F. (1969) *Gut*, **10**, 1031–1034

GREGSON, LORD (1984) *Occupational health and hygiene services*. London: HMSO

GROPP, D. (1958) *Zur atiologie des sogerannten Anilin-Blasenkrebses*. Thesis. Mainz: Gutenberg Universitat

GROSS, E. and KOLSCH, F. (1943) *Archiv fur Gewerbpathologie und Gewerbehygiene*, **12**, 164–170

GRUFFERMAN, S., DUONG, T. and COLE, P. (1976) *Journal of the National Institute of Hygiene*, **57**, 1193–1195

GUIDOTTI, S., WRIGHT, W.E. and PETERS, J.M. (1982) *American Journal of Industrial Medicine*, **3**, 169–171

GUNZ, F.W. and SPEARS, G.F.S. (1968) *British Medical Journal*, **iv**, 604–608

GURALNICK, L. (1962) *Vital Statistics Special Reports*, **53**, 35–43A

GURALNICK, L. (1963a) *Vital Statistics Special Reports*, **53**, 439–612

GURALNICK, L. (1963b) *Vital Statistics Special Reports*, **53**, 343–437

GUTENSOHN, N., LI, F.P., JOHNSON, R.E. and COLE, P. (1975) *New England Journal of Medicine*, **292**, 22–25

HAGUENAUER, J.P., ROMANET, P., DUCLOS, J.C. and GUINCHARD, R. (1977) *Archives des Maladies Professionalles*, **38**, 819–823

HAENSZEL, W. (1961) *Journal of the National Cancer Institute*, **26**, 37–132

HAENSZEL, W., BERG, J.W., SEGI, M., KURIHARA, M. and

LOCKE, F.B. (1973) *Journal of the National Cancer Institute*, **51**, 1765–1779

HAENSZEL, W. and KURIHARA, M. (1968) *Journal of the National Cancer Institute*, **40**, 43–68

HAENSZEL, W., KURIHARA, M., LOCKE, F.B., SHIMUZU, K. and SEGI, M. (1976) *Journal of the National Cancer Institute*, **56**, 265–274

HAGUENDER, J.M., DUBOIS, G., FRIMAT, P., CANTINEAU, A., LEFRANCOIS, H. and FUROND, D. (1981) In *Prevention of Occupational Cancer*. pp. 168–176. Geneva: International Labour Organisation

HAKULINEN, T., SALONEN, T. and TEPPO, L. (1976) *British Journal of Preventive and Social Medicine*, **30**, 138–140

HAKULINEN, T., HOVI, L., KARKINEN-JAASKELAINEN, M., PENTTINEN, K. and SAXEN, L. (1973) *British Medical Journal*, **iv**, 265–267

HAKULINEN, T., LEHTIMAKI, L., LEHTONEN, M. and TEPPO, L. (1974) *Journal of the National Cancer Institute*, **52**, 1711–1714

HALDORSEN, T. and GLATTRE, E. (1976) *Occupational Mortality 1970–73*. Oslo: Central Bureau of Statistics

HAMMOND, E.C. (1977) *Some Negative Findings (Polio, Smallpox, Tetanus and Diphtherial Vaccines; Beauticians) and Evaluation of Risks*. Florida, American Cancer Society 19th Science Writers Seminar

HAMMOND, E.C. and HORN, D. (1958) *Journal of the American Medical Association*, **166**, 1294–1308

HAMMOND, E.C., SELIKOFF, I.J. and CHURG, J. (1965) *Annals of the New York Academy of Science*, **132**, 519–525

HAMMOND, E.C., SELIKOFF, I.J., LAWTHER, P.L. and SEIDMAN, H. (1976) *Annals of the New York Academy of Science*, **271**, 116–124

HAMMOND, E.C., SELIKOFF, I.J. and SEIDMAN, H. (1979) *Annals of the New York Academy of Science*, **330**, 473–490

HANEY, M.J. and McGARITY, W.C. (1971) *Archives of Surgery*, **103**, 69–72

HANIS, N.M., HOLMES, T.M., SHALLENBERGER, L.G. and JONES, K.E. (1982) *Journal of Occupational Medicine*, **24**, 203–212

HANIS, N.M., STAVRAKY, K.M. and FOWLER, J.L. (1979) *Journal of Occupational Medicine*, **21**, 167–174

HANSEN, E.S. (1983) *American Journal of Epidemiology*, **117**, 160–164

HANSEN, J.P., ALLEN, J., BROCK, K., FALCONER, J., HELMS, M.J., SHAVER, G.C. *et al.* (1984) *Journal of Occupational Medicine*, **26**, 29–32

HARDELL, L. (1977) *Lakartidningen*, **74**, 2753–2754

HARDELL, L. (1979) *Lancet*, **i**, 55–56

HARDELL, L. (1981) *Scandinavian Journal of Work and Environmental Health*, **7**, 119–130

HARDELL, L., ERIKSON, M., LENNER, P. and LUNDGREN, E. (1981) *British Journal of Cancer*, **43**, 169–176

HARDELL, L., JOHANSSON, B. and AXELSON, O. (1982) *American Journal of Industrial Medicine*, **3**, 247–257

HARDELL, L. and SANDSTROM, A. (1979) *British Journal of Cancer*, **39**, 711–717

HARDY, H.L., RABE, E.W. and LORCH, S. (1967) *Journal of Occupational Medicine*, **9**, 271–276

HARNES, J.R. (1980) *Journal of Occupational Medicine*, **22**, 364–369

HARRINGTON, J.M., BLOT, W.J., HOOVER, R.N., HOUSWORTH, W.J., HEATH, C.W. and FRAUMENI, J.F. (1978) *Journal of the National Cancer Institute*, **60**, 295–298

HARRINGTON, J.M. and OAKES, D. (1984) *British Journal of Industrial Medicine*, **41**, 188–191

HARRINGTON, J.M. and SHANNON, H.S. (1975) *British Medical Journal*, **iv**, 329–332

HARTING, F.H. and HESSE, W. (1879) *Vierteljabarschrift fur Gerichtliche Medicin und Offentlischs Gesund*, **30**, 296–209; **31**, 102–129, and 313–337

HASHEM, M. (1961) *Journal of the Egypt Medical Association*, **44**, 857–966

HASTERLIK, R.J., FINKEL, A.J. and MILLER, C.E. (1964) *Annals of the New York Academy of Science*, **114**, 832–837

HAYES, R.B., LILIENFELD, A.M. and SNELL, L.M. (1979) *International Journal of Epidemiology*, **8**, 365–374

HEALTH AND SAFETY COMMISSION (1978) *Ionising Radiation: Proposals for Provision of Radiological Protection*. London: HMSO

HEALTH AND SAFETY COMMISSION (1979) *Final Report of the Advisory Committee on Asbestos*. Vols I and II. London: HMSO

HEALTH AND SAFETY EXECUTIVE (1981a) *Formaldehyde: Toxicity Reivew 2*. London: HMSO

HEALTH AND SAFETY EXECUTIVE (1981b) *Styrene: Toxicity Review 1*. London: HMSO

HEALTH AND SAFETY EXECUTIVE (1982a) *Benzene: Toxicity Review 4*. London: HMSO

HEALTH AND SAFETY EXECUTIVE (1982b) *Pentachlorophenol: Toxicity Review 5*. London: HMSO

HEALTH AND SAFETY EXECUTIVE (1982c) *Trichloroethylene: Toxicity Review 6*. London: HMSO

HEALTH AND SAFETY EXECTUVE (1982d) *Carcinogens in the Workplace: the Views of the Health and Safety Executive on a Strategy for Control*. London: HMSO

HEALTH AND SAFETY EXECUTIVE (1983) *Cadmium and its Compounds: Toxicity Review 7*. London: HMSO

HEALTH AND SAFETY EXECUTIVE (1984a) *Employment Medical Advisory Service Report 1981–82*. London: HMSO

HEALTH AND SAFETY EXECUTIVE (1984b) *Asbestos: Control Limits, Measurements of Airborne Dust Concentrations and the Assessment of Control Measures*. London: HMSO

HEALTH AND SAFETY EXECUTIVE (1984c) *Control of Substances Hazardous to Health: Draft Regulations and Draft Approved Codes of Practice*. London: HMSO

HEALTH AND SAFETY AT WORK (1980) *Health and Safety at Work*, March, 1980

HEAREY, C.D., URY, H., SIEGELAUB, A., HO, M.K.P., SALOMON, H. and CELLA, R.L. (1980) *Journal of the National Cancer Institute*, **64**, 1295–1299

HEASMAN, M.A., LIDDELL, F.D.K. and REID, D.D. (1958) *British Journal of Industrial Medicine*, **15**, 141–146

HEASMAN, M.A. and LIPWORTH, L. (1966) *Accuracy of Certification of Cause of Death*. London: HMSO

HEATH, C.W., FALK, H. and CREECH, J.L. (1975) *Annals of the New York Academy of Science*, **246**, 231–236

HELDAAS, S.S., LANGARD, S.L. and ANDERSON, P. (1984) *British Journal of Industrial Medicine*, **41**, 25–30

HELPERIN, W.E., GOODMAN, M., STAYNER, L., ELLIOTT, L.J., KEENLYSIDE, R.A. and LANDRIGAN, P.J. (1983) *Journal of the American Medical Association*, **249**, 510–512

HEMMINKI, K., KYRRONEN, P., NIEMI, M-L., KOSKINEN, K., SALLMEN, M. and VAINIO, H. (1983b) *American Journal of Public Health*, **73**, 32–37

HEMMINKI, K., MUTANEN, P. and NIEMI, M-L. (1983) *British Medical Journal*, **286**, 1976–1977

HEMMINKI, K., MUTANEN, P., SALONIEMI, I., NIEMI, M.-L. and VAINIO, H. (1982) *British Medical Journal*, **285**, 1461–1463

HEMMINKI, K., NIEMI, M.I., KYYRONEN, P., KILPIKARI, I. and VAINIO, H. (1983a) *British Journal of Industrial Medicine,* **40**, 81–86

HEMMINKI, K., SALONIEMI, I., SALONEN, T., PARTANEN, T. and VAINIO, H. (1981) *Journal of Epidemiology and Community Health,* **35**, 11–15

HEMMINKI, K., SORSA, M. and VAINIO, H. (1979) *Scandinavian Journal of Work and Environmental Health,* **5**, 307–327

HEMPLEMANN, L.H., HALL, W.J., PHILIPS, M., COOPER, R.A. and AMES, W.R. (1975) *Journal of the National Cancer Institute,* **55**, 519–530

HENDERSON, B.E., LOVIE, E., JING, J.S., BUELL, P. and GARDNER, M.B. (1976) *New England Journal of Medicine,* **295**, 1101–1106

HENDERSON, B.E., POWELL, D., ROSARIO, I., KEYS, C., HANISCH, R., YOUNG, M. et al. (1974) *Journal of the National Cancer Institute,* **53**, 609–614

HENDERSON, V. and ENTERLINE, P.E. (1973) *Journal of Occupational Medicine,* **15**, 717–719

HENDERSON, V.L. and ENTERLINE, P.E. (1979) *Annals of the New York Academy of Science,* **330**, 117–126

HENDERSON, W.J., JOSLIN, C.A.F., TURNBULL, A.C. and GRIFFITHS, K. (1971) *Journal of Obstetrics and Gynaecology of the British Commonwealth,* **78**, 266–272

HENDRICKS, N.V., BERRY, C.M., LIONE, J.G. and THORPE, J.J. (1959) *Archives of Industrial Health,* **19**, 524–529

HENDRICKS, N.V., LINDEN, N.J., COLLINGS, G.H., DOOLEY, A.E., GARRETT, J.J. and RATHER, J.B. (1962) *Archives of Environmental Health,* **4**, 139–145

HENRY, S.A. (1931) Unpublished report cited by Case and Hosker (1954)

HENRY, S.A. (1946) *Cancer of the Scrotum in Relation to Occupation.* London: Oxford University Press

HENRY, S.A., KENNAWAY, N.M. and KENNAWAY, E.L. (1931) *Journal of Hygiene,* **30**, 125–137

HERBERT, W.E. and BRUSKE, J.S. (1936) *Guy's Hospital Reports,* **86**, 301–308

HERBST, A.L., KURMAN, R.J., SCULLY, R.E. and POSKANZER, D.C. (1972) *New England Journal of Medicine,* **287**, 1259–1264

HERBST, A.L. and SCULLY, R.E. (1970) *Cancer,* **25**, 745–757

HERBST, A.L., ULFELDER, H. and POSKANZER, D.C. (1971) *New England Journal of Medicine,* **284**, 878–881

HERITY, B. (1984) *British Journal of Cancer,* **49**, 371–373

HERITY, B., MORIARTY, M., BOURKE, G.J. and DALY, L. (1981) *British Journal of Cancer,* **43**, 177–182

HERNBERG, S. (1977) In *Origins of Human Cancer.* Eds H.H. Hiatt, J.D. Watson and J.A. Winston. pp. 147–157. New York: Cold Spring Harbour Laboratory

HERNBERG, S., COLLAN, Y., DEGERTH, R., ENGLUND, A., ENGZELL, U., KUOSMA, E. et al. (1983b) *Scandinavian Journal of Work and Environmental Health,* **9** (special number 2), 208–213

HERNBERG, S., WESTERHOLM, P., SCHULTZ-LARSEN, K., DEGERTH, E., KUOSMA, E., ENGLUND, A. et al. (1983a) *Scandinavian Journal of Work and Environmental Health,* **9**, 315–326

HEWER, T., ROSE, E., GHADIRIAN, P., CASTEGNARU, M., MALAVELLE, C., BARTSCH, H. et al. (1978) *Lancet,* ii, 494–496

HICKS, R.M., WALTERS, C.L., ELSEBAI, I., EL AASSER, A.-B., MERZEBANI, M. and GOUGH, T. (1977) *Proceedings of the Royal Society of Medicine,* **70**, 413–417

HIGGINS, I.T.T., GLASSMAN, J.H., OH, M.S. and CORNELL, R.G. (1983) *American Journal of Epidemiology,* **118**, 710–719

HIGGINS, J., WELCH, K., OH, M., BONON, G. and HURWITZ, P. (1981) *American Journal of Industrial Medicine,* **2**, 33–41

HILDICK-SMITH, G.Y. (1976) *British Journal of Industrial Medicine,* **33**, 217–229

HILL, A.B. (1939) *Statistical Report to the Mond Nickel Company Relating to the Incidence of Carcinoma of the Respiratory System at the Clydach Works.* Wales: Mond Nickel Company

HILL, A.B. (1965) *Proceedings of the Royal Society of Medicine,* **54**, 295–300

HILL, A.B. and LEWIS FANING, E. (1948) *British Journal of Industrial Medicine,* **5**, 1–15

HILL, I.D. (1972) *British Journal of Preventive and Social Medicine,* **26**, 132–134

HILL, I.D., DOLL, R. and KNOX, J.F. (1966) *Proceedings of the Royal Society of Medicine,* **59**, 59–60

HILL, J.W. (1977) *Annals of Occupational Health,* **20**, 161–173

HILL, J.W. (1978) *Journal of the Society of Occupational Medicine,* **28**, 134–141

HILL, M., CROWTHER, J.S., DRASAR, B.S., HAWKSWORTH, G., ARIES, V. and WILLIAMS, R.E.O. (1971) *Lancet,* i, 95–100

HILL, M.J., DRASAR, B.S., WILLIAMS, R.E.O., MEADE, T.W., COX, A.G., SIMPSON, J.E.P. et al. (1975) *Lancet,* i, 535–539

HILL, M.J., GODDARD, P. and WILLIAMS, R.E.O. (1971) *Lancet,* ii, 472–473

HILL, W.J. and FERGUSON, W.S. (1979) *Journal of Occupational Medicine,* **21**, 103–106

HILLYARD, C.J., EVANS, I.M.A. and HILL, P.A. (1978) *Lancet,* i, 1009–1011

HINDS, M.W., THOMAS, D.B. and O'REILLY, H.P. (1979) *Cancer,* **44**, 1114–1120

HIROHATA, T. (1968) *Journal of the National Cancer Institute,* **41**, 895–908

HIRST, M., TSE, S., MILLS, D.G. and LEVIN, L. (1984) *Lancet,* i, 186–188

HO, J.H.C., HUANG, D.P. and FONG, Y.Y. (1978) *Lancet,* ii, 626

HO, H.C., KWAN, H.C., WU, P., CHAN, S.K., NG, M.H. and SAW, D. (1978) *Lancet,* ii, 1094–1095

HOAR, S.K., MORRISON, A.L., COLE, P. and SILVERMAN, D.T. (1980) *Journal of Occupational Medicine,* **22**, 722–726

HOAR, S.K. and PELL, S. (1981) *Journal of Occupational Medicine,* **23**, 485–494

HOBBS, M.S.T., WOODWARD, D.S., MURPHY, B., MUSK, A.E. and ELDER, J.E. (1980) In *Biological Effects of Mineral Fibres.* Ed. J.C. Wagner. Vol. 2. pp. 615–625. Lyon: IARC

HOEGERMAN, S.F. and CUMMINS, H.T. (1983) *Health Physics,* **44**, Suppl. I, 365–371

HOFFMAN, W.S., ADLER, H., FISHBEIN, W.I. and BAUER, F.C. (1967) *Archives of Environmental Health,* **15**, 758–765

HOGSTEDT, C., ANDERSON, L., FRENNING, B. and GUSTAVSSON, A. (1982) *Scandinavian Journal of Work and Environmental Health,* **8**, Suppl. 1, 72–78

HOGSTEDT, C., MALMQUIST, N. and WADMAN, B. (1979) *Journal of the American Medical Association,* **241**, 1132–1133

HOGSTEDT, C., ROHLEN, O., BERNDTSSON, B.S., AXELSON, O. and EHRENBERG, L. (1979) *British Journal of Industrial Medicine,* **36**, 276–280

HOGSTEDT, C. and WESTERLAND, B. (1980) *Lakartidningen,* **19**, 1828–1831

HOGUE, W.L. and MALLETTE, F.S. (1949) *Journal of Industrial Hygiene and Toxicology,* **31**, 359–364

HOLDEN, H. (1969) *Lancet,* **ii**, 57

HOLDEN, H. (1980) In *Occupational Exposure to Cadmium.* pp. 23–24. London: Cadmium Association

HOLM, N.V., HAUGE, M. and HARVALD, B. (1980) *Journal of the National Cancer Institute,* **65**, 285–298

HOLMAN, C.D.J., JAMES, I.R., GATTEY, P.H. and ARMSTONG, B.K. (1980) *International Journal of Cancer,* **26**, 703–709

HOLMBERG, P.C. (1977) *Scandinavian Journal of Work and Environmental Health,* **3**, 212–214

HOLMBERG, P.C. (1979) *Lancet,* **ii**, 177–179

HOME OFFICE (1926) *Report of the Departmental Committee Appointed to Consider Evidence as to the Occurrence of Epitheliomatous Ulceration among Mule Spinners.* London: HMSO

HONCHAR, P.A. and HALPERIN, W.E. (1981) *Lancet,* **i**, 268–269

HOOVER, R. (1974) *New England Journal of Medicine,* **291**, 473

HOOVER, R. and FRAUMENI, J.F. (1975) *Environmental Research,* **9**, 196–207

HOOVER, R., GRAY, L.A., COLE, P. and MacMAHON, B. (1976) *New England Journal of Medicine,* **295**, 401–405

HOOVER, R., GRAY, L.A. and FRAUMENI, J.F. (1977) *Lancet,* **ii**, 533–534

HOOVER, R., MASON, T.J., McKAY, F.W. and FRAUMENI, J.F. (1975) In *Persons at High Risk of Cancer.* Ed. J.F. Fraumeni. pp. 343–360. New York: Academic Press

HORNBAK, H. and ASTRUP, F. (1970) *Acta Pathologica Microbiologica Scandinavica,* Suppl. 212, 158–160

HOU, P.C. (1956) *Journal of Pathology and Bacteriology,* **72**, 239–246

HOUTEN, L., BROSS, I.D.J., VIADANA, E. and SONNESSO, G. (1977) *Advances in Experimental Medicine and Biology,* **91**, 93–102

HOWE, G.R., BURCH, J.D., MILLER, A.B., COOK, G.M., ESTEVE, J., MORRISON, B. *et al.* (1980) *Journal of the National Cancer Institute,* **64**, 701–713

HOWE, G.R., CHAMBERS, L., GORDON, P., MORRISON, B. and MILLER, A.B. (1977) *American Journal of Epidemiology,* **106**, 239

HOWE, G.R., FRASER, D., LINDSAY, J., PRESNAL, B. and YU, S.Z. (1983) *Journal of the National Cancer Institute,* **70**, 1015–1019

HOWE, G.R. and LINDSAY, J.P. (1983) *Journal of the National Cancer Institute,* **70**, 37–44

HOWEL-EVANS, W., McCONNELL, R.B., CLARKE, C.A. and SHEPPARD, P.M. (1958) *Quarterly Journal of Medicine,* **27**, 413–431

HUGHES, J. and WEILL, H. (1980) In *Biological Effects of Mineral Fibres.* Ed. J.C. Wagner. Vol. 2. pp. 627–635. Lyon: IARC

HUGUENIN, R., FAUVET, J. and MAZABRAUD, M. (1950) *Archives des Maladies Professionelles,* **11**, 48–51

HUNTER, D. (1975) *The Disease of Occupations.* London: English Universities Press

HUNTER, W.J. (1978) *Journal of the Society of Occupational Medicine,* **28**, 101–108

HUNTER, W.J. (1982) In *Prevention of Occupational Cancer—International Symposium.* pp. 634–636. Geneva: International Labour Office

HURLEY, J.F., ARCHIBALD, R.McL., COLLINGS, P.L., FANNING, D.M., JACOBSEN, M. and STEELE, R.C. (1983) *American Journal of Industrial Medicine,* **4**, 691–704

HUSGAFVEL-PURSIAINEN, K., KALLIOMAKI, P-L and SURSA, M. (1982) *Journal of Occupational Medicine,* **24**, 762–766

HUTCHINSON, J. (1888) *Transactions of the Pathology Society of London,* **39**, 352–363

HUTCHINSON, W.B., THOMAS, D.B., HAMLIN, W.B., ROTH, G.J., PETERSON, A.V. and WILLIAMS, B. (1980) *Journal of the National Cancer Institute,* **65**, 13–20

HYAMS, L. and WYNDER, E.L. (1968) *Journal of Chronic Disease,* **21**, 391–415

IMRE, J. and KOPP, M. (1972) *Thorax,* **27**, 594–598

INDUSTRIAL INJURIES ADVISORY COUNCIL (1982) *Industrial Diseases: a Review of the Schedule and the Question of Individual Proof.* Cmnd 8393. London: HMSO

INFANTE, P.F. (1976) *Annals of the New York Academy of Science,* **271**, 49–57

INFANTE, P.F. (1977) *Environmental Health Perspectives,* **21**, 251–254

INFANTE, P.F. (1978) *Texas Reports on Biology and Medicine,* **37**, 153–161

INFANTE, P.F., EPSTEIN, S.S. and NEWTON, W.A. (1978) *Scandinavian Journal of Work and Environmental Health,* **4**, 137–150

INFANTE, P.F., RINSKY, R.A., WAGONER, J.K. and YOUNG, R.J. (1977) *Lancet,* **ii**, 76–78

INFANTE, P.F., WAGONER, J.K. and SPRINCE, N.L. (1979) In *Dusts and Diseases.* Eds R. Lemen and J.M. Dement. pp. 473–482. Illinois: Pathotox

INFANTE, P.F., WAGONER, J.K. and SPRINCE, N.L. (1980) *Environmental Research,* **21**, 35–43

INFANTE, P.F., WAGONER, J.K., McMICHAEL, A.J., WAXWEILER, R.J. and FALK, H. (1976) *Lancet,* **i**, 734–735

INFANTE, P.F. and WHITE, M.C. (1983) *Environmental Health Perspectives,* **52**, 75–82

INGALLS, H. (1950) *Archives of Industrial Hygiene and Occupational Medicine,* **1**, 662–676

INGALLS, H. and RISQUEZ-IRIBARREN, R. (1961) *Archives of Environmental Health,* **2**, 429–433

INGRAM, J.T. and COMAISH, S. (1967) In *Prevention of Cancer.* Eds R.W. Raven and F.J.C. Roe. pp. 212–215. London: Butterworths

INNES, J.R.M., ULLAND, B.M., VALERIOZ, M.G., PETRUCELLI, L., FISHBEIN, L., HART, E.H. *et al.* (1969) *Journal of the National Cancer Institute,* **42**, 1101–1114

INSTITUTE OF PETROLEUM (1977) *Health and Safety in the Oil Industry.* London: Institute of Petroleum

INSTITUTE OF PETROLEUM (1983) *Health Hazards in a Changing Oil Scene.* London: Institute of Petroleum

INTERNATIONAL AGENCY FOR RESEARCH IN CANCER (1972) *Monograph 1.* Lyon: IARC

INTERNATIONAL AGENCY FOR RESEARCH IN CANCER (1974a) *Monograph 4.* Lyon: IARC

INTERNATIONAL AGENCY FOR RESEARCH IN CANCER (1974b) *Monograph 5.* Lyon: IARC

INTERNATIONAL AGENCY FOR RESEARCH IN CANCER (1976a) *Monograph 11.* Lyon: IARC

INTERNATIONAL AGENCY FOR RESEARCH IN CANCER (1976b) *Monograph 12.* Lyon: IARC

INTERNATIONAL AGENCY FOR RESEARCH IN CANCER (1977a) *Monograph 14.* Lyon: IARC

INTERNATIONAL AGENCY FOR RESEARCH IN CANCER (1977b) *Monograph 15.* Lyon: IARC

INTERNATIONAL AGENCY FOR RESEARCH IN CANCER (1977c) *Lancet,* **ii**, 207–211

INTERNATIONAL AGENCY FOR RESEARCH IN CANCER (1978a) *Monograph 16.* Lyon: IARC

INTERNATIONAL AGENCY FOR RESEARCH IN CANCER (1978b) *Monograph 18.* Lyon: IARC

INTERNATIONAL AGENCY FOR RESEARCH IN CANCER (1978c) *Annual Report.*pp. 32–33. Lyon: IARC

INTERNATIONAL AGENCY FOR RESEARCH IN CANCER (1979a) *Monograph 19.* Lyon: IARC

INTERNATIONAL AGENCY FOR RESEARCH IN CANCER (1979b) *Monograph 20.* Lyon: IARC

INTERNATIONAL AGENCY FOR RESEARCH IN CANCER (1979c) *Monographs, Supplement 1.* Lyon: IARC

INTERNATIONAL AGENCY FOR RESEARCH IN CANCER (1980) *Monograph 23.* Lyon: IARC

INTERNATIONAL AGENCY FOR RESEARCH IN CANCER (1981) *Monograph 25.* Lyon: IARC

INTERNATIONAL AGENCY FOR RESEARCH IN CANCER (1982a) *Monograph 27.* Lyon: IARC

INTERNATIONAL AGENCY FOR RESEARCH IN CANCER (1982b) *Monograph 28.* Lyon: IARC

INTERNATIONAL AGENCY FOR RESEARCH IN CANCER (1982c) *Monograph 29.* Lyon: IARC

INTERNATIONAL AGENCY FOR RESEARCH IN CANCER (1982d) *Monographs, Supplement 4.* Lyon: IARC

INTERNATIONAL AGENCY FOR RESEARCH IN CANCER (1983a) *Monograph 30.* Lyon: IARC

INTERNATIONAL AGENCY FOR RESEARCH IN CANCER (1983b) *Annual Report for 1982.* Lyon: IARC

INTERNATIONAL AGENCY FOR RESEARCH IN CANCER (1984) *Monograph 33.* Lyon: IARC

INTERNATIONAL LABOUR OFFICE (1977) *Occupational Exposure Limits for Airborne Toxic Substances.* Geneva: ILO

INTERNATIONAL LABOUR OFFICE (1982) *Prevention of Occupational Cancer.* Geneva: ILO

INTERNATIONAL LABOUR ORGANISATION (1934) *Workmens' Compensation (Occupational Diseases) Convention (Revised) 1934: Convention 42.* Geneva: ILO

IRONSIDE, P. and MATTHEWS, J. (1975) *Cancer,* **36,** 1115–1121

ISHIMARU, T., OKADA, H., TOMIYASU, T., TSUCHIMOTO, T., HOSHINO, T. and ICHIMARU, M. (1971) *American Journal of Epidemiology,* **93,** 157–165

ISOMAKI, H., HAKULINEN, T. and JOUTSENLAHTI, U. (1979) *Lancet,* i, 392

JABLON, S. (1975) In *Persons at High Risk of Cancer.* Ed. J.F. Fraumeni. pp. 151–165. New York: Academic Press

JABLON, S. and KATO, H. (1972) *Radiation Research,* **50,** 649–698

JABLON, S. and MILLER, R.W. (1978) *Radiology,* **126,** 677–679

JABLON, S., TACHIKAWA, K., BELSKY, J.L. and STEER, A. (1971) *Lancet,* i, 927–931

JACOBSEN, M. (1976) *Dust Exposure, Lung Disease and Coal Miners' Mortality.* PhD thesis, Edinburgh University

JARVHOLM, B. and LAVENIUS, B. (1981) *Scandinavian Journal of Work and Environmental Health,* 7, 179–184

JARVHOLM, B., LILLIENBERG, L., SALLSTEN, G., THRINGER, G. and AXELSON, O. (1981) *Journal of Occupational Medicine,* **23,** 333–337

JARVHOLM, B., THIRINGER, G. and AXELSON, O. (1982) *British Journal of Industrial Medicine,* **39,** 196–197

JEDLICKA, V.L., HERMANSKA, Z., SMIDA, I. and KOUBA, A. (1958) *Acta Medica Scandinavica,* **161,** 447–451

JENSEN, O.M. (1979) *International Journal of Cancer,* **23,** 454–463

JENSEN, O.M. (1980) *Lancet,* ii, 480–481

JENSEN, O.M. (1982) *Lancet,* ii, 935

JENSEN, O.M. and ANDERSEN, S.K. (1982) *Lancet,* i, 913

JENSEN, O.M., OLSEN, J.H. and ØSTERLIND, A. (1984) *Lancet,* i, 794

JIRASEK, L., KALENSKY, J., KUBECK, K., PAZDEROVA, J. and LUKAS, E. (1974) *Ceskoslovenska Dermatologie,* **49,** 145–147

JOHANSSON, S., ANGERVALL, L., BENGTSSON, U. and WAHLQVIST, L. (1974) *Cancer,* **33,** 743–753

JOHNSON, E.S. and FISCHMAN, H.R. (1982) *Lancet,* i, 913–914

JOHNSON, F.E., KUGLER, M.A. and BROWN, S.M. (1981) *Lancet,* ii, 40

JOHNSON, F.L., FEAGLER, J.R., LERNER, K.G., MAJERUS, P.W., SIEGEL, M., HARTMANN, J.R. et al. (1972) *Lancet,* **ii,** 1273–1276

JOHNSTONE, T. (1981) *British Medical Journal,* **282,** 1550

JONES, H.B. and GRENDON, A. (1975) *Cosmetology and Toxicology,* **18,** 251–268

JONES, J.G. (1961) *Annals of Occupational Hygiene,* **3,** 264–271

JONES, J.S.P., SMITH, P.G., POOLEY, F.D., BERRY, G., SAWLE, G.W., WIGNALL, B.K. et al. (1980) In *Biological Effects of Mineral Fibres.* Ed. J.C. Wagner. pp. 637–653. Lyon: IARC

JOYNER, R.E. (1964) *Archives of Environmental Health,* **8,** 700–710

KABAT, G.C. and WYNDER, E.L. (1984) *Cancer,* **53,** 1214–1221

KALLEN, B., MALMQVIST, G. and MORITZ, I.J. (1982) *Archives of Environmental Health,* **37,** 81–85

KAMINSKI, R., GIESSERT, K.S. and DACEY, E. (1980) *Journal of Occupational Medicine,* **22,** 183–189

KANG, H.K., INFANTE, P.F. and CARRA, J.S. (1980) *Science,* **207,** 935–936

KANTOR, A.F., HARTGE, P., HOOVER, R.N., NARAYANA, A.S., SULLIVAN, J.W. and FRAUMENI, J.F. (1984) *American Journal of Epidemiology,* **119,** 510–515

KANTOR, A.F., McCREA, M.G., WISTER MEIGS, J. and FLANNERY, J.T. (1979) *Journal of Epidemiology and Community Health,* **33,** 253–256

KAPLAN, I. (1959) *Journal of the American Medical Association,* **151,** 2039–2043

KAPLAN, S.D. (1983) *Mortality Study of Petroleum Refinery Workers: Up-date of Follow-up.* New York: American Petroleum Institute

KARMODY, A.J. and KYLE, J. (1969) *British Journal of Surgery,* **56,** 362–364

KARPAS, A., WREGHITT, T.G. and NAGINGTON, J. (1978) *Lancet,* ii, 1016–1019

KATSNELSON, B.A. and MOKRONOSOVA, K.A. (1979) *Journal of Occupational Medicine,* **21,** 15–20

KAWAI, M., ARMAMOTO, H. and HARADA, K. (1967) *Archives of Environmental Health,* **14,** 859–864

KELLERMANN, G., SHAW, C.R. and LUYTEN-KELLERMANN, M. (1973) *New England Journal of Medicine,* **289,** 934–937

KENNAWAY, E.L. (1925) *Journal of Industrial Hygiene,* **8,** 69–93

KENNAWAY, E.L. and KENNAWAY, N.M. (1946) *Cancer Research,* **6,** 49–53

KENNAWAY, E.L. and KENNAWAY, N.M. (1947) *British Journal of Cancer,* **1,** 260–298

KENNAWAY, E.L. and KENNAWAY, N.M. (1953) *British Journal of Cancer,* **7,** 10–18

KENNAWAY, N.M. and KENNAWAY, E.L. (1936) *Journal of Hygiene,* **36,** 236–267

KENNEDY, J. and SPIRTAS, R. (1977) *Occupational Characteristics of Disabled Female Workers.* Washington DC:

Annual Meeting of the American Public Health Association

KERSEY, J., SPECTOR, B. and GOOD, R.A. (1973) *International Journal of Cancer*, **12**, 333–347

KESSLER, I.I. (1970) *Journal of the National Cancer Institute*, **44**, 673–686

KHACHATRYAN, E.A. (1972a) *Voprosy Onkologii*, **18**, 85–86

KHACHATRYAN, E.A. (1972b) *Gigiena Truda i Professionalnye Zabolevaniia*, **16**, 54–55

KHLEBNIKOVA, M.I., GLADKOVA, E.V., KURENKO, L.T., PSHENITSYN, A.V. and SHALIN, B.M. (1970) *Gigiena Truda i Professionalnye Zabolevaniia*, **14**, 7–10

KIESSELBACH, N., KORALLUS, U., LANGE, H.J., NEISS, A. and ZWINGERS, T. (1979) *Zentralblatt fur Arbeitsmedizin*, **10**, 257–259

KILPATRICK, S.J. (1962) *Population Studies*, **16**, 175–187

KILPIKARI, I., PUKKALA, E., LEHTONEN, M. and HAKAMA, M. (1982) *International Archives of Occupational and Environmental Health*, **51**, 65–71

KINLEN, L.J. (1983) *British Medical Journal*, **287**, 1017–1019

KINLEN, L.J., BADARACCO, M.A., MOFFETT, J. and VESSEY, M.P. (1974) *Journal of Obstetrics and Gynaecology of the British Empire*, **81**, 849–855

KINLEN, L.J., EASTWOOD, J.B., KEER, D.N.S., MOORHEAD, J.F., OLIVER, D.O., ROBINSON, B.H.B. *et al.* (1980) *British Medical Journal*, **280**, 1401–1403

KINLEN, L.J., HARRIS, R., GARROD, A. and RODRIGUEZ, K. (1977) *British Medical Journal*, **ii**, 366–368

KINLEN, L.J., SHEIL, A.G.R., PETO, R. and DOLL, R. (1979) *British Medical Journal*, **ii**, 1461–1466

KINNEAR, J., ROGERS, J., FINN, O.A. and MAIR, A. (1955) *British Journal of Industrial Medicine*, **12**, 36–42

KIPLING, M.D. (1968) *Oil and the Skin*. Annual Report of the Chief Inspector of Factories, 1967. London: HMSO

KIPLING, M.D. (1971) *Transactions of the Society of Occupational Medicine*, **21**, 73–78

KIPLING, M.D. and WALDRON, H.A. (1976) *Preventive Medicine*, **5**, 262–278

KIPLING, M.D. and WATERHOUSE, J.A.H. (1967) *Lancet*, **i**, 730–731

KJELLSTROM, T., FRIBERG, L. and RAHNSTER, B. (1979) *Environmental Health Perspectives*, **28**, 199–204

KLATSKIN, G. (1977) *Gastroenterology*, **73**, 386–394

KLAUBER, M.R. and LYON, J.L. (1978) *Cancer*, **41**, 2355–2358

KLEPP, O. and MAGNUS, K. (1979) *International Journal of Cancer*, **23**, 482–486

KLIENFELD, M., GIEL, C.P., MAJERANOWSKI, J.F. and MESSITE, J. (1963) *Archives of Environmental Health*, **i**, 107–115

KLIENFELD, M., MESSITE, J. and KOOYMAN, O. (1967) *Archives of Environmental Health*, **15**, 177–180

KLIENFELD, M., MESSITE, J., KOOYMAN, O. and ZAKI, M.H. (1967) *Archives of Environmental Health*, **14**, 663–667

KLIENFELD, M., MESSITE, J. and ZAKI, M.H. (1974) *Journal of Occupational Medicine*, **16**, 345–349

KNEALE, G.N., MANCUSO, T.F. and STEWART, A.M. (1984a) *British Journal of Industrial Medicine*, **41**, 6–8

KNEALE, G.N., MANCUSO, T.F. and STEWART, A.M. (1984b) *British Journal of Industrial Medicine*, **41**, 9–14

KNEALE, G.W. and STEWART, A.M. (1982) *British Journal of Industrial Medicine*, **39**, 201–202

KNILL-JONES, R.P., MOIR, D.D., RODRIGUES, L.V. and SPENCE, A.A. (1972) *Lancet*, **ii**, 1326–1328

KNILL-JONES, R.P., NEWMAN, B.J. and SPENCE, A.A. (1975) *Lancet*, **ii**, 807–809

KNOWLES, R.S. and VIRDEN, J.E. (1980) *British Medical Journal*, **281**, 589–591

KNOX, G. (1964) *British Journal of Preventive and Social Medicine*, **18**, 17–24

KNOX, J.F., DOLL, R. and HILL, I.D. (1965) *Annals of the New York Academy of Science*, **132**, 526–535

KNOX, J.F., HOLMES, S., DOLL, R. and HILL, I.D. (1968) *British Journal of Industrial Medicine*, **25**, 293–303

KOBUSCH, A.-B., SIMARD, A., FELDSTEIN, M., VAUCLAIR, R., GIBBS, G.W., BERGERON, F. *et al.* (1984) *Journal of Chronic Disease*, **37**, 599–607

KOLONEL, L.N. (1976) *Cancer*, **37**, 1782–1787

KOLONEL, L.N., HIROHATA, T., CHAPPELL, B.V., VIOLA, F.V. and HARRIS, D.E. (1980) *Journal of the National Cancer Institute*, **64**, 739–743

KOLONEL, L.N. and WINKELSTEIN, W. (1977) *Lancet*, **ii**, 566–567

KONO, S., TOKUDOME, S., IKEDA, M., YOSHIMURA, T. and KURATSUNE, M. (1983) *Journal of the National Cancer Institute*, **70**, 443–446

KOSKELA, R.S., HERNBERG, S., KARAVA, R., JARVINEN, E. and NURMINEN, M. (1976) *Scandinavian Journal of Work and Environmental Health*, **2**, Suppl. 1, 73–89

KOSS, L.G., MELAMED, M.R. and KELLY, R.E. (1969) *Journal of the National Cancer Institute*, **43**, 233–243

KOSS, L.G., MELAMED, M.R., RICCI, A., MELICK, W.F. and KELLY, R.E. (1965) *New England Journal of Medicine*, **272**, 767–770

KRAUS, A.S., LEVIN, M.L. and GERHARDT, P.R. (1957) *American Journal of Public Health*, **47**, 961–970

KRISTOFERSEN, L. (1979) *Occupational Mortality*. Oslo: Central Bureau of Statistics

KUNZ, E., SEVI, J., PLACET, V. and HORACEK, J. (1979) *Health Physics*, **36**, 699–706

KURATSUNE, M., TOKUDOME, S., SHIRAKUSA, T., YOSHIDA, M., TOKUMITSU, Y., HAYANO, T. *et al.* (1974) *International Journal of Cancer*, **13**, 552–558

KURODA, S. and KAWAHATA, K. (1936) *Zeitschrift fur Krebsforschung*, **45**, 36–39

KURPPA, K., KOSKELA, R.S. and GUDBERGSSON, H. (1982) *Lancet*, **ii**, 150

KUSCHNER, M. (1981) *Environmental Health Perspectives*, **40**, 101–105

KVALE, G., HOIBY, E.A. and PEDERSON, E. (1979) *International Journal of Cancer*, **23**, 593–597

KWA, S-L. and FINE, L.J. (1980) *Journal of Occupational Medicine*, **22**, 792–794

LAMPERTH-SEILER, E. (1974) *Schweizerische Medizinische Wochenschrift*, **104**, 1655–1659

LANCASTER, H.O. and NELSON, J. (1951) *Medical Journal of Australia*, **44**, 452–456

LANCET (1965) **ii**, 1173

LANCET (1968) **i**, 76–77

LANCET (1970) **ii**, 758–759

LANCET (1971) **i**, 787–788

LANCET (1976) **i**, 944–945

LANCET (1977) **i**, 1348–1349

LANCET (1979a) **ii**, 1114–1115

LANCET (1979b) **i**, 1121–1122

LANCET (1983a) **i**, 511–512

LANCET (1983b) **ii**, 26

LANCET (1984a) **i**, 203

LANCET (1984b) **i**, 1221–1222

LANCET (1984c) **i**, 1390–1391

LANGARD, S., ANDERSON, A. and GYLSETH, B. (1980) *British Journal of Industrial Medicine*, **37**, 114–120

LANGARD, S. and NORSETH, T. (1975) *British Journal of Industrial Medicine*, **32**, 62–65

LANGARD, S. and VIGANDER, T. (1983) *British Journal of Industrial Medicine*, **40**, 71–74

LANGE, C.-E., JUHE, S., STEIN, G. and VELTMAN, G. (1975) *Annals of the New York Academy of Science*, **246**, 18–21

LANGER, A.M. and McCAUGHEY, W.T.E. (1982) *Lancet*, **ii**, 1102–1103

LAROUZE, B., LONDON, W.T., SAIMOT, G., WERNER, B.G., LUSTBADER, E.D., PAYET, M. *et al.* (1976) *Lancet*, **ii**, 534–538

LARSSON, L.G. and DAMBER, I. (1982) *Cancer Detection and Prevention*, **5**, 385–389

LARSSON, L., SANDSTROM, A. and WESTLING, P. (1975) *Cancer Research*, **35**, 3308–3316

LEA, A.J. (1964) *Annals of Rheumatic Disease*, **23**, 480–484

LEA, A.J. (1965) *Annals of the Royal College of Surgeons*, **37**, 169–176

LECK, I., SIBARY, K. and WAKEFIELD, J. (1978) *Journal of Epidemiology and Community Health*, **32**, 108–110

LECK, I. and STEWARD, J.K. (1972) *British Medical Journal*, **iv**, 631–634

LEE, T. (1980) *Times*, 13/11/80

LEE, W.R., ALDERSON, M.R. and DOWNES, J.E. (1972) *British Journal of Industrial Medicine*, **29**, 188–195

LEE, A.M. and FRAUMENI, J.F. (1969) *Journal of the National Cancer Institute*, **42**, 1045–1052

LEE, F.I. and HARRY, D.S. (1974) *Lancet*, **ii**, 1316–1318

LEE-FELDSTEIN, A. (1983) *Journal of the National Cancer Institute*, **70**, 601–610

LEICHER, F. (1954) *Archiv Gewerbepathologie und Gewerbehygiene*, **13**, 382–392

LEMEN, R. and DEMENT, J.M. (1979) *Dusts and Diseases.* Illinois: Pathotox

LEMEN, R.A., LEE, J.S., WAGONER, J.K. and BLEJER, H.P. (1976) *Annals of the New York Academy of Science*, **271**, 273–279

LERCH, I. (1980) *New Scientist*, 3/1/80, 8–11

LERER, T.J., REDMOND, C.K., BRESLIN, P.P., SALVIN, L. and RUSH, A.W. (1974) *Journal of Occupational Medicine*, **16**, 608–614

LETTERER, E., NEIDHART, K. and KLETT, H. (1944) *Archiv fur Gewerbepathologie und Gewerbehygiene*, **12**, 323–361

LEVENE, A. (1976) *Lancet*, **ii**, 475

LEVIN, M.L., KRESS, L.C. and GOLDSTEIN, H. (1942) *New York State Journal of Medicine*, **42**, 1737–1744

LEVINE, R.J., ANDJELKOVICH, D.A., SHAW, L.K. AND DALCORSO, R.D. (1983c) In *Formaldehyde: Toxicology, Epidemiology, Mechanisms.* Eds. J.J. Clary, J.E. Gibson and R.S. Waritz. pp. 127–140. New York: Marcel Dekker

LEVINE, R.J., BLUNDEN, P.B., DALCORSO, R.D., STARR, T.B. and ROSS, C.E. (1983a) *Journal of Occupational Medicine*, **25**, 591–597

LEVINE, R.J., DALCORSO, R.D., BLUNDEN, P.B. and BATIGELLI, M.C. (1983b) In *Formaldehyde Toxicity.* Ed. J.E. Gibson. pp. 212–226. New York: Hemisphere

LEVINSON, C. (1981) *Ethylene Oxide: New Findings Deepen Cancer Suspicion.* Geneva: Internationale Federation von Chemie Energie und Fabrikarbeiteverbanden

LEVY, S. (1972) *British Journal of Industrial Medicine*, **29**, 196–200

LEW, E.W. (1979) *Anesthesiology*, **51**, 195–199

LEWIS, A.C.W. and DAVISON, B.C.C. (1969) *Lancet*, **ii**, 235–237

LEWIS, E.B. (1963) *Science*, **142**, 1492–1494

LI, F.P., CASSADY, J.R. and JAFFE, N. (1975) *Cancer*, **35**, 1230–1235

LI, F.P., FRAUMENI, J.F., MANTEL, N. and MILLER, R.W. (1969) *Journal of the National Cancer Institute*, **43**, 1159–1164

LI, F.P., RAPPORT, A.H., FRAUMENI, J.F. and JENSEN, R.D. (1970) *Journal of the American Medical Association*, **214**, 1559–1561

LIDDELL, D. and MILLER, K. (1983) *Scandinavian Journal of Work and Environmental Health*, **9**, 1–8

LIDDELL, F.D.K. (1960) *British Journal of Industrial Medicine*, **17**, 228–233

LIDDELL, F.D.K. (1973) *British Journal of Industrial Medicine*, **30**, 15–24

LIDDELL, F.D.K. (1975) *Archives of Environmental Health*, **30**, 266–267

LIDDELL, F.D.K., McDONALD, J.C. and THOMAS, D.C. (1977) *Journal of the Royal Statistical Society, series A*, **140**, 469–491

LIEBEN, J. and PISTAWKA, H. (1967) *Archives of Environmental Health*, **14**, 559–563

LILIS, R. and NICHOLSON, W.J. (1976) In *Proceeding of NIOSH Styrene Butadiene Briefing.* Cincinnati: US Department of Health, Education and Welfare

LIN, R. and KESSLER, I. (1981) *Journal of the American Medical Association*, **245**, 147–152

LINDAHL, O. (1972) *Lakartidnigen*, **69**, 2945–2948

LINDQUIST, C. and TEPPO, L. (1978) *British Journal of Cancer*, **37**, 983–989

LINOS, A., KYLE, R.A., O'FALLON, W.M. and KURLAND, L.T. (1980) *International Journal of Epidemiology*, **9**, 131–135

LIONE, J.G. and DENHOLM, J.S. (1959) *Archives of Industrial Health*, **19**, 530–539

LIPKIN, I.L. (1972) In *Some Results of a Study of Pollution of the Environment with Carcinogenic Substances.* Ed. L.M. Shabad. pp. 107–111. Moscow: Ministry of Public Health

LIPPMANN, M. and GOLDSTEIN, D.G. (1970) *Archives of Environmental Health*, **21**, 591–599

LITTLEFIELD, L.G. and GOH, K.O. (1973) *Cytogenetics and Cell Genetics*, **12**, 17–22

LLOYD, D.C., PURROTT, R.J., PROSSER, J.S., EDWARDS, A.A., DOLPHIN, G.W., WHITE, A.D. *et al.* (1978) *Doses in Radiation Accidents Investigated by Chromosome Aberration Analysis.* London: HMSO

LLOYD, J.W. (1971) *Journal of Occupational Medicine*, **13**, 53–68

LLOYD, J.W. (1975) *Journal of Occupational Medicine*, **17**, 333–334

LLOYD, J.W. and CIOCCO, A. (1969) *Journal of Occupational Medicine*, **11**, 299–310

LLOYD, J.W., DECOUFLE, P. and SALVIN, L.G. (1977) *Journal of Occupational Medicine*, **19**, 543–550

LLOYD, J.W., LUNDIN, F.E., REDMOND, C.K. and GEISER, P.B. (1970) *Journal of Occupational Medicine*, **12**, 151–157

LLOYD, O.LL. (1978) *Lancet*, **i**, 318–320

LLOYD, O.LL., SCLARE, G., LLOYD, M.M. and YULE, F.A. (1982) In *Cancer Epidemiology.* Ed. E. Grundman. pp. 103–114. Stuttgart: Gustav Fischer Verlag

LLOYD DAVIES, T.A. (1971) *Respiratory Disease in Foundrymen.* London: HMSO

LOBE, L-P. and EHRHARDT, H-P. (1978) *Deutsch Gesundheitswes*, **33**, 1037–1040

LOCKWOOD, K. (1961) *Acta Pathologica Microbiologica Scandinavica*, **51**, Suppl. 145, 1–166

LOGAN, W.P.D. (1982) *Cancer Mortality by Occupation and Social Class 1851–1971.* London: HMSO

LOGUE, J.N., KOONTZ, M.D. and HATTWICK, M.A. (1982) *Journal of Occupational Medicine,* **24**, 398–408

LORENZ, E. (1944) *Journal of the National Cancer Institute,* **5**, 1–15

LUBIN, J.H., POTTERN, L.M., BLOT, W.J., TOKUDOME, S., STONE, B.J. and FRAUMENI, J.F. (1981) *Journal of Occupational Medicine,* **23**, 779–784

LUEPKER, R.V. and SMITH, M.L. (1978) *Journal of Occupational Medicine,* **20**, 677–682

LUMLEY, K.P.S. (1976) *British Journal of Industrial Medicine,* **33**, 108–114

LUNDIN, F.E., LLOYD, J.W., SMITH, E.M., ARCHER, V.E. and HOLADAY, D.A. (1969) *Health Physics,* **16**, 571–578

LUNDIN, F.W., WAGONER, J.K. and ARCHER, V.E. (1971) *Radon Daughter Exposure and Respiratory Cancer.* NIOSH–NIEHS joint monograph 1. Springfield: Illinois

LYNCH, H.T., LARSEN, A.L., MAGNUSON, C.W. and KRUSH, A.J. (1966) *Cancer,* **19**, 1891–1897

LYNCH, J., HANIS, N.M., BIRD, M.G., MURRAY, J.M. and WALSH, J.P. (1979) *Journal of Occupational Medicine,* **21**, 333–341

LYNCH, K.M. and SMITH, W.A. (1935) *American Journal of Cancer,* **24**, 56–64

LYNGE, E., ANDERSEN, O. and KRISTENSEN, T.S. (1983) *Lancet,* **i**, 527–528

LYON, J.L., FILLMORE, J.L. and KLAUBER, M.R. (1977) *Lancet,* **ii**, 869

LYON, J.L., GARDNER, J.W. and KLAUBER, M.R. (1976) *Lancet,* **i**, 1243

LYON, J.L., KLAUBER, M.R., GARDNER, J.W. and SMART, C.R. (1976) *New England Journal of Medicine,* **294**, 129–133

MACBETH, R. (1965) *Journal of Laryngology,* **79**, 592–612

McCALLUM, R.I., WOOLEY, V. and PETRIE, A. (1983) *British Journal of Industrial Medicine,* **40**, 384–389

McCAUGHAN, G., PARSONS, C. and GALLAGHER, N.D. (1979) *Medical Journal of Australia,* **i**, 304–306

McCREA CURNEN, M.G., VARMA, A.A.D., CHRISTINE, B.W. and TURGEON, L.R. (1974) *Journal of the National Cancer Institute,* **53**, 943–947

McCULLAGH, S.F. (1980) *Journal of the Society of Occupational Medicine,* **30**, 153–156

MACDONALD, E. (1956) *Proceedings of the Third National Cancer Congress.* pp. 181–185. Philadelphia: Lippincott

McDONALD, A.D. and FRY, J.S. (1982) *Scandinavian Journal of Work and Environmental Health,* **8**, Suppl. 1, 53–58

McDONALD, A.D., FRY, J.S., WOOLEY, A.J. and McDONALD, J.C. (1983a) *British Journal of Industrial Medicine,* **40**, 361–367

McDONALD, A.D., FRY, J.S., WOOLEY, A.J. and McDONALD, J.C. (1983b) *British Journal of Industrial Medicine,* **40**, 368–374

McDONALD, A.D., FRY, J.S., WOOLEY, A.J. and McDONALD, J.C. (1984) *British Journal of Industrial Medicine,* **41**, 151–157

McDONALD, A.D. and McDONALD, J.C. (1978) *Environmental Research,* **17**, 340–346

McDONALD, A.D. and McDONALD, J.C. (1980) *Cancer,* **46**, 1650–1656

McDONALD, J.A., LI, F.P. and MEHTA, C.R. (1979) *Journal of Occupational Medicine,* **21**, 811–813

McDONALD, J.C., BECKLAKE, M.R., GIBBS, G.W., McDONALD, A.D. and ROSSITER, C.E. (1974) *Archives of Environmental Health,* **28**, 61–68

McDONALD, J.C., LIDDELL, F.D.K., GIBBS, G.W., EYSSEN, G.E. and McDONALD, A.D. (1980) *British Journal of Industrial Medicine,* **37**, 11–24

McDONALD, J.C., McDONALD, A.D., GIBBS, G.W., SIEMATYCKI, J. and ROSSITER, C.E. (1971) *Archives of Environmental Health,* **22**, 677–686

McDONALD, J.C., ROSSITER, C.E., EYSSEN, G. and McDONALD, A.D. (1973) In *Proceedings of the IVth International Pneumoconiosis Conference* (Bucharest, 1971). pp. 232–237. Bucharest: Apimondia

McDOWALL, M. (1983) *Lancet,* **i**, 246

McDOWALL, M. and BALARAJAN, R. (1984) *Lancet,* **i**, 510–511

McDOWALL, M.E. (1984) *British Journal of Industrial Medicine,* **41**, 179–182

McELHENY, V.K. (1981) In *Quantification of Occupational Cancer.* Eds R. Peto and M. Schneidermann. pp. 689–694. New York: Cold Spring Harbour Laboratory

McGINTY, L. (1978) *Chemistry in Britain,* **14**, 508–514

McGOOGAN, E. and CAMERON, H. (1978) *Scottish Medical Journal,* **23**, 19–22

MacINTYRE, I. (1975) *Journal of Occupational Medicine,* **17**, 23–26

MacKENZIE, I. (1965) *British Journal of Cancer,* **19**, 1–8

McLAUGHLIN, A.I.G. and HARDING, H.E. (1956) *Archives of Industrial Health,* **14**, 350–378

McLAUGHLIN, J.K., BLOT, W.J., MANDEL. J.S., SCHUMAN, L.M., MEHL, E.S. and FRAUMENI, J.F. (1983) *Journal of the National Cancer Institute,* **71**, 287–291

MACLEAN, J.T. and FOWLER, V.B. (1965) *Journal of Urology,* **75**, 384–423

MACMAHON, B. (1962) *Journal of the National Cancer Institute,* **28**, 1173–1191

MACMAHON, B., COLE, P., LIN, T.M., LOWE, C.R., MIRRA, A.P., RAVNIHAR, B. *et al.* (1970b) *Bulletin of the World Health Organisation,* **43**, 209–221

MACMAHON, B., LIN, T.M., LOWE, C.R., MIRRA, A.P., RAVNIHAR, B., SALBER, E.J. *et al.* (1970a) *Bulletin of the World Health Organisation,* **42**, 185–194

McMICHAEL, A.J. (1976) *Journal of Occupational Medicine,* **18**, 165–168

McMICHAEL, A.J., ANDJELKOVIC, D.A. and TYROLER, H.A. (1976) *Annals of the New York Academy of Science,* **271**, 125–137

McMICHAEL, A.J. and HARTSHORNE, J.M. (1982) *Medical Journal of Australia,* **i**, 253–256

McMICHAEL, A.J., HAYNES, S.G. and TYROLER, H.A. (1975) *Journal of Occupational Medicine,* **17**, 128–131

McMICHAEL, A.J. and JOHNSON, H.M. (1982) *Journal of Occupational Medicine,* **24**, 375–378

McMICHAEL, A.J., SPIRTAS, R., GAMBLE, J.F. and TOUSEY, P.M. (1976) *Journal of Occupational Medicine,* **18**, 178–185

McMICHAEL, A.J., SPIRTAS, R. and KUPPER, L.L. (1974) *Journal of Occupational Medicine,* **16**, 458–464

McMICHAEL, A.J., SPIRTAS, R., KUPPER, L.L. and GAMBLE, J.F. (1975) *Journal of Occupational Medicine,* **17**, 234–239

McMILLAN, G.H.G., PETHYBRIDGE, R.J. and SHEERS, G. (1980) *British Journal of Industrial Medicine,* **37**, 268–272

McNULTY, J.C. (1962) *Medical Journal of Australia,* **ii**, 935–955

MABUCHI, K., LILIENFELD, A.M. and SNELL, L.M. (1979) *Archives of Industrial Health,* **34**, 312–320

MABUCHI, K., LILIENFELD, A.M. and SNELL, L.M. (1980) *Preventive Medicine,* **9**, 51–77

MACHLE, W. and GREGORIUS, F. (1948) *Public Health Reports,* **63**, 1114–1127

MACK, T.M. and PAGANINI-HILL, A. (1981) *Cancer,* **47,** 1471–1483

MADISON, R., AFIFI, A.A. and MITTMAN, C. (1984) *Journal of Chronic Disease,* **37,** 167–176

MAGNUS, K., ANDERSEN, A. and HOGETVEIT, A.C. (1982) *International Journal of Cancer,* **30,** 681–685

MAILLARD, J.M. (1980) *Pneumon et Coeur,* **36,** 41–48

MALCOLM, D. and BARNETT, H.A.R. (1982) *British Journal of Industrial Medicine,* **39,** 410–410

MALEK, B., KREMAROVA, B. and RODOVA, O. (1980) *Lekarske Prace,* **31,** 124–126

MALKER, H.R., MALKER, B.K. and BLOT, W.J. (1983) *Lancet,* **ii,** 858

MALKER, H.R., MALKER, B.K., McLAUGHLIN, J.K. and BLOT, W.J. (1984) *Lancet,* **i,** 56

MALKER, H. and WEINER, J. (1984) *Arbete och Halsa,* **9,** 1–107

MANCUSO, T. (1963) *Acta Unio International Contra Cancrum,* **19,** 488–489

MANCUSO, T. (1970) *Environmental Research,* **3,** 251–275

MANCUSO, T. (1975) In *Proceedings of the International Conference on Heavy Metals in the Environment.* Ed. T.C. Hutchinson. pp. 343–356. Toronto: Institute for Environmental Studies

MANCUSO, T.F. (1979) In *Dusts and Diseases.* Eds R. Lemen and J.M. Dement. pp. 463–471. Illinois: Pathotox

MANCUSO, T.F. (1980) *Environmental Research,* **21,** 48–55

MANCUSO, T.F. (1983) *American Journal of Industrial Medicine,* **4,** 510–513

MANCUSO, T.F. and BRENNAN, M.J. (1970) *Journal of Occupational Medicine,* **12,** 333–341

MANCUSO, T.F., CIOCCO, A. and EL-ATTAR, A.A. (1968) *Journal of Occupational Medicine,* **10,** 213–232

MANCUSO, T.F. and COULTER, E.J. (1959) *American Journal of Public Health,* **49,** 1525–1536

MANCUSO, T.F. and COULTER, E.J. (1963) *Archives of Environmental Health,* **6,** 210–226

MANCUSO, T.F. and EL-ATTAR, A.A. (1966) *Industrial Medicine and Surgery,* **35,** 1059–1067

MANCUSO, T.F. and EL-ATTAR, A.A. (1967a) *Journal of Occupational Medicine,* **9,** 277–285

MANCUSO, T.F. and EL-ATTAR, A.A. (1967b) *Journal of Occupational Medicine,* **9,** 147–162

MANCUSO, T.F. and EL-ATTAR, A.A. (1969) *Journal of Occupational Medicine,* **11,** 422–434

MANCUSO, T.F. and HUEPER, W.C. (1951) *Industrial Medicine and Surgery,* **20,** 358–363

MANCUSO, T.F., STEWART, A. and KNEALE, G. (1977) *Health Physics,* **33,** 369–385

MANNING, K.P., SKEGG, D.C.G., STELL, P.M. and DOLL, R. (1981) *Clinical Otolaryngology,* **6,** 165–170

MANTEL, N. and STARK, C.R. (1968) *Biometrics,* **24,** 997–1005

MARAM, E.M., LUDWIG, J. and KURLAND, L.T. (1979) *American Journal of Epidemiology,* **109,** 152–157

MARCH, H.C. (1950) *American Journal of Medical Science,* **220,** 282–286

MARONI, M., COLOMBI, A., ARBOSTI, G., CANTONI, S. and FOA, V. (1981) *British Journal of Industrial Medicine,* **38,** 55–60

MARSH, G.M. (1982) *British Journal of Industrial Medicine,* **39,** 313–322

MARSH, G.M. (1983a) In *Formaldehyde Toxicity.* Ed. J.E. Gibson. pp. 237–255. New York: Hemisphere

MARSH, G.M. (1983b) *Journal of Occupational Medicine,* **25,** 219–230

MARSH, G.M. and ENTERLINE, P.E. (1979) *Journal of Occupational Medicine,* **21,** 665–670

MARTINEZ, I. (1969) *Journal of the National Cancer Institute,* **42,** 1069–1094

MARTINSCHNIG, K.M., NEWELL, D.J., BARNSLEY, W.C., COWAN, W.K., FEINMAN, E.L. and OLIVER, E. (1977) *British Medical Journal,* **i,** 746–749

MARTLAND, H.S. (1929) *Journal of the American Medical Association,* **92,** 466–473

MARTLAND, H.S., CONLON, P. and KNEE, J.P. (1925) *Journal of the American Medical Association,* **85,** 1769–1776

MARUCHI, N., BRIAN, D., LUDWIE, J., ELVEBACK, L.R. and KURLAND, L.T. (1979) *Mayo Clinic Proceedings,* **54,** 245–249

MASON, T.J. (1975) *Environmental Health Perspectives,* **11,** 79–84

MASON, T.J. (1976) *Annals of the New York Academy of Science,* **270,** 370–376

MASON, T.J., FRAUMENI, J.F. and McKAY, F.W. (1972) *Journal of the National Cancer Institute,* **49,** 661–664

MASTROMATTEO, E. (1955) *British Journal of Industrial Medicine,* **12,** 240–243

MASTROMATTEO, E. (1967) *Journal of Occupational Medicine,* **9,** 127–136

MATANOSKI, G.M., SARTWELL, P.E. and ELLIOTT, E.A. (1975) *Lancet,* **i,** 926–927

MATANOSKI, G.M., SELTSER, R., SARTWELL, P.E., DIAMOND, E.L. and ELLIOTT, E.A. (1975a) *American Journal of Epidemiology,* **101,** 188–198

MATANOSKI, G.M., SELTSER, R., SARTWELL, P.E., DIAMOND, E.L. and ELLIOTT, E.A. (1975b) *American Journal of Epidemiology,* **101,** 199–210

MATANOSKI, G.M., LANDAU, E., TONASCIA, J., LAZAR, C., ELLIOTT, E.A., McENROE, W. et al. (1981) *Environmental Research,* **25,** June, 8–28

MATOLO, N.M., KLAUBER, M.R., FORISHEK, W.M. and DIXON, J.A. (1972) *Cancer,* **29,** 733–737

MATSUNAGA, E. (1980) *Journal of the National Cancer Institute,* **65,** 47–51

MAUPAS, P., WERNER, B., LAROUZE, B., MILLMAN, I., LONDON, W.T., O'CONNELL, A. et al. (1975) *Lancet,* **ii,** 9–11

MAXWELL, K.J. and ELWOOD, J.M. (1983) *Lancet,* **ii,** 579

MAY, G. (1982) *British Journal of Industrial Medicine,* **39,** 128–135

MAZUMDAR, S., REDMOND, C., SOLLECITO, W. and SUSSMAN, N. (1975) *Journal of Air Pollution Control Association,* **25,** 382–389

MEDICAL RESEARCH COUNCIL (1973) *British Medical Journal,* **i,** 213–216

MEINHARDT, T.J., YOUNG, R.J. and HARTLE, R.W. (1978) *Scandinavian Journal of Work and Environmental Health,* **4,** Suppl. 2, 240–246

MELAMED, M.R., KOSS, L.G., RICCI, A. and WHITMORE, W.F. (1960) *Cancer,* **13,** 67–74

MELICK, W.F., ESCUE, H.M., NARYKA, J.J., MEZERA, R.A. and WHEELER, E.P. (1955) *Journal of Urology,* **74,** 760–766

MELICK, W.F., NARYKA, J.J. and KELLY, R.E. (1971) *Journal of Urology,* **106,** 220–226

MENCK, H.R. and HENDERSON, B.E. (1976) *Journal of Occupational Medicine,* **18,** 797–801

MENCK, H.R., PIKE, M.C., HENDERSON, B.E. and JING, J.S. (1977) *Journal of the National Cancer Institute,* **59,** 1423–1425

MERCHANT, J.A. and ORTMEYER, C. (1981) *Chest,* **79,** Supplement, 6S–11S

MERETOJA, T., JARVENTAUS, H., SORSA, M. and VAINIO, H. (1978) *Scandinavian Journal of Work and Environmental Health*, **4**, 259–264

MEREWETHER, E.R.A. (1949) *Annual Report of the Chief Inspector of Factories for the Year 1947.* pp. 79–81. London: HMSO

MERLER, E., CARNEVALE, F., D'ANDREA, F. and SOLARI, P.L. (1982) In *Prevention of Occupational Cancer.* pp. 268–272. Geneva: ILO

METTLER, F.A., HEMPLEMANN, L.H., DUTTON, A.M., PIFER, J.W., TOYOOKA, E.T. and AMES, W.R. (1969) *Journal of the National Cancer Institute*, **43**, 803–811

MEURMAN, L.O., KIVILUOTO, R. and HAKAMA, M. (1974) *British Journal of Industrial Medicine*, **31**, 105–112

MEURMAN, L.O., KIVILUOTO, R. and HAKAMA, M. (1979) *Annals of the New York Academy of Science*, **330**, 491–495

MEYER, W.H. and CHURCH, F.W. (1961) *Medical Bulletin*, **21**, 256–265

MICHEL-BRIAND, C. and SIMONIN, M. (1977) *Archives Maladies Professionelles*, **38**, 1001–1013

MILHAM, S. (1971) *American Journal of Epidemiology*, **94**, 307–310

MILHAM, S. (1974a) *New England Journal of Medicine*, **290**, 1329

MILHAM, S. (1974b) *A Study of the Mortality Experience of the AFL–CIO United Brotherhood of Carpenters and Joiners of America, 1969–70.* Springfield VA: National Technical Information Service

MILHAM, S. (1976) *Occupational Mortality in Washington State, 1950–71.* Vols 1–3. Cincinatti, Ohio: US Department of Health, Education and Welfare

MILHAM, S. (1979) *Journal of Occupational Medicine*, **21**, 475–480

MILHAM, S. (1982a) *Lancet*, **i**, 690

MILHAM, S. (1982b) *New England Journal of Medicine*, **307**, 249

MILHAM, S. (1982c) *Lancet*, **i**, 1464–1465

MILHAM, S. (1983) *Occupational Mortality in Washington State, 1950–79.* Cincinatti, Ohio: US Department of Health and Human Services

MILHAM, S. and HESSER, J.E. (1967) *Lancet*, **ii**, 136–137

MILHAM, S. and STRONG, T. (1974) *Environmental Research*, **7**, 176–182

MILLER, A.B. (1977) *Cancer Research*, **37**, 2939–2942

MILLER, A.B. (1983) *Journal of Occupational Medicine*, **25**, 439–442

MILLER, A.B., KELLY, A., CHOI, N.W., MATTHEWS, V., MORGAN, R.W., MUNAN, L. *et al.* (1978) *American Journal of Epidemiology*, **108**, 499–509

MILLER, B.G., JACOBSEN, M. and STEELE, R.C. (1981) *Coalminers' Mortality in Relation to Radiological Category, Lung Function, and Exposure to Airborne Dust.* Edinburgh: Institute of Occupational Medicine

MILLER, R.W. and JABLON, S. (1970) *Radiology*, **96**, 269–276

MILLS, P.K., NEWELL, G.R. and JOHNSON, D.E. (1984) *Lancet*, **i**, 207–211

MILNE, J.E.H. (1976a) *British Journal of Industrial Medicine*, **33**, 115–122

MILNE, J. (1976b) *British Journal of Industrial Medicine*, **33**, 47–48

MINER, J.K., ROM, W.N., LIVINGSTON, G.K. and LYON, J.L. (1983) *Journal of Occupational Medicine*, **25**, 30–33

MITTRA, I. and HAYWARD, J.L. (1974) *Lancet*, **i**, 885–891

MODAN, B., RON, E. and WERNER, A. (1977) *Radiology*, **123**, 741–744

MOGHISSI, K.S., MACK, H.C. and PORZAK, J.P. (1968) *American Journal of Obstetrics and Gynaecology*, **100**, 607–614

MOLE, R.H. (1982) *British Journal of Industrial Medicine*, **39**, 200–201

MOLINA, G., HOLMBERG, B., ELOFSSON, S., HOLMLUND, L., MOOSINE, R. and WESTERHOLM, P. (1981) *Environmental Health Perspectives*, **41**, 145–151

MOMMSEN, S., ASGAARD, J. and SELL, A. (1982) *European Journal of Cancer*, **18**, 1205–1210

MONAGHAN, J.M. and SIRISENA, L.A.W. (1978) *British Medical Journal*, **i**, 1588–1590

MONSON, R.R. and FINE, L.J. (1978) *Journal of the National Cancer Institute*, **61**, 1047–1053

MONSON, R. and NAKANO, K.K. (1976a) *American Journal of Epidemiology*, **103**, 284–296

MONSON, R.R. and NAKANO, K.K. (1976b) *American Journal of Epidemiology*, **103**, 297–303

MONSON, R.R., PETERS, J.M. and JOHNSON, M.N. (1974) *Lancet*, **ii**, 397–398

MONTESANO, R. and TOMATIS, L. (1977) *Cancer Research*, **37**, 310–316

MOORE, S.R.W. (1969) *British Journal of Industrial Medicine*, **26**, 25–46

MORGAN, J.G. (1958) *British Journal of Industrial Medicine*, **15**, 224–234

MORGAN, R.W., CLAXTON, K.W., DIVINE, B.J., KAPLAN, S.D. and HARRIS, V.B. (1981) *Journal of Occupational Medicine*, **23**, 767–770

MORGAN, R.W. and JAIN, M.G. (1974) *Canadian Medical Association Journal*, **iii**, 1067–1070

MORGAN, R.W., KAPLAN, S.D. and BRATSBERG, J.A. (1981) *Archives of Environmental Health*, **36**, 179–183

MORGAN, R.W., KAPLAN, S.D. and GAFFEY, W.R. (1981) *Journal of Occupational Medicine*, **23**, 13–21

MORI, M., KIYOSAWA, H. and MIYAKE, H. (1984) *Cancer*, **53**, 2746–2752

MORI, W. (1967) *Cancer*, **20**, 627–631

MORINGA, K., OSHIMA, A. and HARA, I. (1982) *American Journal of Industrial Medicine*, **3**, 243–246

MORIYAMA, I.M. (1984) *American Journal of Public Health*, **74**, 621

MORIYAMA, I.M., BAUM, W.S., HAENSZEL, W.M. and MATTISON, B.F. (1958) *American Journal of Public Health*, **48**, 1376–1387

MORRISON, A.S. (1976) *Journal of the National Cancer Institute*, **56**, 731–733

MORRISON, A.S. and COLE, P. (1976) *Urological Clinics of North America*, **3**, 13–29

MOSBECH, J. and ACHESON, E.D. (1971) *Danish Medical Bulletin*, **18**, 34–35

MOSBECH, J. and VIDEBAEK, A. (1950) *British Medical Journal*, **ii**, 390–394

MOSES, M. and SELIKOFF, I.J. (1981) *Lancet*, **i**, 1370

MOSS, E. and LEE, W.R. (1974) *British Journal of Industrial Medicine*, **31**, 224–232

MOSS, E., SCOTT, T.S. and ATHERLEY, G.R.C. (1972) *British Journal of Industrial Medicine*, **29**, 1–14

MOULD, R.F. and BAKOWSKI, M.T. (1976) *Lancet*, **ii**, 1134–1135

MOVSHOVITZ, M. and MODAN, B. (1973) *Journal of the National Cancer Institute*, **51**, 777–779

MOWER, H.F., RAY, R.M., SHOFF, R., STEMMERMAN, G.M., NOMURA, A., GLOBER, G.A. *et al.* (1979) *Cancer Research*, **39**, 328–331

MULVIHILL, J.J. (1975) In *Persons at High Risk of Cancer.*

Ed. J.F. Fraumeni. pp. 1–35. New York: Academic Press

MUSICCO, M., FILIPPINI, G., BORDO, B.M., MELOTTO, A., MORELLO, G. and BERRINO, F. (1982) *American Journal of Epidemiology,* **116**, 782–790

MUSTACCHI, P. and MILLIMORE, D. (1976) *Journal of the National Cancer Institute,* **56**, 717–720

NAJARIAN, T. and COLTON, T. (1978) *Lancet,* i, 1018–1020

NAJEM, G.R., LOURIA, D.B., SEEBODE, J.J., THIND, I.S., PRUSAKOWSKI, J.M., AMBROSE, R.B. and FERNICOLA, A.R. (1982) *International Journal of Epidemiology,* **11**, 212–217

NASCA, P.C., LAWRENCE, C.E., GREENWALD, P., CHOROST, S., ARBUCE, J.T. and PAULSON, A. (1980) *Journal of the National Cancer Institute,* **64**, 23–28

NATIONAL BOARD OF HEALTH AND WELFARE (1980) *The Swedish Cancer–Environment Registry.* Stockholm: National Board of Health

NATIONAL INSTITUTE FOR OCCUPATIONAL SAFETY AND HEALTH (1977) *A Retrospective Survey of Cancer in Relation to Occupation.* PHS Publication 77-178. Washington: Government Printing Office

NATIONAL RADIOLOGICAL PROTECTION BOARD (1978) *Annual Research and Development Report.* London: HMSO

NELSON, W.C., LYKINS, M.H., MACKEY, J., NEWILL, V.V., FINKLER, J.F. and HAMMER, D.I. (1973) *Journal of Chronic Disease,* **26**, 105–118

NESS, G.O., DEMENT, J.M., WAXWEILER, R.J. and WAGONER, J.K. (1979) In *Dust and Diseases.* Eds R. Lemen and J.M. Dement. pp. 233–249. Illinois: Pathotox

NEUBAUER, O. (1947) *British Journal of Cancer,* **1**, 192–251

NEUBERGER, M., KUNDI, M., HAIDER, M. and GRUNDORFER, W. (1982) In *Prevention of Occupational Cancer.* pp. 235–241. Geneva: ILO

NEWELL, G.R., RAWLINS, W., KINNEAR, B.K., CORREA, P., HENDERSON, B.E., DWORSKY, R. et al. (1973) *Journal of the National Cancer Institute,* **51**, 1437–1441

NEWHOUSE, M. (1973) In *Biological Effects of Asbestos.* Eds P. Bogovski, J.C. Gilson, V. Timbrell and J.C. Wagner. pp. 203–208. Lyon: IARC

NEWHOUSE, M.L. (1969) *British Journal of Industrial Medicine,* **26**, 294–301

NEWHOUSE, M.L. (1978) *Annals of Occupational Hygiene,* **21**, 293–296

NEWHOUSE, M.L. and BERRY, G. (1973) *Lancet,* ii, 615

NEWHOUSE, M.L. and BERRY, G. (1976) *British Journal of Industrial Medicine,* **33**, 147–151

NEWHOUSE, M.L. and BERRY, G. (1979) *Annals of the New York Academy of Science,* **330**, 53–60

NEWHOUSE, M.L., BERRY, G. and SKIDMORE, J.W. (1982) *Annals of Occupational Hygiene,* **26**, 899–909

NEWHOUSE, M.L., BERRY, G., WAGNER, J.C. and TUROK, M.E. (1972) *British Journal of Industrial Medicine,* **29**, 134–141

NEWHOUSE, M.L., GREGORY, M.M. and SHANNON, H. (1980) In *Biological Effects of Mineral Fibres.* Ed. J.C. Wagner. Vol. 2. pp. 687–695. Lyon: IARC

NEWHOUSE, M.L., MILLER, B.F. and MOORE, W.K.S. (1976) Paper given at Seminar on *Biology of Talc used in Health Products,* Cardiff, May 1976

NEWHOUSE, M.L., PEARSON, R.M., FULLERTON, J.M., BOESEM, E.A.M. and SHANNON, H.S. (1977) *British Journal of Preventive and Social Medicine,* **31**, 148–153

NEWHOUSE, M.L. and THOMPSON, H. (1965) *British Journal of Industrial Medicine,* **22**, 261–266

NEWMAN, D. (1890) *Glasgow Medical Journal,* **33**, 469–470

NEWMAN, J.A., ARCHER, V.E., SACCOMANNO, G., KUSCHNER, M., AUERBACH, O., GRONDAHL, R.D. et al. (1976) *Annals of the New York Academy of Science,* **271**, 260–268

NEWSHOLME, A. (1903) *British Medical Journal,* ii, 1529–1531

NICHOLLS, J.C. (1974) *British Journal of Surgery,* **61**, 244–249

NICHOLSON, W.J., HAMMOND, E.C., SEIDMAN, H. and SELIKOFF, I.J. (1975) *Annals of the New York Academy of Science,* **246**, 225–230

NICHOLSON, W.J., PERKEL, G. and SELIKOFF, I.J. (1982) *American Journal of Industrial Medicine,* **3**, 259–311

NICHOLSON, W.J., SEIDMAN, H,. HOOS, D. and SELIKOFF, I.J. (1981) *The Mortality Experience of New York City Newspaper Pressmen, 1950–76.* New York: Mount Sinai School of Medicine

NICHOLSON, W.J., SELIKOFF, I.J. and SEIDMAN, H. (1978) *Scandinavian Journal of Work and Environmental Health,* **4**, Suppl. 2, 247–252

NICHOLSON; W.J., SELIKOFF, I.J., SEIDMAN, H., LILIS, R. and FORMBY, P. (1979) *Annals of the New York Academy of Science,* **330**, 11–21

NORDSTROM, S., BIRKE, E. and GUSTAVSSON, L. (1983) *Bioelectromagnetics,* **4**, 91–101

NORELL, S., AHLBOM, A., LIPPING, H. and OSTERBLOM, L. (1983) *Lancet,* i, 462–463

NORMAN, J.E. (1975) *Journal of the National Cancer Institute,* **54**, 311–317

NORMAN, J.E., ROBINETTE, C.D. and FRAUMENI, J.F. (1981) *Journal of Occupational Medicine,* **23**, 818–822

NORPRA, H., SORSA, M., VAINIO, H., GROHN, P., HEINONEN, E., HOLSTI, L. et al. (1980) *Scandinavian Journal of Work and Environmental Health,* **6**, 299–301

NORSETH, T. (1981) *Environmental Health Perspectives,* **40**, 121–130

NOVOTNA, E., DAVID, A. and MALEK, B. (1979) *Prace Lekarske,* **31**, 121–123

NURMINEN, M. and HERNBERG, S. (1984) *Journal of Occupational Medicine,* **26**, 341

O'BERG, M.T. (1980) *Journal of Occupational Medicine,* **22**, 245–252

OCCUPATIONAL SAFETY AND HEALTH ADMINISTRATION (1980) *Identification, Classification and Regulation of Occupational Carcinogens.* 45 Federal Register 5001

O'DONNELL, W.M., MANN, R.H. and GROSH, J.L. (1966) *Cancer,* **19**, 1143–1147

O'DONOVAN, W.J. (1924) *British Journal of Dermatology,* **36**, 477–481

OFFICE OF POPULATION CENSUSES AND SURVEYS (1973) *Cohort Studies, New Developments.* London: HMSO

OGLE, W. (1885) *Supplement to the 45th Annual Report of the Registrar General.* London: HMSO

OHSAKI, Y., ABE, S., KIMURA, K., TSUNETA, Y., MIKAMI, H. and MURAO, M. (1978) *Thorax,* **33**, 372–374

OKUBO, T. and TSUCHYA, K. (1977) *Keio Journal of Medicine,* **26**, 171–177

OLDHAM, P.D. and ROSSITER, C.E. (1965) *British Journal of Industrial Medicine,* **22**, 92–100

OLIN, R. (1976) *Lancet,* ii, 916

OLIN, R. (1978) *American Industrial Hygiene Journal,* **39**, 557–562

OLIN, R. and AHLBOM, A. (1980) *Environmental Research,* **22**, 154–161

OLSEN, J.H. and JENSEN, O.M. (1983) *Ugeskrift for Laeger,* **145**, 2951–2956

OLSEN, J.H. and JENSEN, O.M. (1984) *Lancet*, **ii**, 47–48

OLSEN, J. and SABROE, S. (1979) *International Journal of Epidemiology*, **8**, 375–382

OLSEN, J. and SABROE, S. (1984) *Journal of Epidemiology*, **38**, 117–121

OLSEN, J., SABROE, S. and LAJERS, M. (1984) *European Journal of Cancer and Clinical Oncology*, **20**, 639–643

OLSON, C. (1974) *Journal of the American Veterinary Medical Association*, **165**, 630–632

OLSSON, H. and BRANDT, L. (1979) *British Medical Journal*, **ii**, 580–581

OLSSON, H. and BRANDT, L. (1981) *Lancet*, **ii**, 579

OLSSON, H. and BRANDT, L. (1983) *Lancet*, **i**, 583

ORTMEYER, C.E., COSTELLO, J., MORGAN, W.K.C., SWECKER, S. and PETERSON, M. (1974) *Archives of Environmental Health*, **29**, 67–72

OSBORNE, R.H. and DE GEORGE, F.V. (1963) *American Journal of Human Genetics*, **15**, 380–388

OSBURN, H.S. (1957) *Central African Journal of Medicine*, **3**, 215–223

OSBURN, H.S. (1969) *South African Medical Journal*, **43**, 1307–1312

OTT, M.G., FISHBECK, W.A., TOWNSEND, J.C. and SCHNEIDER, E.J. (1976) *Journal of Occupational Medicine*, **18**, 735–738

OTT, M.G., HOLDER, B.B. and GORDON, H.G. (1974) *Archives of Environmental Health*, **29**, 250–255

OTT, M.G., HOLDER, B.B. and LANGER, R.R. (1976) *Journal of Occupational Medicine*, **18**, 171–177

OTT, M.G., HOLDER, B.B. and OLSON, R.D. (1980) *Journal of Occupational Medicine*, **22**, 47–50

OTT, M.G., KOLEESAR, R.C., SCHARNWEBER, E.J., SCHNEIDER, E.J. and WENABLE, J.R. (1980) *Journal of Occupational Medicine*, **22**, 445–460

OTT, M.G. and LANGNER, R.R. (1983) *Journal of Occupational Medicine*, **25**, 763–768

OTT, M.G., LANGNER, R.R. and HOLDER, B.B. (1975) *Archives of Environmental Health*, **30**, 333–339

OTT, M.G., SCHWARNWEBER, H.C. and LANGNER, R.R. (1980) *British Journal of Industrial Medicine*, **37**, 163–168

OTT, M.G., TOWNSEND, J.C., FISHBECK, W.A. and LANGNER, R.R. (1978) *Archives of Environmental Health*, **33**, 3–10

OTTERLAND, A. (1960) *Acta Medica Scandinavica*, supplement 357, 1–300

PADDLE, G.M. (1976) *Lancet*, **i**, 1079

PADDLE, G.M. (1980) *Archives of Toxicology*, supplement 3, 263–269

PADDLE, G.M. (1981) In *Quantification of Occupational Cancer*. Eds R. Peto and M. Schneiderman. pp. 177–186. New York: Cold Spring Harbour Laboratory

PAFFENBARGER, R.S., WING, A.L. and HYDE, T.R. (1977) *Journal of the National Cancer Institute*, **58**, 1489–1491

PAGANINI-HILL, A., GLAZER, E., HENDERSON, B.E. and ROSS, R.K. (1980) *Journal of Occupational Medicine*, **22**, 542–544

PAGE, R.C. (1955) *Archives of Industrial Health*, **2**, 126–131

PAGNOTTO, L.D., ELKINS, H.B. and BRUGSH, H.G. (1979) *American Industrial Hygiene Association Journal*, **40**, 137–146

PAGNOTTO, L.D., ELKINS, H.B., BRUGSH, H.G. and WALKLEY, E. (1961) *Industrial Hygiene*, **22**, 417–421

PALMER, W.G. and SCOTT, W.D. (1981) *American Industrial Hygiene Journal*, **42**, 329–340

PANEL ON NITRATES OF THE COORDINATING COMMITTEE FOR SCIENTIFIC AND TECHNICAL ASSESSMENTS OF ENVIRONMEN-TAL POLLUTANTS (1978) Washington: National Academy of Sciences

PARIS, J.A. (1825) *Pharmacologia*. London: Phillips

PARK, A.T. (1965–66) *Journal of Statistical and Social Inquiry of Ireland*, **21**, 24–42

PARKES, H.G. (1984) *Health and Safety at Work*, June, 1984

PARKES, H.G., VEYS, C.A., WATERHOUSE, J.A.H. and PETERS, A. (1982) *British Journal of Industrial Medicine*, **39**, 209–220

PARKINSON, G.S. (1971) *Annals of Occupational Hygiene*, **14**, 145–153

PARMEGGIANI, L. (1983) *Encyclopedia of Occupational Safety and Health*. 3rd edn. Vols 1 and 2. Geneva: ILO

PASTERNACK, B. and ERLICH, L. (1972) *Archives of Environmental Health*, **25**, 286–294

PASTERNAK, B.S., DUBIN, N. and MOSESON, M. (1983) *Lancet*, **i**, 704

PASTERNAK, B.S., SHORE, R.E. and ALBERT, R.E. (1977) *Journal of Occupational Medicine*, **19**, 741–746

PAYMASTER, J.C. and GANGADHARAN, P. (1967) *Journal of Urology*, **97**, 110–113

PAZDEROVA-VEJLUPKOVA, J., LUKAS, E., NEMCOVA, M., PICKOVA, J. and JIRASEK, L. (1981) *Archives of Environmental Health*, **36**, 5–11

PEARSON, E.S. and HARTLEY, H.O. (1970) *Biometrica Tables for Statisticians*, 3rd edn. Vol. 1. Cambridge: Cambridge University Press

PEDERSEN, E., HOGETVEIT, A.C. and ANDERSEN, A. (1973) *International Journal of Cancer*, **12**, 32–41

PEERS, F.G. and LINDSELL, C.A. (1973) *British Journal of Cancer*, **27**, 473–484

PELL, S. (1978) *Journal of Occupational Medicine*, **20**, 21–29

PELL, S., O'BERG, M.T. and KARRH, B.W. (1978) *Journal of Occupational Medicine*, **20**, 725–740

PERKEL, G., MAZZOCCHI, A. and BELICZKY, L. (1975) *Annals of the New York Academy of Science*, **246**, 311–312

PERRY, K., BOWLER, R.G., BUCKELL, H.M., DRUETT, H.A. and SCHILLING, R.S.F. (1948) *British Journal of Occupational Medicine*, **5**, 6–15

PERSHAGEN, G., ELINDER, C.G. and BOLANDER, A.M. (1977) *Environmental Health Perspectives*, **19**, 133–137

PETERSEN, G.R. and MILHAM, S. (1974) *Journal of the National Cancer Institute*, **53**, 957–958

PETERSEN, G.R. and MILHAM, S. (1980) *Occupational Mortality in California, 1959–61*. NIOSH Publication 80–104. Washington DC: US Government Printing Office

PETROVIC, S., TOMIC, M. and MUTAVOZIC, M. (1966) *Journal of Urology and Nephrology*, **72**, 429–444

PETO, J. (1978) *Lancet*, **i**, 484–489

PETO, J., DOLL, R., HOWARD, S.V., KINLEN, L.J. and LEWINSOHN, H.C. (1977) *British Journal of Industrial Medicine*, **34**, 169–173

PETO, J., SEIDMAN, H. and SELIKOFF, I.J. (1982) *British Journal of Cancer*, **45**, 124–135

PHAROAH, P.O.D., ALBERMAN, E., DOYLE, P. and CHAMBERLAIN, G. (1977) *Lancet*, **i**, 34–36

PHILLIPS, R.L. (1975) *Cancer Research*, **35**, 3513–3522

PICKLE, L.W. and GOTTLIEB, M.S. (1980) *American Journal of Public Health*, **70**, 256–259

PINTO, S.S. and BENNETT, B.M. (1963) *Archives of Environmental Health*, **7**, 583–591

PINTO, S.S., ENTERLINE, P.E., HENDERSON, V. and VARNER, M.O. (1977) *Environmental Health Perspectives*, **19**, 127–130

PINTO, S.S., HENDERSON, V. and ENTERLINE, P.E. (1978) *Archives of Environmental Health*, **33**, 325–331

POCHIN, E.E. (1960) *British Medical Journal*, ii, 1545–1550

POCHIN, E.E. (1967) *Clinical Radiology*, **18**, 113–125

POCHIN, E.E. (1975) *British Medical Bulletin*, **31**, 184–190

POCHIN, E.E. (1978) *Journal of the Royal College of Physicians*, **12**, 210–218

POCHIN, E.E. (1983) *The Biological Bases of the Assumptions made by NRPB in the Calculation of Health Effects: Proof of Evidence*. Chilton: NRPB

POKROVSKAYA, L.V. and SHABYNINA, N.H. (1973) *Gigiena Truda i Professionalnye Zabolevaniia*, **10**, 23–26

POLE, D.J., McCALL, M.G., READER, R. and WOODINGS, T. (1977) *Journal of Chronic Disease*, **30**, 19–27

POLEDNAK, A.P. (1978) *Journal of the National Cancer Institute*, **60**, 77–82

POLEDNAK, A.P. (1981) *Archives of Environmental Health*, **36**, 235–242

POLEDNAK, A.P., STEHNEY, A.F. and LUCAS, H.E. (1983) *Health Physics*, **44**, Suppl. 1, 239–251

POLEDNAK, A.P., STEHNEY, A.F. and ROWLAND, R.E. (1978) *American Journal of Epidemiology*, **107**, 179–195

PORTAL, R.W. (1961) *British Journal of Industrial Medicine*, **18**, 153–156

POTT, P. (1775) *Chirurgical Observations Relative to the Cataract, the Polypus of the Nose, the Cancer of the Scrotum, the Different Kinds of Ruptures, and the Mortification of the Toes and Feet*. London: Hawse Clark and Collins

POTTS, C.L. (1965) *Annals of Occupational Hygiene*, **8**, 55–61

POUR, P. and GHADIRIAN, P. (1974) *Cancer*, **33**, 1649–1652

PRESTON-MARTIN, S., HENDERSON, B.E. and PIKE, M.C. (1982) *Cancer*, **49**, 2201–2207

PRESTON-MARTIN, S., PAGANINI-HILL, A., HENDERSON, B.E., PIKE, M.C. and WOOD, C. (1980) *Journal of the National Cancer Institute*, **65**, 67–73

PRICE, C.H.G. (1962) *Journal of Bone and Joint Surgery*, **44b**, 366–376

PRIESTER, W.A. and MASON, T.J. (1974) *Journal of the National Cancer Institute*, **53**, 43–49

PRIESTER, W.A., OLEINICK, A. and CONNOR, G.H. (1970) *Lancet*, i, 367–368

PUFFER, R. and GRIFFITH, G.W. (1967) *Patterns of Urban Mortality*. Washington DC: Pan American Health Organization

PUNNONEN, R., GRONROOS, M. and PELTONEN, R. (1974) *Lancet*, ii, 949

PUTONI, R., VERCELLI, M., MERLO, F., VALERIO, F. and SANTI, L. (1979) *Annals of the New York Academy of Science*, **330**, 353–377

PYE-SMITH, R.J. (1913) *Proceedings of the Royal Society of Medicine*, **6**, Clinical section, 229–236

RADFORD, E.P. (1976) *Annals of the New York Academy of Science*, **271**, 228–238

RADFORD, E.P. and RENARD, K.G.STC. (1984) *New England Journal of Medicine*, **310**, 1485–1494

RADOWSKI, J.L., DEICHMANN, W.B. and CLIZER, E.E. (1968) *Food and Cosmetic Toxicology*, **6**, 209–224

RAMPEN, F.H.J. and MULDER, J.H. (1980) *Lancet*, i, 562–565

RAVICH, A. and RAVICH, R.A. (1951) *New York State Journal of Medicine*, **51**, 1519–1520

RAZIS, D.V., DIAMOND, H.D. and CRAVER, L.F. (1959) *Annals of Internal Medicine*, **51**, 933–971

REDMOND, C.K. and BRESLIN, P.P. (1975) *Journal of Occupational Medicine*, **17**, 313–317

REDMOND, C.K., CIOCCO, A., LLOYD, J.W. and RUSH, H.W. (1972) *Journal of Occupational Medicine*, **14**, 621–629

REDMOND, C.K., SMITH, E.M. and LLOYD, J.W. (1969) *Journal of Occupational Medicine*, **11**, 513–521

REDMOND, C.K., STROBINO, B.R. and CYPRESS, R.H. (1976) *Annals of the New York Academy of Science*, **271**, 102–115

REEVE, G.R., BOND, G.G., LLOYD, J.W., COOK, R.R., WAXWEILER, R.J. and FISHBECK, W.A. (1983) *Journal of Occupational Medicine*, **25**, 387–393

REEVE, G.R., THOMAS, T.L., KELLY, V.F., WAXWEILER, R.J. and ITAYA, S. (1982) *Annals of the New York Academy of Science*, **381**, 54–61

REGISTRAR GENERAL (1855) *14th Annual Report of the Registrar General of Births, Marriages, and Deaths in England*. London: HMSO

REGISTRAR GENERAL (1971) *Registrar General's Decennial Supplement, England and Wales, 1961, Occupational Mortality*. London: HMSO

REGISTRAR GENERAL (1978) *Registrar General's Decennial Supplement, England and Wales, 1971, Occupational Mortality*. London: HMSO

REGISTRAR GENERAL, SCOTLAND (1981) *Occupational Mortality, 1969–1973*. Edinburgh: General Register Office

REHN, L. (1895) *Archiv für Klinische Chirurgie*, **50**, 588–600

REID, D.D. and BUCK, C. (1956) *British Journal of Industrial Medicine*, **13**, 265–268

REID, D.D. and ROSE, G.A. (1964) *British Medical Journal*, ii, 1437–1439

REID, R., LAVERTY, C., COPPLESTON, M., ISARANGKUL, W. and HILLS, E. (1980) *Obstetrics and Gynaecology*, **55**, 476–483

REIMER, R.R., CLARK, W.H., GREENE, M.H., AINSWORTH, A.M. and FRAUMENI, J.F. (1978) *Journal of the American Medical Association*, **239**, 744–746

REISSLAND, J.A. (1978) *An Assessment of the Mancuso Study*. NRPB—79. London: HMSO

RENCHER, A.C., CARTER, M.W. and McKEE, M.W. (1977) *Journal of Occupational Medicine*, **19**, 754–758

REYNOLDS, P., AUSTIN, D. and THOMAS, J. (1982) *American Journal of Epidemiology*, **116**, 570

RIGEL, D.S., FRIEDMAN, R.J., LEVENSTEIN, M. and GREENWALD, D.J. (1983) *Lancet*, i, 704

RIIHIMAKI, V., ASP, S. and HERNBERG, S. (1982) *Scandinavian Journal of Work and Environmental Health*, **8**, 37–42

RIMINGTON, J. (1968) *British Medical Journal*, i, 732–734

RIMINGTON, J. (1971) *British Medical Journal*, ii, 373–375

RINSKY, R.A., YOUNG, R.J. and SMITH, A.B. (1981) *American Journal of Industrial Medicine*, **2**, 217–245

RINSKY, R.A., ZUMWALDE, R.D., WAXWEILER, R.J., MURRAY, W.E., BIERBAUM, P.J., LANDRIGAN, P.J. et al. (1981) *Lancet*, i, 231–235

RISBERG, B., NICKELS, J. and WAGERMARK, J. (1980) *Cancer*, **45**, 2422–2427

ROACH, S.A. (1970) *Annals of Occupational Hygiene*, **13**, 7–15

ROBBINS, A. (1982) *Annals of the New York Academy of Science*, **381**, xi

ROBENS, LORD (1972) *Safety and Health at Work*. Cmnd 5034. London: HMSO

ROBERTSON, J.McD. and INGALLS, T.H. (1980) *Archives of Industrial Health*, **35**, 181–186

ROBINETTE, C.D., HRUBEC, Z. and FRAUMENI, J.F. (1979) *American Journal of Epidemiology*, **109**, 687–700

ROBINSON, C.E., CEMENT, J.M., NESS, G.O. and WAXWEILER, R.J. (1982) *British Journal of Industrial Medicine*, **39**, 45–53

ROBINSON, C.E., LEMEN, R. and WAGONER, J.K. (1979) In *Dusts and Diseases*. Eds R. Lemen and J.M. Dement. pp. 131–143. Illinois: Pathotox

ROBINSON, H. (1969) *Journal of Occupational Medicine*, **11**, 411–416

ROBINSON, J.S., THOMPSON, J.M., BELCHER, R. and STEPHEN, W.I. (1976) *British Medical Journal*, ii, 815

ROBINSON, T.R. (1976) *Journal of Occupational Medicine*, **18**, 31–40

ROCHE, J., FOURNET, J., HOSTEIN, J., PANH, M. and BONNET-EYMARD, J. (1978) *Gastroenterologie Clinique et Biologique*, ii, 669–678

ROCKETTE, H.E. (1977) *Journal of Occupational Medicine*, **19**, 795–801

ROCKETTE, H.E. and ARENA, V.C. (1983) *Journal of Occupational Medicine*, **25**, 549–557

RODRICKS, J.V., ANDERSON, E.L., GAYLOR, D.W., HELLER, R.A., KELLER, R.A., KOVER, F. *et al.* (1979) *Scientific Bases for Identifying Potential Carcinogens and Estimating their Risks*. Washington: Interagency Regulating Liaison Group

ROE, F.J.C. (1978) *Annals of Occupational Hygiene*, **21**, 323–326

ROE, F.J.C. (1979) *Lancet*, ii, 744

ROJEL, J. (1953) *Acta Pathologica Microbiologica Scandinavica, Supplement* **97**, 1–82

ROSDAHL, N., LARSEN, S.O. and CLEMMESEN, J. (1974) *British Medical Journal*, ii, 253–256

ROSENBAUM, S. (1963) *British Medical Journal*, i, 169–170

ROSENBERG, H.M. (1981) In *Quantification of Occupational Cancer*. Eds R. Peto and M. Schneiderman. pp. 317–331. New York: Cold Spring Harbour Laboratory

ROSS, R., DWORSKY, R., NICHOLLS, P., PAGANINI-HILL, A., WRIGHT, W., KOSS, M. *et al.* (1982) *Lancet*, ii, 1118–1120

ROSS, R.K., McCURTIS, J.W., HENDERSON, B.E., MENICK, H.R., MACK, T.M. and MARTIN, S.P. (1979) *British Journal of Cancer*, **39**, 284–292

ROSSITER, C.E. and COLES, R.M. (1980) In *Biological Effects of Mineral Fibres*. Ed. J.C. Wagner. Vol. 1. pp. 713–721. Lyon: IARC

ROTH, F. (1959) *Zentralblatt für Allgemeine Pathologie und Pathologische Anatomie*, **100**, 529–530

ROTHMAN, K.J. (1982) In *Cancer Epidemiology and Prevention*. Eds D. Schottenfeld and J.F. Fraumeni. pp. 15–22. Philadelphia: Saunders

ROTHSCHILD, LORD (1978) *Times*, 24/11/78

ROTHSCHILD, H. and MOLVEY, J.J. (1982) *Journal of the National Cancer Institute*, **68**, 755–760

ROTKIN, I.D. (1967) *American Journal of Public Health*, **57**, 815–829

ROTKIN, I.D. (1977) *Cancer Treatment Reports*, **61**, 173–180

ROUSH, G.C., KELLY, J.A., MEIGS, J.W. and FLANNERY, J.T. (1982) *American Journal of Epidemiology*, **116**, 76–85

ROUSH, G.C., MEIGS, J.W., KELLY, J.A., FLANNERY, J.T. and BURDO, H. (1980) *American Journal of Epidemiology*, **111**, 183–193

ROUSH, G.C., SCHYMURA, M.J. and FLANNERY, J.T. (1984) *Cancer*, **54**, 596–601

ROUSSEL, J., PERNOT, C., SCHOUMACHER, P., PERNOT, M. and KESSLER, Y. (1964) *Journal de Radiologie et d'Electrologie*, **45**, 541–546

ROWE, V.K. (1975) *Annals of the New York Academy of Science*, **246**, 306–310

ROWLAND, R.E. (1975) In *Radiation Research*. Eds O.F. Nygaard, H.I. Adler and W.K. Sinclair. pp. 146–155. New York: Academic Press

ROWLAND, R.E., STEHNEY, A.F. and LUCAS, H.F. (1978) *Radiation Research*, **76**, 368–383

ROYAL COLLEGE OF PATHOLOGISTS AND PHYSICIANS (1982) *Journal of the Royal College of Physicians, London*, **16**, 202–218

ROYAL COLLEGE OF PHYSICIANS (1970) *Air Pollution and Health*. London: Pitman Medical

ROYAL SOCIETY (1983) *Risk Assessment*. London: Royal Society

ROYLE, H. (1975) *Environmental Research*, **10**, 39–53

RUBINO, G.F., PIOLATTO, G., NEWHOUSE, M.L., SCANSETTI, G., ARESINI, G.A. and MURRAY, R. (1979b) *British Journal of Industrial Medicine*, **36**, 187–194

RUBINO, G.F., SCANSETTI, G., PIOLATTO, G. and GAY, G. (1979c) In *Dusts and Diseases*. Eds R. Lemen and J.M. Dement. pp. 357–363. Illinois: Pathotox

RUBINO, G.F., SCANSETTI, G., PIOLATTO, G. and PIRA, E. (1979a) *Arkiv Hygijenu Radai Toksikologiju*, **30**, Supplement, 627–632

RUBINO, G.F., SCANSETTI, G., PIOLATTO, G. and ROMANO, C.A. (1976) *Journal of Occupational Medicine*, **18**, 186–193

RUSHTON, L. (1982) *Lancet*, i, 1421

RUSHTON, L. and ALDERSON, M.R. (1981a) *British Journal of Industrial Medicine*, **38**, 225–234

RUSHTON, L. and ALDERSON, M.R. (1981b) *British Journal of Cancer*, **43**, 77–84

RUSHTON, L. and ALDERSON, M.R. (1983) *British Journal of Industrial Medicine*, **40**, 330–339

RUSHTON, L., ALDERSON, M.R. and NAGARAJAH, C.R. (1983) *British Journal of Industrial Medicine*, **40**, 340–345

RUTSTEIN, D.D., MULLAN, R.J., FRAZIER, T.M., HALPERIN, W.E., MELIUS, J.M. and SESTITO, J.P. (1983) *American Journal of Public Health*, **73**, 1054–1062

SACCOMANNO, G., ARCHER, V.E., AURBACH, O., KUSCHNER, M., SAUNDERS, R.P. and KLEIN, M.G. (1971) *Cancer*, **27**, 515–523

SADEGHI, A. and BEHMARD, S. (1978) *Cancer*, **42**, 353–356

SADOFF, L., WINKLEY, J. and TYSON, S. (1973) *Oncology*, **27**, 244–257

SAGERMAN, R.H., CASSADY, J.R., TRETTER, P. and ELLSWORTH, R.M. (1969) *American Journal of Roentgenology*, **105**, 529–535

SAKABE, H. (1973) *Industrial Health*, **11**, 145–148

SAKABE, H. and FUKUDA, K. (1977) *Industrial Health*, **15**, 173–174

SAKABE, H., MATSUSHITA, H. and KOSHI, S. (1976) *Annals of the New York Academy of Science*, **271**, 67–70

SAMET, J.M., KUTVIRT, D.M., WAXWEILER, R.J. and KEY, C.R. (1984) *New England Journal of Medicine*, **310**, 1481–1484

SANDERSON, K.V. (1984) In *Precancerous States*. Ed. R.L. Carter. pp. 74–92. London: Oxford University Press

SANGHVI, L.D., RAO, K.C.M. and KHANOLKAR, V.R. (1955) *British Medical Journal*, i, 1111–1114

SANOTSKII, I.V. (1976) *Environmental Health Perspectives*, **17**, 85–93

SARACCI, R. (1981) In *Recent Advances in Occupational Health*. Ed. J.C. McDonald. pp. 119–128. London: Churchill Livingstone

SARIC, M., KULCAR, Z., ZORICA, M. and GELIC, L. (1976) *Environmental Health Perspectives*, **17**, 189–192

SARTOR, F.A. (1982) *American Journal of Epidemiology*, **115**, 144–145

SAULI, H. (1979) *Occupational Mortality, 1971–1975*. Helsinki: Statistics Office of Finland

SAUNDERS, C.M. (1978) *The Management of Terminal Disease*. London: Arnold

SAVAGE, J.R.K. (1979) *Nature*, **277**, 512–513

SAXEN, E.A. and SAXEN, L.O. (1954) *Documenta de Medicina Geographia et Tropica*, **6**, 335–341

SCHILLING, R.S. (1956) *Lancet*, **ii**, 261–265

SCHILLING, R.S. (1971) *British Journal of Industrial Medicine*, **28**, 27–35

SCHIMKE, R.N. (1976) *Advances in Internal Medicine*, **21**, 249–265

SCHIMKE, R.N. (1978) *Genetics and Cancer in Man*. Edinburgh: Churchill Livingstone

SCHIMPFF, S.C., BRAGER, D.M., SCHIMPFF, C.R., COMSTOCK, G.W. and WIERNIK, P.H. (1976) *Annals of Internal Medicine*, **84**, 547–550

SCHNEIDER, R. and RIGGS, J.L. (1973) *Journal of the American Veterinary Medical Association*, **162**, 217–219

SCHOENBERG, J.B., STEMHAGEN, A., MOGIELNICKI, A.P., ALTMAN, R., ABE, T. and MASON, T.J. (1984) *Journal of the National Cancer Institute*, **72**, 973–981

SCHOTTENFELD, D., BERG, J.W. and VITSKY, B. (1971) *Journal of the National Cancer Institute*, **46**, 161–170

SCHOTTENFELD, D., WARSHAVER, M.E., ZAUBER, A.G., MEICKLE, J.G. and HART, B.R. (1981) In *Quantification of Occupational Cancer*. Eds R. Peto and M. Schneiderman. pp. 247–260. New York: Cold Spring Harbour Laboratory

SCHRAUZER, G.N. (1976) *Medical Hypotheses*, **2**, 39–49

SCHREEK, R. (1944) *Cancer Research*, **4**, 433–437

SCHUMANN, L.M., MANDEL, J., BLACKARD, C., BAUER, H., SCARLETT, J. and McHUGH, R. (1977) *Cancer Treatment Reports*, **61**, 181–186

SCOTT, A. (1922) *British Medical Journal*, **ii**, 1108–1109

SCOTT, T.S. (1962) *Carcinogenic and Chronic Toxic Hazards of Aromatic Amines*. Amsterdam: Elsevier

SCOTT, T.S. and WILLIAMS, M.H.C. (1957) *British Journal of Industrial Medicine*, **14**, 150–163

SEARLE, C.E., WATERHOUSE, J.A.H., HENMAN, B.A., BARTLETT, D. and McCOMBIE, S. (1978) *British Journal of Cancer*, **38**, 192–193

SEIDMAN, H. (1970) *Environmental Research*, **3**, 234–249

SEIDMAN, H., LILIS, R. and SELIKOFF, I.J. (1976) In *Prevention and Detection of Cancer*. Ed. H.E. Nieburgs. Vol. 1. pp. 943–960. New York: Marcel Dekker

SEIDMAN, H., SELIKOFF, I.J. and HAMMOND, E.C. (1979) *Annals of the New York Academy of Science*, **330**, 61–90

SELEVAN, S.G., DEMENT, J.M., WAGONER, J.K. and FROINES, J.R. (1979a) *Journal of Environmental Pathology and Toxicology*, **2**, 273–284

SELEVAN, S.G., DEMENT, J.M., WAGONER, J.K. and FROINES, J.R. (1979b) In *Dusts and Diseases*. Eds R. Lemen and J.M. Dement. pp. 379–388. Illinois: Pathotox

SELIKOFF, I.J., BADER, R., BADER, M.E. and HAMMOND, E.C. (1967) *American Journal of Medicine*, **42**, 487–496

SELIKOFF, I.J., CHURG, J. and HAMMOND, E.C. (1964) *Journal of the American Medical Association*, **188**, 142–146

SELIKOFF, I.J., CHURG, J. and HAMMOND, E.C. (1965) *New England Journal of Medicine*, **272**, 560–565

SELIKOFF, I.J. and HAMMOND, E.C. (1964) *Journal of the American Medical Association*, **188**, 142–146

SELIKOFF, I.J. and HAMMOND, E.C. (1975) In *Persons at High Risk of Cancer*. Ed. J.F. Fraumeni. pp. 467–483. New York: Academic Press

SELIKOFF, I.J. and HAMMOND, E.C. (1979) *Annals of the New York Academy of Science*, **330**, i

SELIKOFF, I.J. and HAMMOND, E.C. (1982) *Annals of the New York Academy of Science*, **381**, 1–364

SELIKOFF, I.J., HAMMOND, E.C. and CHURG, J. (1968) *Journal of the American Medical Association*, **204**, 104–110

SELIKOFF, I.J., HAMMOND, E.C. and CHURG, J. (1972) *Archives of Environmental Health*, **25**, 183–186

SELIKOFF, I.J., HAMMOND, E.C. and SEIDMAN, H. (1973) In *Biological Effects of Asbestos*. Eds P. Bagovski, J.C. Gilson, V. Timbrell, J.C. Wagner and W. Davies. pp. 209–216. Lyon: IARC

SELIKOFF, I.J., HAMMOND, E.C. and SEIDMAN, H. (1979) *Annals of the New York Academy of Science*, **330**, 91–116

SELIKOFF, I.J., LILIS, R. and NICHOLSON, W.J. (1979) *Annals of the New York Academy of Science*, **330**, 295–311

SELIKOFF, I.J. and SEIDMAN, H. (1981) *Cancer*, **47**, 1469–1473

SELIKOFF, I.J., SEIDMAN, H. and HAMMOND, E.C. (1980) *Journal of the National Cancer Institute*, **65**, 507–513

SELTZER, C.C. and JABLON, S. (1974) *American Journal of Epidemiology*, **100**, 367–372

SEXTON, R.J. (1960) *Archives of Environmental Health*, **1**, 208–231

SHANK, R.C. (1977) In *Environmental Toxicology*. Eds H.F. Kraybill and M.A. Mehlman. pp. 291–318. London: Hemisphere Press

SHANNON, H.S., HAYES, M., JULIAN, J.A. and MUIR, D.C.F. (1984) *British Journal of Industrial Medicine*, **41**, 35–38

SHANNON, H.S., WILLIAMS, M.K. and KING, E. (1976) *British Journal of Industrial Medicine*, **33**, 236–242

SHAW, G., LAVEY, R., JACKSON, R. and AUSTIN, D. (1984) *American Journal of Epidemiology*, **119**, 788–795

SHEERS, G. and TEMPLETON, A.R. (1968) *British Medical Journal*, **ii**, 574–579

SHEFFET, A., THIND, I., MILLER, A.M. and LOURIA, D.B. (1982) *Archives of Environmental Health*, **37**, 44–52

SHENNAN, D.H. and BISHOP, D.S. (1974) *West Indian Medical Journal*, **23**, 44–53

SHEPHERD, J.H., DEWHURST, J. and PRYSE-DAVIES, J. (1979) *British Medical Journal*, **ii**, 246

SHERWOOD, R.J. (1971) *Annals of Occupational Hygiene*, **14**, 125–135

SHETTIGARA, P.T. and MORGAN, R.W. (1975) *Archives of Environmental Health*, **30**, 517–519

SHILLING, S. and LALICH, N.R. (1984) *Public Health Reports*, **99**, 152–161

SHILS, M.E. and BRAMNICK, J. (1983) *Bulletin of the New York Academy of Medicine*, **59**, 863–1163

SIEBER, S.M. and ADAMSON, R.H. (1976) *Advances in Cancer Research*, **22**, 57–155

SIEMATYCKI, J., DAY, N.E., FABRY, J. and COOPER, J.A. (1981) *Journal of the National Cancer Institute*, **66**, 217–225

SILVERMAN, D.T., HOOVER, R.N., ALBERT, S. and GRAFF, K.M. (1983) *Journal of the National Cancer Institute*, **70**, 237–245

SIMARD, A., VAUCLAIR, R., COLE, P., PERRET, C., NAULT, M. and PAQUETTE, G. (1983) *Journal of Chronic Disease*, **36**, 617–623

SIMLER, M., MAURER, M. and MANDARD, J.C. (1964) *Strasbourg Medicine*, **15**, 910–918

SIMON, D., YEN, S. and COLE, P. (1975) *Journal of the National Cancer Institute*, **54**, 587–591

SMITH, A.H., FISHER, D.O., PEARCE, N. and TEAGUE, C.A. (1982) *Community Health Studies*, **6**, 114–119

SMITH, A.H., WAXWEILER, R.J. and TYROLER, H.A. (1980) *American Journal of Epidemiology,* **112**, 787–797

SMITH, D. (1976) *Journal of Social and Occupational Medicine,* **26**, 92–94

SMITH, P.G. and DOLL, R. (1976) *British Journal of Radiology,* **49**, 224–232

SMITH, P.G. and DOLL, R. (1981) *British Journal of Radiology,* **54**, 187–194

SMITH, P.G., KINLEN, L.J. and DOLL, R. (1974) *Lancet,* **ii**, 525

SMITH, P.G., KINLEN, L.J., WHITE, G.C., ADELSTEIN, A.M. and FOX, A.J. (1980) *British Journal of Cancer,* **41**, 422–428

SMITH, P.G., PIKE, M.C., KINLEN, L.J., JONES, A. and HARRIS, R. (1977) *Lancet,* **ii**, 59–62

SMITH, P.M., CROSSLEY, I.R. and WILLIAMS, D.M.J. (1976) *Lancet,* **ii**, 602–604

SMITH, P.R. and LICKISS, J.N. (1980) *Lancet,* **i**, 719

SMITH, R.J. (1981) *Science,* **211**, 556–557

SNEGIREFF, L.S. and LOMBARD, O.M. (1951) *Archives of Industrial Hygiene,* **4**, 199–205

SOMERVILLE, S.M., DAVIES, J.M., HENDRY, W.F. and WILLIAMS, G. (1980) *British Medical Journal,* **i**, 540–542

SOMMERS, S.C. and McMANUS, R.G. (1953) *Cancer,* **6**, 347–359

SONAKUL, D., KOOMPIROCHANA, C., CHINDRA, K. and STITNIMANKARN, T. (1978) *South East Asian Journal of Tropical Medicine and Public Health,* **9**, 215–219

SORAHAN, T. and WATERHOUSE, J.A.H. (1983) *British Journal of Industrial Medicine,* **40**, 293–300

SORAHAN, T., WATERHOUSE, J.A.H., COOKE-SMITH, E.M.B., JACKSON, J.R. and TEMKIN, L. (1983) *Annals of Occupational Hygiene,* **27**, 173–182

SOUTHAM, A.H. and WILSON, S.R. (1922) *British Medical Journal,* **ii**, 971–973

SPARKS, P.J. and WEGMAN, D.H. (1980) *Journal of Occupational Medicine,* **22**, 733–736

SPENCE, A.A., COHEN, E.N., BROWN, B.W., KNILL-JONES, R.P. and HIMMELBERGER, D.U. (1977) *Journal of the American Medical Association,* **238**, 955–959

SPENCE, A.A. and KNILL-JONES, R.P. (1978) *British Journal of Anaesthesia,* **50**, 713–719

SPIERS, P.S. (1969) *Public Health Reports,* **84**, 385–388

SPIERS, F.W., LUCAS, H.F., RUNDO, J. and ANAST, G.A. (1983) *Health Physics,* **44**, Suppl. 1, 65–72

SPIRTAS, R. (1977) In *Proceedings of the NIOSH Styrene Butadiene Briefing.* Ed. L. Ede. pp. 9–12. Cincinnati: US Department of Health, Education and Welfare (NIOSH 77–129)

SPIRTAS, R. and KAMINSKI, R. (1978) *Journal of Occupational Medicine,* **20**, 427–429

SPITZER, W.O., HILL, G.B., CHAMBERS, L.W., HELLIWELL, B.F. and MURPHY, H.B. (1975) *New England Journal of Medicine,* **293**, 419–424

STAIANO, N., GALLELI, J.F., ADAMSON, R.H. and THORGEIRSSON, S. (1981) *Lancet,* **i**, 615–616

STARR, C. (1969) *Science,* **165**, 1232–1238

STARR, T.B. and LEVINE, R.J. (1983) *American Journal of Epidemiology,* **118**, 897–904

STATISTIKA CENTRALBYRAN (1981) *Dodsfallsregister 1961– 1970.* Orebro: Statistika Centralbryan

STEINBECK, G., CARSTENSEN, J., WIKLUND, K. and EKLUND, G. (1983) *Lancet,* **ii**, 1503

STELL, P.M. and McGILL, T. (1973) *Lancet,* **ii**, 416–417

STEMHAGEN, A., SLADE, J., ALTMAN, R. and BILL, J. (1983) *American Journal of Epidemiology,* **117**, 443–454

STEPHENSON, J.H. and GRACE, W.J. (1954) *Psychosomatic Medicine,* **16**, 287–294

STERN, E. and DIXON, W.J. (1961) *Cancer,* **14**, 153–160

STEWART, A., WEBB, J. and HEWITT, D. (1958) *British Medical Journal,* **i**, 1495–1508

STEWART, H.L., DUNHAM, L.J., DORN, H.F., THOMAS, L.B., EDGCOMB, J.H. and SYMEONIDIS, A. (1966) *Journal of the National Cancer Institute,* **37**, 1–95

STEVENSON, T.H.C. (1923) *Biometrika,* **15**, 382–400

STILLE, W.T. and TABERSHAW, I.R. (1982) *Journal of Occupational Medicine,* **24**, 480–484

STOCKS, P. (1938) *Journal of the Royal Statistical Society, series A,* **101**, 669–696

STOCKS, P. (1952) *British Journal of Cancer,* **6**, 99–111

STOCKS, P. (1960) *British Journal of Cancer,* **14**, 397–418

STOCKS, P. (1961) *British Journal of Cancer,* **15**, 701–711

STOCKS, P. (1962) *British Journal of Cancer,* **16**, 592–598

STOCKS, P. (1970) *British Journal of Cancer,* **24**, 215–225

STRANDBERG, M., SANDBACK, K., AXELSON, O. and SUNDELL, L. (1978) *Lancet,* **i**, 384–385

STROECKLE, J.D., HARDY, H.L. and WEBER, A.L. (1969) *American Journal of Medicine,* **46**, 543–561

STUKONIS, M. and DOLL, R. (1969) *International Journal of Cancer,* **4**, 248–254

STUMPHIUS, J. (1979) *Annals of the New York Academy of Science,* **330**, 317–322

STUTMAN, O. (1976) *Advances in Cancer Research,* **22**, 261–422

SUNDERMAN, F.W. (1976) *Preventive Medicine,* **5**, 279–294

SWANSON, G.M., SCHWARTZ, A.G. and BURROWS, R.W. (1984) *American Journal of Public Health,* **74**, 464–467

SWERDLOW, A.J. (1979) *British Medical Journal,* **ii**, 1324–1327

SYMONS, M.J., ANDJELKOVIC, D.A., SPIRTAS, R. and HERMAN, D.R. (1982) *Annals of the New York Academy of Science,* **381**, 146–159

TABERSHAW, I.R. and COOPER, W.C. (1974) *A Mortality Study of Petroleum Refinery Workers.* Washington: American Petroleum Institute

TABERSHAW, I.R. and COOPER, W.C. (1975) *A Mortality Study of Petroleum Workers: Social Security Follow-up.* Washington: American Petroleum Institute

TABERSHAW, I.R. and GAFFEY, W.R. (1974) *Journal of Occupational Medicine,* **16**, 508–518

TABERSHAW, I.R. and LAMM, S.H. (1977) *Lancet,* **ii**, 867–868

TABOR, E., GERETY, R.J., VOGEL, C.L., BAYLEY, A.C., ANTHONY, P.P., CHAN, C.H. *et al.* (1977) *Journal of the National Cancer Institute,* **58**, 1197–1200

TAREEF, E.M., KONTCHALOVSKAYA, N.M. and ZORINA, L.A. (1963) *Acta Unio Contra Cancrum,* **19**, 751–755

TATHAM, J. (1902) In *Dangerous Trades.* Ed. T. Oliver. p. 121. London: Murray

TATHAM, J. (1908) *Supplement to the 65th Annual Report of the Registrar General in England and Wales.* p. xiii. London: HMSO

TAULBEE, J., ANDJELKOVIC, D., WILLIAMS, T., GAMBLE, J.F. and WOLF, P. (1977) In *Proceedings of the NIOSH Styrene Butadiene Briefing.* pp. 113–162. Cincinnatti: US Department of Health, Education and Welfare

TAYLOR, F.H. (1966) *American Journal of Public Health,* **56**, 218–228

TEASDALE, C., FORBES, J.F. and BAUM, M. (1976) *Lancet,* **i**, 360–361

TEMPLETON, A.C. (1975) In *Persons at High Risk of Cancer.* Ed. J.F. Fraumeni. pp. 69–83. New York: Academic Press

TERRIS, M. and OALMANN, M.C. (1960) *Journal of the American Medical Association,* **174**, 1847–1851

TETA, M.J., LEWINSOHN, H.C., MEIGS, J.W., VIDONE, R.A., MOWARD, L.Z. and FLANNERY, J.T. (1983) *Journal of Occupational Medicine*, **25**, 749–756

TETA, M.J., WALRATH, J., MEIGS, J.W. and FLANNERY, J.T. (1984) *Journal of the National Cancer Institute*, **72**, 1051–1057

THACKRAH, C.T. (1832) *The Effects of Arts, Trades, and Professions, and of the Civic States and Habits of Living, on Health and Longevity, with Suggestions for the Removal of Many Agents which Produce Disease.* London: Longman

THERIAULT, G. and ALLARD, P. (1981) *Journal of Occupational Medicine*, **23**, 671–676

THERIAULT, G. and GOULET, L. (1979) *Journal of Occupational Medicine*, **21**, 367–370

THERIAULT, G., TREMBLAY, C., CORDIER, S. and GINGAM, S. (1984) *Lancet*, **i**, 947–950

THIESS, A.M. and FLEIG, I. (1978) *Archives of Toxicology*, **41**, 149–152

THIESS, A.M. and FRENTZEL-BEYME, R. (1978) cited by IARC (1977b)

THIESS, A.M., FRENTZEL-BEYME, R. and PENNING, E. (1979) cited by IARC (1979a)

THIESS, A.M., FRENTZEL-BEYME, R., LINK, R. and WILD, H. (1980) *Zentralblatt für Arbeitsmedizin Arbeitsschutz Prophylaxe*, **30**, 259–267

THIESS, A.M., FRENTZEL-BEYME, R., LINK, R. and STOCKER, W.G. (1982) In *Prevention of Occupational Cancer.* pp. 249–259. Geneva: ILO

THIESS, A.M., HEY, W. and ZELLER, H. (1973) *Zentralblatt für Arbeitsmedizin Arbeitsschutz Prophylaxe*, **23**, 97–102

THIESSEN, E.U. (1974) *Cancer*, **34**, 1102–1107

THOMAS, H.F., BENJAMIN, I.T., ELWOOD, P.C. and SWEETNAM, P.M. (1982) *British Journal of Industrial Medicine*, **39**, 273–276

THOMAS, L.B., POPPER, H., BERK, P.D., SELIKOFF, I. and FALK, H. (1975) *New England Journal of Medicine*, **292**, 17–22

THOMAS, T.L. (1982) *International Journal of Epidemiology*, **11**, 175–180

THOMAS, T.L. and DECOUFLE, P. (1979) *Journal of Occupational Medicine*, **21**, 619–623

THOMAS, T.L., DECOUFLE, P. and MOURE-EVASO, R. (1980) *Journal of Occupational Medicine*, **22**, 97–103

THOMAS, T.L., WAXWEILER, R.J., CRANDALL, M.S., WHITE, D.W., MOURE-ERASO, R. and FRAUMENI, J.F. (1984) *American Journal of Industrial Medicine*, **6**, 3–16

THOMAS, T.L., WAXWEILER, R.J., MOURE-ERASO, R., ITAYA, S. and FRAUMENI, J.F. (1982) *Journal of Occupational Medicine*, **24**, 135–141

THORPE, J.J. (1974) *Journal of Occupational Medicine*, **16**, 375–382

TIMONEN, T.T.T. and ILVONEN, M. (1978) *Lancet*, **i**, 350–352

TOKUDOME, S. and KURATSUNE, M. (1976) *International Journal of Cancer*, **17**, 310–317

TOKUHATA, G.K. and LILIENFELD, A.M. (1963) *Journal of the National Cancer Institute*, **30**, 289–319

TOLA, S., HERNBERG, S., COLAN, Y., LINDERBORG, H. and KORKALA, M.L. (1980a) *International Archives of Occupational and Environmental Health*, **46**, 79–85

TOLA, S., KOSKELA, R.S., HERNBERG, S. and JARVINEN, E. (1979) *Journal of Occupational Medicine*, **21**, 753–760

TOLA, S., VILHUNEN, R., JARVINEN, E. and KORKALA, M.L. (1980b) *Journal of Occupational Medicine*, **22**, 737–740

TOLLEY, H.D., MARKS, S., BUCHANAN, J.A. and GILBERT, E.S. (1983) *Radiation Research*, **95**, 211–213

TOMLIN, P.J. (1979) *British Medical Journal*, **i**, 779–784

TON THAT, T., TRAN THI, A., NGUYEN DANG, T., PHAM HUANG, P., NGUYEN NHU, B., TON THAT, B. *et al.* (1973) *Chirurgie*, **99**, 427–436

TOUGH, I.M. and COURT BROWN, W.M. (1965) *Lancet*, **i**, 684

TOUGH, I.M., SMITH, P.G., COURT BROWN, W.M. and HARNDEN, D.G. (1970) *European Journal of Cancer*, **6**, 49–55

TOWNSEND, J.C., OTT, M.G. and FISHBECK, W.A. (1978) *Journal of Occupational Medicine*, **20**, 543–548

TRACEY, J.P. and SHERLOCK, P. (1968) *New York State Journal of Medicine*, **68**, 2202–2204

TRELL, E., KORSGAARD, R., HOOD, B., KITZING, P., NORDIC, G. and SIMONSSON, B.G. (1976) *Lancet*, **ii**, 140

TRICHOPOULOS, D., TABOR, E., GERETY, R.J., XIROUCHAXI, E., SPARROS, L., MUNOZ, N. *et al.* (1978) *Lancet*, **ii**, 1217–1219

TRUHAUT, R. and MURRAY, R. (1978) *International Archives of Occupational and Environmental Health*, **41**, 65–76

TSAI, S.T., WEN, C.P., WEISS, N.S., WONG, O., McCLELLAN, W.A. and GIBSON, R.L. (1983) *Journal of Occupational Medicine*, **25**, 685–692

TSUCHIYA, K. (1965) *Cancer*, **18**, 136–144

TSUCHIYA, K., OKUBO, T. and ISHIZU, S. (1975) *British Journal of Industrial Medicine*, **32**, 203–209

TURBITT, M.L., PATRICK, R.S., GOUDIE, R.B. and BUCHANAN, W.M. (1977) *Journal of Clinical Pathology*, **30**, 1124–1128

TURNER, H.G. and GRACE, H.G. (1938) *British Journal of Hygiene*, **38**, 90–103

TURNER WARWICK, M. (1977) *British Journal of Diseases of the Chest*, **71**, 219–220

TUYNS, A.J., PEQUIGNOT, G. and JENSEN, O.M. (1977) *Bulletin of Cancer*, **64**, 45–60

TYROLER, II.A., ANDJELKOVIC, D., HARRIS, R., LEDNAR, W. and McMICHAEL, A. (1976) *Environmental Health Perspectives*, **17**, 13–20

TYRRELL, A.M., McCAUGHEY, W.T.E. and MacAIRT, J.G. (1971) *Journal of the Irish Medical Association*, **64**, 213–217

UN SCIENTIFIC COMMITTEE ON THE EFFECTS OF ATOMIC RADIATION (1972) *Ionizing Radiation: Levels and Effects.* Vols I and II. New York: United Nations

UN SCIENTIFIC COMMITTEE ON THE EFFECTS OF ATOMIC RADIATION (1977) *Sources and Effects of Ionizing Radiation.* New York: United Nations

UN SCIENTIFIC COMMITTEE ON THE EFFECTS OF ATOMIC RADIATION (1982) *Ionizing Radiation: Sources and Biological Effects.* New York: United Nations

UNITED STATES DEPARTMENT OF LABOR (1978) *Occupational Exposure to Acrylonitrile. Proposed Standard and Notice of Hearing.* Federal Register, 48, 2586–2621

VAGERO, D. and OLIN, R. (1983) *British Journal of Industrial Medicine*, **40**, 188–192

VAISMAN, A.I. (1967) *Eksperimentalni Khirurgie Anesteziologe*, **3**, 44–49

VALERIO, F., RAFFETTO, G., PUTONI, M. and VERCELLI, M. (1982) *Cancer Detection and Prevention*, **5**, 335–341

VENA, J.E., BYERS, T., SWANSON, M. and COOKFAIR, D. (1982) *Lancet*, **ii**, 713

VENITT, S., CROFTON-SLEIGH, C., HUNT, J., SPEECHLEY, V. and BRIGGS, K. (1984) *Lancet*, **i**, 74–77

VERSLUYS, J.J. (1949) *British Journal of Cancer*, **3**, 161–185

VESSEY, M.P., KAY, C.R., BALDWIN, J.A., CLARKE, J.A. and MacLEOD, I.B. (1977) *British Medical Journal*, **i**, 1064–1065

VEYS, C.A. (1969) *Journal of the National Cancer Institute*, **43**, 219–226

VEYS, C.A. (1974) *British Journal of Industrial Medicine*, **31**, 65–71

VEYS, C.A. (1981) *Journal of the Society of Occupational Medicine*, **31**, 19–26

VIADANA, E., BROSS, I.D. and HOUTEN, L. (1976) *Journal of Occupational Medicine*, **18**, 787–792

VIANNA, N.J., GREENWALD, P. and DAVIES, J.N.P. (1971) *Lancet*, **i**, 1209–1211

VIANNA, N.J. and POLAN, A.K. (1973) *New England Journal of Medicine*, **289**, 499–502

VIANNA, N.J. and POLAN, A.K. (1978) *Lancet*, **i**, 1061–1063

VIANNA, N.J. and POLAN, A. (1979) *Lancet*, **i**, 1394–1395

VIANNA, N.J., POLAN, A.K., KEOGH, M.D. and GREENWALD, P. (1974) *Lancet*, **ii**, 131–133

VIGLIANI, E.C. (1976) *Annals of the New York Academy of Science*, **271**, 143–151

VIGLIANI, E.C. and BARSOTTI, M. (1961) *Medicina del Lavora*, **52**, 241–250

VIGLIANI, E.C. and FORNI, A. (1976) *Environmental Research*, **11**, 122–127

VILLIERS, A.J.DE and WINDISH, J.P. (1964) *British Journal of Industrial Medicine*, **21**, 94–109

VINEIS, P., TERRACINI, B., COSTA, G., MERLATTI, F. and SEGNAN, N. (1982) In *Prevention of Ocupational Cancer*. pp. 327–331. Geneva: ILO

VINNI, K. and HAKAMA, M. (1980) *British Journal of Industrial Medicine*, **37**, 180–184

VOBECKY, J., DEVROEDE, G., LACAILLE, J. and WATIER, A. (1978) *Gastroenterology*, **75**, 221–223

VOGEL, C.L., ANTHONY, P.P., MODY, N. and BARKER, L.F. (1970) *Lancet*, **ii**, 621–624

VON HEY, W., THIESS, A.M. and ZELLER, H. (1974) *Zentralblatt für Arbeitsmedizin*, **24**, 71–77

VORWALD, A.J. and KARR, J.W. (1938) *American Journal of Pathology*, **14**, 49–57

WADA, S., MIYANISHI, M., NISHIMOTO, Y., KAMBE, S. and MILLER, R.W. (1968) *Lancet*, **i**, 1161–1163

WADE, L. (1963) *Archives of Environmental Health*, **6**, 730–735

WAGNER, J.C., BERRY, G. and POOLEY, F.D. (1982) *British Medical Journal*, **285**, 603–606

WAGNER, J.C., SLEGGS, C.A. and MARCHAND, P. (1960) *British Journal of Industrial Medicine*, **17**, 260–271

WAGONER, J.K., ARCHER, V.E., CARROLL, B.E., HOLADAY, D.A. and LAWRENCE, P.A. (1964) *Journal of the National Cancer Institute*, **32**, 787–801

WAGONER, J.K., ARCHER, V.E., LUNDIN, F.E., HOLADAY, D.A. and LLOYD, J.W. (1965) *New England Journal of Medicine*, **273**, 181–188

WAGONER, J.K., INFANTE, P.F. and BAYLISS, D.L. (1980) *Environmental Research*, **21**, 15–34

WAGONER, J.K., INFANTE, P.F. and MANCUSO, T. (1978) *Science*, **201**, 298–303

WAGONER, J.K., INFANTE, P.F. and SARACCI, R. (1976) *Lancet*, **ii**, 194–195

WAGONER, J.K., JOHNSON, W.M. and LEMEN, R. (1973) *Congressional Record of the US Senate*, 14 March 1973, S 4660

WAGONER, J.K., MILLER, R.W., LUNDIN, F.W., FRAUMENI, J.F. and HAIJ, M.E. (1963) *New England Journal of Medicine*, **269**, 284–289

WAHLBERG, J.E. (1974) *Acta Dermatovener*, **54**, 471–474

WAHNER, H.W., CUELLO, C., CORREA, P., URIBE, L.F. and GAITAN, E. (1966) *American Journal of Medicine*, **40**, 58–66

WALD, N., BOREHAM, J., DOLL, R. and BONSALL, J. (1984) *British Journal of Industrial Medicine*, **41**, 31–34

WALD, N., IDLE, M., BOREHAM, J. and BAILEY, A. (1980) *Lancet*, **ii**, 813–815

WALDRON, H.A. (1977) *Journal of the Society of Occupational Medicine*, **27**, 45–49

WALDRON, H.A. (1979) *Lecture notes on occupational medicine*. Oxford: Blackwell

WALDRON, H.A. (1983) *British Journal of Industrial Medicine*, **40**, 390–401

WALKER, A.M. (1984) *Journal of Occupational Medicine*, **26**, 422–426

WALL, S. (1980) *International Journal of Epidemiology*, **9**, 73–87

WALLACE, D.C., EXTON, L.A. and McLEOD, S.R.C. (1971) *Cancer*, **27**, 1262–1266

WALLER, R.E. (1967) In *Prevention of Cancer*. Eds R.W. Raven and F.J.C. Roe. pp. 181–186. London: Butterworths

WALLER, R.E. (1981) *Environment International*, **5**, 479–493

WALRATH, J. (1983) *American Journal of Epidemiology*, **118**, 432

WALRATH, J. and FRAUMENI, J.F. (1983a) *International Journal of Cancer*, **31**, 407–411

WALRATH, J. and FRAUMENI, J.F. (1983b) In *Formaldehyde Toxicity*. Ed. J.E. Gibson. pp. 227–236. New York: Hemisphere Press

WANG, H.H. and GRUFFERMAN, S. (1981) *Journal of Occupational Medicine*, **23**, 364–366

WANG, H.H. and MacMAHON, B. (1979a) *Journal of Occupational Medicine*, **21**, 745–748

WANG, H.H. and MacMAHON, B. (1979b) *Journal of Occupational Medicine*, **21**, 741–744

WANG, J.D., WEGMAN, D.H. and SMITH, J.J. (1983) *British Journal of Industrial Medicine*, **40**, 177–181

WANG, O. and DECOUFLE, P. (1982) *Journal of Occupational Medicine*, **24**, 299–304

WARREN, S. (1956) *Journal of the American Medical Association*, **162**, 464–468

WATANABE, C. and FUKUCHI, Y. (1975) *International Congress of Occupational Health*, **18**, 149–150

WATERHOUSE, J.A.H. (1971) *Annals of Occupational Hygiene*, **14**, 161–170

WATERHOUSE, J.A.H. (1972) *Annals of Occupational Hygiene*, **15**, 43–44

WATERHOUSE, J.A.H. (1975) *British Journal of Cancer*, **32**, 262

WATERHOUSE, J.A.H. (1979) In *Advances in Medical Oncology, Research, and Education*. Ed. G.M. Birch. Vol. 3. pp. 97–105. Oxford: Pergamon

WAXWEILER, R.J., ALEXANDER, V., LEFFINGWELL, S.S., HARING, M. and LLOYD, J.W. (1983) *Journal of the National Cancer Institute*, **70**, 75–81

WAXWEILER, R.J., SMITH, A.H., FALK, H. and TYROLER, H.A. (1981) *Environmental Health Perspectives*, **41**, 159–165

WAXWEILER, R.J., STRINGER, W., WAGONER, J.K. and JONES, J. (1976) *Annals of the New York Academy of Science*, **271**, 40–48

WEGELIN, C. (1928) *Cancer Review*, **iii**, 297–313

WEGMAN, D.H., PETERS, J.M., BOUNDY, M.G. and SMITH, J.J. (1982) *British Journal of Industrial Medicine*, **39**, 233–238

WEIL, C.S., SMYTH, H.F. and NALE, T.W. (1952) *Archives of Industrial Hygiene and Occupational Medicine*, **5**, 535–540

WEILL, H., HUGHES, J. and WAGGENSPACK, C. (1979) *American Review of Respiratory Disease*, **120**, 345–354

WEISS, A. (1953) *Medizinische*, **3**, 93–94

WEISS, W. (1976) *Journal of Occupational Medicine*, **18**, 194–199

WEISS, W. (1977a) *Journal of Occupational Medicine*, **19**, 611–614

WEISS, W. (1977b) *Journal of Occupational Medicine*, **19**, 737–740

WEISS, W. (1980) *Journal of Occupational Medicine*, **22**, 527–529

WEISS, W. and BOUCOT, K.R. (1975) *Journal of the American Medical Association*, **234**, 1139–1142

WEISS, W. and FIGUEROA, W.G. (1976) *Journal of Occupational Medicine*, **18**, 623–627

WEISS, W., MOSER, R.I. and AUERBACH, O. (1979) *American Review of Respiratory Disease*, **120**, 1031–1037

WELTON, J.C., MARR, J.S. and FRIEDMAN, S.M. (1979) *Lancet*, **i**, 791–794

WEN, C.P. and TSAI, S.P. (1979) *Gastroenterology*, **76**, 656–657

WEN, C.P., TSAI, S.P., GIBSON, R.L. and McLELLAN, W.A. (1984) *Journal of Occupational Medicine*, **26**, 118–127

WEN, C.P., TSAI, S.P., McLELLAN, W.A. and GIBSON, R.L. (1983) *American Journal of Epidemiology*, **118**, 526–642

WENNSTROM, J., PIERCE, E.R. and McCUSICK, V.A. (1974) *Cancer*, **34**, 850–857

WERNER, J.B. and CARTER, J.T. (1981) *British Journal of Industrial Medicine*, **38**, 247–253

WERTHEIMER, N. and LEEPER, E. (1979) *American Journal of Epidemiology*, **109**, 273–284

WERTHEIMER, N. and LEEPER, E. (1982) *International Journal of Epidemiology*, **11**, 345–355

WEST, R.D. (1966) *Cancer*, **19**, 1001–1007

WESTERHOLM, P. (1980) *Scandinavian Journal of Work and Environmental Health*, Suppl. 2, **6**, 1–86

WHITAKER, C.J., LEE, W.R. and DOWNES, J.E. (1979) *British Journal of Industrial Medicine*, **36**, 43–51

WHITAKER, C.J., MOSS, E., LEE, W.R. and CUNLIFFE, S. (1979) *British Journal of Industrial Medicine*, **36**, 292–298

WHITNEY, J.S. (1934) *Death Rates by Occupation: Based on Data of the US Bureau of Census, 1930*. New York: National Tuberculosis Association

WHITTEMORE, A.S. and McMILLAN, A. (1983) *Journal of the National Cancer Institute*, **71**, 489–499

WHITWELL, F., SCOTT, J. and GRIMSHAW, M. (1977) *Thorax*, **32**, 377–386

WHORTON, D., MILBY, T.H., KRAUS, R.M. and STUBBS, H.A. (1979) *Journal of Occupational Medicine*, **21**, 161–166

WHORTON, M.D. (1983) *American Journal of Public Health*, **73**, 1031–1032

WHORWELL, P.J., FOSTER, K.J., ALDERSON, M.R. and WRIGHT, R. (1976) *Lancet*, **ii**, 113–114

WICKEN, A.J. (1966) *Environmental and Personal Factors in Lung Cancer and Chronic Bronchitis in Northern Ireland, 1960–1962*. London: Tobacco Research Council

WIGNALL, B.K. and FOX, A.J. (1982) *British Journal of Industrial Medicine*, **39**, 34–38

WIKLUND, K. (1983) *Cancer*, **51**, 566–568

WILLIAMS, E.H., DAY, N.E. and GESER, A.G. (1974) *Lancet*, **ii**, 19–22

WILLIAMS, E.H., SMITH, P.G., DAY, N.E., GESER, A., ELLICE, J. and TURKI, P. (1978) *British Journal of Cancer*, **37**, 109–119

WILLIAMS, R.R. (1976) *Lancet*, **i**, 996–999

WILLIAMS, R.R. and HORM, J.W. (1977) *Journal of the National Cancer Institute*, **58**, 525–547

WILLIAMS, R.R., STEGENS, N.L. and GOLDSMITH, J.R. (1977) *Journal of the National Cancer Institute*, **59**, 1147–1185

WILLIAMS, R.R., STEGENS, N.L. and HORM, J.L. (1977) *Journal of the National Cancer Institute*, **58**, 518–524

WILSON, S.R. (1910) *Cancer of the Scrotum*. Tom Jones essay prize. Manchester: University of Manchester

WINGRAVE, S.J., BERAL, V., ADELSTEIN, A.M. and KAY, C.R. (1981) *Journal of Epidemiology and Community Health*, **35**, 51–58

WINKLSTEIN, W. and KANTOR, S. (1969) *Archives of Environmental Health*, **18**, 544–557

WINN, D.M., BLOT, W.J., SHY, C.M. and FRAUMENI, J.R. (1982) *American Journal of Industrial Medicine*, **3**, 161–167

WINN, D.M., BLOT, W.J., SHY, C.M., PICKLE, L.W., TOLEDO, A. and FRAUMENI, J.F. (1981) *New England Journal of Medicine*, **304**, 745–749

WOLF, O. (1978) *Zeitschrift für de Gesamte Hygiene*, **24**, 174–177

WOLF, P.H., ANDJELKOVIC, D., SMITH, A. and TYROLER, H. (1981) *Journal of Occupational Medicine*, **23**, 103–108

WONG, O. (1981) In *Quantification of Occupational Cancer*. Eds R. Peto and M. Schneiderman. pp. 359–378. New York: Cold Spring Harbour Laboratory

WONG, O. (1983) In *Formaldehyde Toxicity*. Ed. E. Gibson. pp. 256–272. New York: Hemisphere Press

WONG, O., BROCKER, W., DAVIS, H.V. and NAGLE, G.S. (1984) *British Journal of Industrial Medicine*, **41**, 15–24

WONG, O. and DECOUFLE, P. (1982) *Journal of Occupational Medicine*, **24**, 299–304

WORLD HEALTH ORGANISATION (1974) *Report EHE/75.1* Geneva: WHO

WORLD HEALTH ORGANISATION (1977) *Methods used in Establishing Permissible Levels in Occupational Exposures to Harmful Agents*. Geneva: WHO

WORLD HEALTH ORGANISATION (1978) *Steroid Contraception and the Risk of Neoplasia*. Geneva: WHO

WORLD HEALTH ORGANISATION (1982) *Recommended Health-based Limits in Occupational Exposure to Pesticides*. Geneva: WHO

WRIGHT, W.E., PETERS, J.M. and MACK, J.M. (1982) *Lancet*, **ii**, 1160–1161

WRIGHT, W.E., PETERS, J.M. and MACK, J.M. (1983) *American Journal of Industrial Medicine*, **4**, 577–581

WRIGHT, W.E., SHERWIN, R.P., DICKSON, E.A., BERNSTEIN, L., FROMM, J.B. and HENDERSON, D.B.E. (1984) *British Journal of Industrial Medicine*, **41**, 39–45

WYNDER, E.L. and BROSS, I.J. (1957) *British Medical Journal*, **i**, 1137–1143

WYNDER, E.L., BROSS, I.J. and DAY, E. (1956) *Journal of the American Medical Association*, **160**, 1384–1391

WYNDER, E.L., CORNFIELD, J., SCHROFF, P.D. and DURARSWAMI, K.R. (1954) *American Journal of Obstetrics and Gynecology*, **68**, 1016–1047

WYNDER, E.L., COVEY, L.S., MABUCHI, K. and MUSHINSKI, M. (1976) *Cancer*, **38**, 1591–1601

WYNDER, E.L. and GOLDSMITH, R. (1977) *Cancer*, **40**, 1246–1268

WYNDER, E.L., HULTBERG, S., JACOBSSON, F. and BROSS, I.J. (1957) *Cancer*, **10**, 470–487

WYNDER, E.L., KMET, J., DUNGAL, N. and SEGI, M. (1963) *Cancer*, **16**, 1461–1496

WYNDER, E.L., MABUCHI, K., MARUCHI, N. and FORTNER, J.G. (1973) *Cancer*, **31**, 641–648

WYNDER, E.L., MABUCHI, K. and WHITMORE, W.F. (1971) *Cancer,* **28,** 344–360

WYNDER, E.L., ONDERDONK, J. and MANTEL, N. (1963) *Cancer,* **16,** 1388–1407

WYNNE GRIFFITH, G. (1982) *Lancet,* **i,** 399

YOSHIDA, O. and MIYAKAWA, M. (1972) In *Third International Symposium of Princess Takamatsu Cancer Research Fund.* Eds. W. Nakahara, T. Hirayama, K. Nishioka and H. Sugamo. Baltimore: University Park Press

YOUNG, M., RUSSELL, W.T., BROWNLEE, J. and COLLIS, E.L. (1926) *An Investigation into the Statistics of Cancer in Different Trades and Professions.* London: HMSO

ZACK, J.A. and SUSKIND, R.R. (1980) *Journal of Occupational Medicine,* **22,** 11–14

ZACK, M., CANNON, S., LLOYD, O., HEATH, C.W., FALLETA, J.M., JONES, B. *et al.* (1980) *American Journal of Epidemiology,* **111,** 329–336

ZACK, M., HEATH, C.W., ANDREWS, M.D., GRIVAS, A.S. and CHRISTINE, B.W. (1977) *Journal of the National Cancer Institute,* **59,** 1343–1349

ZAKELJ, M.P., FRASER, P. and INSKIP, H. (1984) *Lancet,* **i,** 510

ZAVON, M.R., HOEGG, U. and BINGHAM, E. (1973) *Archives of Environmental Health,* **27,** 1–7

ZEIGEL, R.F., ARYA, S.K., HOOSZEWICZ, J.S. and CARTER, W.A. (1977) *Oncology,* **34,** 29–44

ZIELHUIS, R.R. (1979) *New Findings on Health Hazards in Occupational Exposure to Styrene.* Lecture given to Occupational Circle in Amsterdam, 15/5/79

ZOBER, A. (1979) *International Archives of Occupational and Environmental Health,* **43,** 107–121

ZUR HAUSEN, J. (1976) *Cancer Research,* **36,** 794

Index

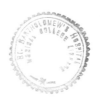